fractures

A HISTORY AND ICONOGRAPHY OF THEIR TREATMENT

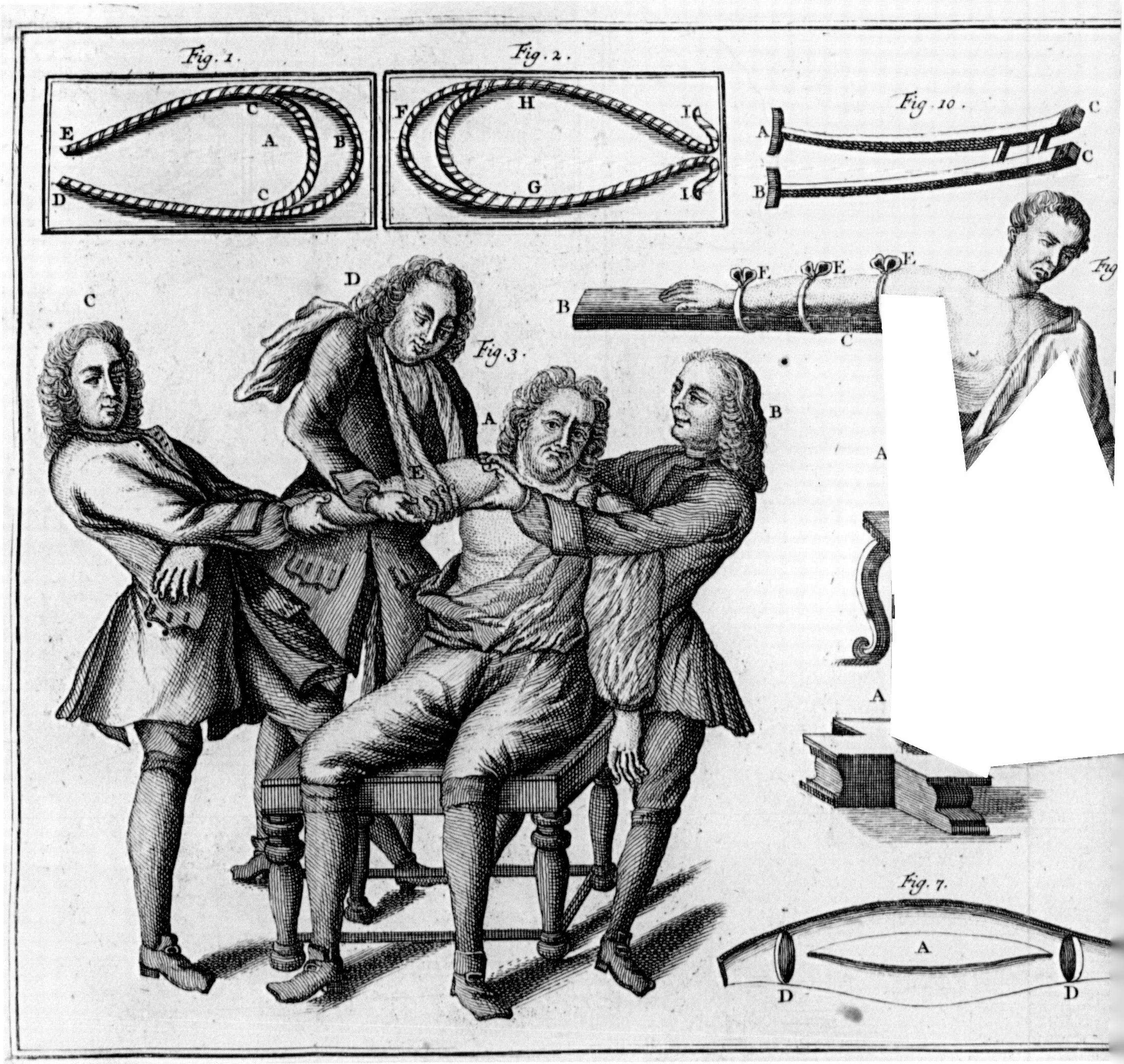

Treatment of dislocations from Lorenz Heister, *A General System of Surgery*, London: W. Innys, 1750, plate 10.

An Explanation of the Tenth Table.

Fig. 1. Is a Sling which may be used to make an Extension in Luxations of the Head. See the Chapter on Luxations of the Head.
Fig. 2. Is another Sling, to retain the Patient's Body firm in the same Case.
Fig. 3. Shews the most commodious Method of reducing a recent Luxation of the Humerus.
A is the Patient, seated ready to undergo the Operation.
B Is the Assistant that holds the Patient firm in his Seat.
C Is the Assistant that extends the dislocated Humerus.
D The Surgeon, reducing the dislocated Humerus.
E A Napkin, whereby the Surgeon elevates the Arm in order to its Reduction.
Fig. 4. Is a Machine commonly called the Ambe of Hippocrates, used formerly to reduce Luxations of the Humerus: It consists of the Fulcrum A A, to which is fastened the moveable Lever B C, joined to each other by a Sort of moveable Articulation D.
Fig. 5. Shews how the former Instrument is to be applied to a Luxation of the Humerus. There is some Difference between the Structure of this and the former, at the Joint C D. Some think this is preferable to the last.
A A is the Fulcrum, B C the Lever, to which the luxated Arm is fastened by the three Ligatures E E E. D the Place where the Fulcrum and Lever are fastened together by a moveable Joint. When the End of the Lever B is pressed downwards, the luxated Arm is extended, and lifted up near its Scapula.
Fig. 6. Is Petit's Machine for reducing Luxations for the Humerus, and several other Luxations.
a a are two Arms of Horns by which the Patient, and particularly his Scapula, is held firm, from giving way in the Extension; B the other End of it, resting upon the Ground or Floor; C C Pulleys of the Machine; d d the Rope, by winding up which, an Extension is made;

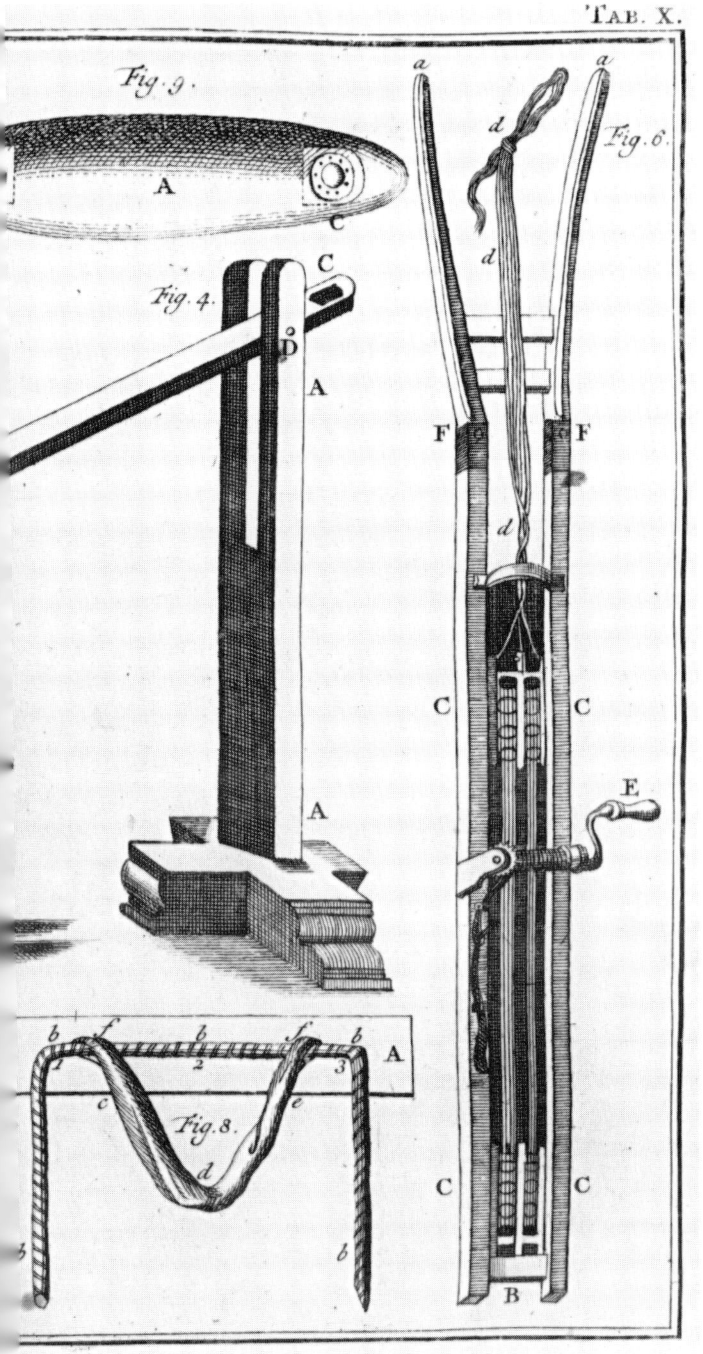

E the Handle, which being turned round, draws the Rope Tight, and extends the Limb; F F the Place where the two Horns are joined to the Body of the Machine.
Fig. 7. Is A Retinaculum or Supporter, to be used in a Luxation for the Humerus. A an Opening or Slit in the Machine; B the Form of it at each End; D D two Apertures, through which the two Legs or Horns a a of the instrument Fig. 6. are to be passed.
Fig. 8. Is a particular Sling of Mr. Petit's, proper for extending luxated Limbs. A A the Part made with Leather; b b b a Silk Ligature, sewed to the Leather in three Places at 1, 2, 3. The Part A A is fastened round the Arm; c d e is a strong Loop fastened to the Silk Ligature at f f so as to be moveable.
[Fig. 9 is not mentioned in the English text.]
Fig. 10. Is an Instrument recommended by Petit for the Reduction of a luxated Femur when dislocated forwards. It is to be fastened at F F in the Machine Fig. 6. instead of the two Arms a a. The Part A is applied to the Os Ileum, and the Part B to the Middle of the Thigh; but C C are fixed into the Machine Fig. 6. at F F.

fractures

A HISTORY AND ICONOGRAPHY OF THEIR TREATMENT

LEONARD F. PELTIER, M.D.

NORMAN PUBLISHING
SAN FRANCISCO
1990

Published by Norman Publishing
442 Post Street
San Francisco, California 94102–1579

Library of Congress Cataloging-in-Publication Data

Peltier, Leonard F.
Fractures: a history and iconography of their treatment / by Leonard F. Peltier.
p. cm.
ISBN 0–930405–16–1 (alk. paper)
1. Fractures—Treatment—History. I. Title.
RD101.P43 1989 89-12946
617.1'5'09—dc20 CIP

This book is printed on acid-free paper, and its binding materials have been chosen for strength and durability.

Norman Orthopedic Series, No. 1
Norman Surgery Series, No. 3

Manufactured in the United States of America.

TO OWEN H. WANGENSTEEN

Contents

Illustrations

CHAPTER FIVE

CHAPTER SEVEN

CHAPTER EIGHT

CHAPTER NINE

CHAPTER TEN

APPENDIX B

Abbreviations

Abh Geistes social Klasse Jahrgang *Abhandlungen des Geistes und socialwissenschaftlichen Klasse Jahrgang*
Acta anesthesiol scand *Acta anaesthesiologica scandinavica*
Acta chir austrica *Acta chirurgica austrica*
Acta chir scand *Acta chirugica scandinavica*
Acta morpho Acad sci Hung *Acta morphological Academia scientarium Hungary*
Acta orthop scand *Acta orthopaedica scandinavica*
AMA Arch Surg *The American Medical Association's Archives of Surgery*
Am Anthro *American Anthropologist*
Am J Med Sci *The American Journal of Medical Science*
Am J Orthop Surg *The American Journal of Orthopedic Surgery*
Am J Sports Med *The American Journal of Sports Medicine*
Am J Surg *The American Journal of Surgery*
Am Med Rec *The American Medical Recorder*
Am Med Times *American Medical Times*
Am Surg *American Surgeon*
Anat Rec *Anatomical Record*
Ann Med Hist *Annals of Medical History*
Ann sci nat *Annales des sciences naturelles*
Ann Surg *Annals of Surgery*
Annuaire méd-chir hôp Par *Annuaire médico-chirurgical des hôpitaux de Paris*
Arch klin Chir *Archiv für klinische Chirurgie*
Arch Neurol Psychiat *Archives of Neurology and Psychiatry*
Arch ortho Unfall-Chir *Archiv fuer orthopaedische und Unfall-Chirurgie*
Archs gén méd *Archives génerales de médecine*
Archs méd pharm nav *Archives de médecine et pharmacie navales*
Archs Mus Hist nat *Archives du Muséum d'Histoire naturelle*
Assoc Med J *Association Medical Journal*
Berl klin Wschr *Berlin klinische Wochenschrift*
Boston Med Surg J *Boston Medical and Surgical Journal*
Brit J Radiol *British Journal of Radiology*
Brit J Surg *British Journal of Surgery*
Brit Med J *British Medical Journal*

Brooklyn Med J *Brooklyn Medical Journal*
Bruns Beitr klin Chir *Bruns' Beiträge zur klinischen Chirurgie*
Bull Am Coll Surg *Bulletin of the American College of Surgeons*
Bull Hist Med *Bulletin of the History of Medicine*
Bull Johns Hopkins Hosp *Bulletin, Johns Hopkins Hospital*
Bull mém soc chir Paris *Bulletin et mémoires de la société de chirurgiens de Paris*
Bull NY Acad Med *Bulletion of the New York Academy of Medicine*
Bull Soc Med Hist *Bulletin of the Society of Medical History of Chicago*
Can J Surg *Canadian Journal of Surgery*
Chin Med J *Chinese Medical Journal*
Chir org mov *Chirurgia degli organi di movimento*
Clinica chir *Clinica chirurgica*
Clin J *Clinical Journal*
Clin J. B. Murphy *The Clinics of John B. Murphy, M.D.*
Clin Orthop *Clinical Orthopaedics and Related Research*
Congrès méd France *Congrès médical de France*
Dtsch Ges Chir *Deutsche Gesellschaft für Chirurgie*
Dtsch Klin-Berl *Deutsch Klinik-Berlin*
Dtsch med Wschr *Deutsche medizinische Wochenschrift*
Dtsch Zeit Chir *Deutsche Zeitschrift für Chirurgie*
Edinb Med Surg J *Edinburgh Medical and Surgical Journal*
Ergeb Chir Orthop *Ergebnisse der Chirurgie und Orthopädie*
Fortschr Geb Röntgenstr *Fortschritte auf dem Gebiete der Röntgenstrahlen*
G Accad Med Torino *Giornale R. Accademia di Medicina di Torino*
Gaz hôp civ milit *Gazette des hôpitaux civils et militaires de l'Empire Ottoman*
Helv chir acta *Helvetica chirurgica acta*
Helv med acta *Helvetica medica acta*
Indian Med J *Indian Medical Journal*
Injury *Injury; British Journal of Accident Surgery*
JAMA *Journal of the American Medical Association*
J Bone Joint Surg *Journal of Bone and Joint Surgery (Boston or London)*
J chir (Paris) *Journal de chirurgie (Paris)*
J compl dict sci méd *Journal complémentaire du dictionnaire des sciences médicales*
Jena Zeit Naturw *Jenaische Zeitschrift für Naturwissenschaft*
J Hist Med Allied Sci *Journal of the History of Medicine and Allied Sciences*
J Int Coll Surg *Journal of the International College of Surgeons*
J MO State Med Assoc *Journal of the Missouri State Medical Association*
J Neurosurg *Journal of Neurosurgery*

J Orthop Res *Journal of Orthopaedic Research*
J Trauma *Journal of Trauma*
Klin Wschr *Klinische Wochenschrift*
Lancet *The Lancet*
Liverpool Med-Chir J *Liverpool Medico-Chirurgical Journal*
Lyon chir *Lyon chirurgical*
Mayo Clin Proc *Mayo Clinic Proceedings*
Med-Chir Rev London *The Medico-Chirurgical Review and Journal of Practical Medicine - London*
Med Comms Mass Med Soc *Medical Communications of the Massachusetts Medical Society*
Med Exam *The Medical Examiner*
Med J Australia *The Medical Journal of Australia*
Med News *Medical News*
Med Record (NY) *Medical Record (New York)*
Med Repository *The Medical Repository*
Med Surg Reg *The Medical and Surgical Register*
Med Trib *The Medical Tribune*
Mém Acad chir (Paris) *Mémoires de l'Académie de chirurgie (Paris)*
Mém Acad roy sci *Mémoires de l'Académie royale des sciences*
Montpellier chir *Montpellier chirurgical*
Münch med Wschr *Münchener medizinische Wochenschrift*
N Am Vet *The North American Veterinarian*
N Eng J Med *The New England Journal of Medicine*
New Orl Med Surg J *The New Orleans Medical and Surgical Journal*
NH J Med *The New Hampshire Journal of Medicine*
Nord Med Ark *Nordiskt Medicinskt Arkiv*
NY Med J *The New York Medical Journal*
NY Med Phys J *New York Medical and Physical Journal*
NY Quart J Med Surg *The New York Quarterly Journal of Medicine and Surgery*
Orthop Rev *Orthopaedic Review*
Paris chir *Paris chirurgical*
Phila J Med Phys Sci *The Philadelphia Journal of Medical and Physical Sciences*
Philos Trans Roy Soc London *Philosophical Transactions of the Royal Society of London*
Piedmont Hosp Bull *The Piedmont Hospital Bulletin (Atlanta)*
Presse méd *La presse médicale*
Proc Roy Soc Edinb *Proceedings of the Royal Society of Edinburgh*
Proc Roy Soc Med *Proceedings of the Royal Society of Medicine*
Rev méd-chir Paris *Revue médico-chirurgicale de Paris*
Rev ortop traumatol *Revista de ortopedia y traumatologia*
Russ Samm Naturw Heilk *Russische Sammlung für Naturwissenschaft und Heilkunst*
St. Bartholomew's Hosp Rep *St. Bartholomew's Hospital Report*

San Fran Med Press *San Francisco Medical Press*
Sber phys-med Ges Würzb *Sitzungsberichte der physicalisch-medizinischen Gesellschaft zu Würzburg*
Scalpel *Le Scalpel*
Sci med ital *Scientia medica italica*
SGO *Surgery, Gynecology, and Obstetrics*
South Med J *Southern Medical Journal*
South Med Surg J *Southern Medical and Surgical Journal*
South Surg *The Southern Surgeon*
Surg Clin North Am *The Surgical Clinics of North America*
Surg Forum *Surgical Forum*
Trans Am Med Assoc *Transactions of the American Medical Association*
Trans Am Surg Assoc *Transactions of the American Surgical Association*
Trans Clin Soc London *Transactions of the Clinical Society of London*
Trans NY Acad Med *Transactions of the New York Academy of Medicine*
Transplant Proc *Transplant Proceedings*
Trans South Surg Assoc *Transactions of the Southern Surgical Association*
Trans State MO Med Assoc *Transactions of the State of Missouri Medical Association*
Verh dtsch Ges Chir *Verhandlungen der deutsche Gesellchaft für Chirurgie*
Veröff Geb Milit-Sanitwes *Veröffentlichungen aus dem Gebiete des Militär-Sanitätswesens*
Virchows Arch path Anat Physiol *Virchow's Archiv für pathologische Anatomie und Physiologie und klinische Medizin*
Wien klin Wschr *Wiener klinische Wochenschrift*
Wis Med J *Wisconsin Medical Journal*
Wschr ges Heilk Berlin *Wochenschrift für die gesammte Heilkunde Berlin*
Zeit ärtzl Landprax *Zeitschrift für ärztliche Landpraxis*
Zeit Chir Osterode *Zeitschrift für Chirurgen von Chirurgen Osterode*
Zeit orthop Chir *Zeitschrift für orthopädische Chirurgie, einschliesslich der Heilgymnastik und Massage*
Zentralbl Chir *Zentralblatt für Chirurgie*

Preface

There has been no attempt to address the history of the treatment of fractures since the monumental works of Malgaigne and Gurlt were published in the middle of the nineteenth century. Since that time, progress has occurred at almost a logarithmic rate with the introduction of anesthesia; antiseptic-aseptic surgical technique; the discovery of X rays and antibiotics; and in metallurgy and bioengineering, to name only a few of the major advances.

The history of the diagnosis and treatment of most diseases is made difficult by their continual variation and evolution. Not only do their incidence and manifestations vary, but the diseases themselves may disappear entirely and be replaced by newly discovered conditions. For example, the decade of the 1970s marked the disappearance of smallpox and the recognition of "Legionnaire's disease," and the early 1980s marked the recognition of acquired immune deficiency syndrome (AIDS). In contrast to the mutability of such disease processes is the constancy or immutability of the effects of trauma. The problems posed by burns, contusions, lacerations, fractures, and dislocations have not changed since the beginning of recorded history. The skeletal injuries treated by Imhotep, Hippocrates, and Galen were similar to those treated by Paré, Pott and Cooper, Watson-Jones, and Böhler. It is easy, therefore, for us to identify with these surgeons of the past as we face the problems of the management of such cases.

The purpose of this account is to review briefly the history of the treatment of fractures and dislocations up to approximately the middle of the twentieth century—briefly, because an enormous amount of literature on the subject has accumulated throughout the years. I have tried to select those individual achievements that are significant, to define basic trends in the evolution of methods of treatment, and to comment on the peripheral events that have affected this development.

Acknowledgments

It was Owen Harding Wangensteen who first stimulated my interest in the history of medicine. This interest was encouraged and nourished by Wallace H. Cole and Ralph H. Major. My colleagues in the Sections of Orthopedic Surgery at the University of Kansas Medical Center, Kansas City, Kansas, and at the University Medical Center in Tucson, Arizona, have all given me information, advice, constructive criticism and helpful suggestions. This project would have been impossible without the support that I received from the Library of the College of Medicine of the University of Arizona and its dedicated staff, particularly Zo Deane Knipe and Kathy Tower, and especially Nguyen Thi Nga. The Louise Darling Biomedical Library at the University of California, Los Angeles, the Loren D. Carlson Health Sciences Library at the University of California, Davis, the Lane Medical Library at Stanford University, the New York Academy of Medicine Library, and, of course, the National Library of Medicine, History of Medicine Division, Bethesda, Maryland, have all generously shared their resources with me. For this reason I can say that I have not referred to any sources that I have not actually seen. All translations from the German and French, not otherwise attributed, are my own, and I am of course responsible for any errors of interpretation. I would like to especially acknowledge the help of my secretaries, Janolyn Berry and Roberta Leo, who aided significantly in the preparation of the manuscript, and that of my colleague, Dr. Donald P. Speer, who looked over my shoulder with a keen editorial eye during the entire project.

Leonard F. Peltier, M.D.

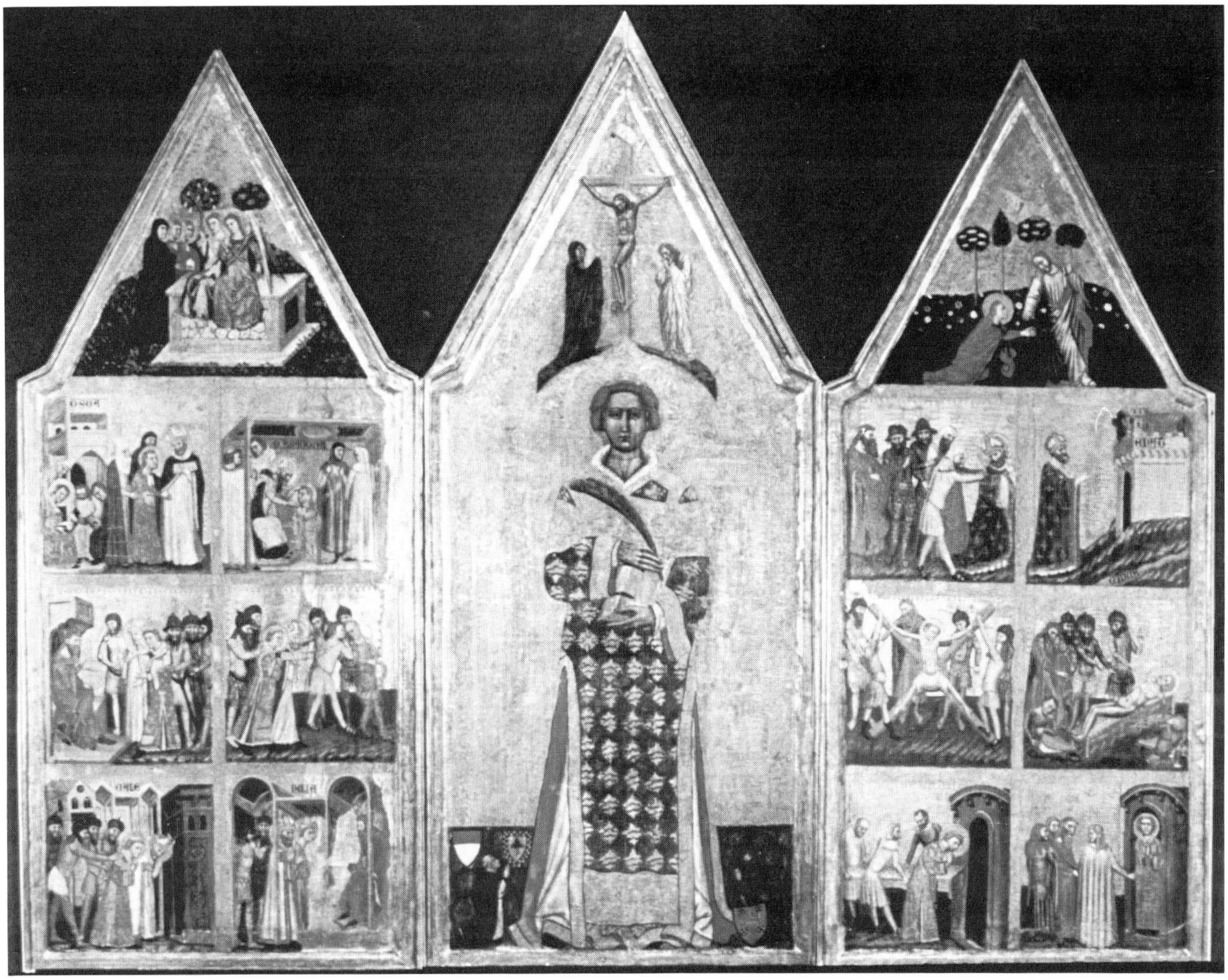

St. Vincent of Zaragosa

The Jesuit missionary to northern Mexico, Juan de Esteyneffer, had a most interesting medical hagiology, listing 153 different saints who were related to medical problems or diseases.* One of these was the patron saint of fractures, St. Vincent of Zaragosa.

St. Vincent was ordained by St. Valerius, Bishop of Zaragosa, and served as his deacon. In 304 a.d., during the persecution of the Christians by Diocletian and Maximian, the two were arrested, imprisoned, and tortured. Valerius eventually was released, but after having his joints dislocated on the rack and undergoing other cruel torture, Vincent died. Several miracles were attributed to St. Vincent and he was elevated to sainthood. In Spain, he became associated with fractures and dislocations, presumably because of his sufferings on the rack. In France, he is associated with vintners. His saint's day is the 22nd of January.**

This is a photograph of a triptych in the Museu d'Art de Catalunya in Barcelona of St. Vincent of Zaragosa. The center figure is that of St. Vincent holding the palm branch indicative of his martyrdom. The panels on either side depict incidents of his trial, torture, and sainthood.

* Juan de Esteyneffer, *Florilegio medicinal de todas enfermas*, new edition with commentary by Carmen Anzures y Bolanos (Mexico: Academia Nacional de Medicina, 1978).

** *Butler's Lives of the Saints*, complete edition, edited, revised, and supplemented by Herbert Thurston, S. J., and Donald Atwater, Vol. I (New York: P. J. Kennedy & Sons, 1981).

CHAPTER ONE

Bone-Setting

*Huat hanat isto pista sista domiabo damnaustra et luxato.**
—*Cato*

THE PRACTICE OF folk medicine is as old as man himself. It arose in response to the medical needs of a society in which there were no educated physicians, and it persists throughout the world today in areas that lack physicians and medical facilities, among groups without access to regular medical care, and among those who would rather be treated by a folk medicine practitioner than a regular physician. Traditionally, practitioners of folk medicine have been specialists, and medical care in primitive communities has been fragmented among a surprisingly large number of specialists: shamans, midwives, herbalists, and bone-setters, to name but a few. For example, the early Hawaiians had priests who were diagnosticians, *kahuna haha;* herbalists, *kahuna lapaau;* masseurs, *kahuna lomilomi;* obstetricians, *kahuna hoohanau;* psychotherapists, *kahuna nui;* and bone-setters, *kahuna haihai.*[1] This tendency toward specialization was apparent to Herodotus in the fifth century B.C. and is noted in his account of the practice of medicine in ancient Egypt:

> *The practice of medicine they split up into separate parts, each doctor being responsible for the treatment of only one disease. There are, in consequence, innumerable doctors, some specializing in disease of the eyes, others of the teeth, others of the stomach, and so on.*[2]

In Europe, the persistence of itinerant surgical practitioners was favored by canons promulgated by the Church in the eleventh and twelfth centuries; these canons forbade clerics, many of whom were physicians, to perform operations (*Ecclesia abhorret a sanguine.*). The Church thus left the field of surgery open to exploitation by

* An incantation to be used while reducing a dislocation. See W. B. McDaniel "A Sempiternal Superstition," *Classical J* 45 (1950): 171–76, 233–36.

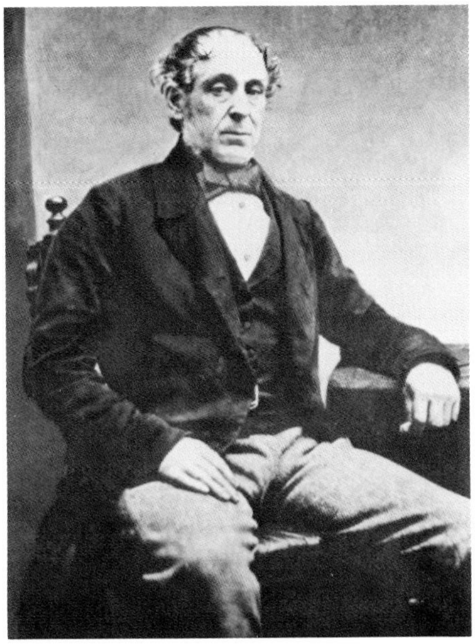

Figure 1.1 Evan Thomas (1804–1884), Liverpool bone-setter and father of Hugh Owen Thomas. From David LeVay, *The Life of Hugh Owen Thomas* (Edinburgh and London: E. & S. Livingstone, 1956), facing p. 8.

empirics. Among the itinerant practitioners in fifteenth-century France, Joseph-François Malgaigne lists incisors for stone, herniotomists, couchers for cataracts, tooth-pullers, drug vendors, dosers, and bone-setters.[3] Most sorts of folk practitioners have disappeared as the practice of medicine has grown and developed, but bone-setters can still be found in practice today.

A bone-setter is an empiric practitioner who claims the power of diagnosing and setting fractures, reducing dislocations, and relieving painful and stiff joints. The bone-setter differs from the cultist in that his craft is entirely empirical; bone-setters have made no effort to elaborate a theory to support or justify their practice. Manipulation is applied directly to the limb or joint, and no systemic or distantly removed effects are predicated.

In France, a bone-setter is called a *rebouter* or *bailleuil*, after Jean de Bailleuil, abbot of Joyenval and a noted practitioner of bone-setting; in Holland, they are called *scherpregeter ledenzetter*; in Germany, *knocheneinrichter*; in Italy, *concia-ossi*. In Spain, bone-setters are called *algebrista*, from the Arabic *al-jahr*, *aljebr*, the reunion of broken parts—the same root from which the word *algebra* is derived.

Bone-setters consider their craft to be a natural gift or "knack," and both men and women may be so endowed. Individuals born "feet first" by breech delivery or who have been struck by lightning are thought to have such a gift.[4] The knack can be inherited and as a consequence runs in families, some of which are well known.

For example, the nineteenth-century surgeon Hugh Owen Thomas came from a family of Welsh bone-setters which had a rather romantic origin. Sometime between 1730 and 1745, two small boys were cast upon a beach on the Isle of Anglesey in Wales during a storm. The origin of the ship from whose loss they were the sole survivors is unknown. One of the boys was adopted by a local farmer and given the name Evan Thomas. He became the progenitor of a line of bone-setters. Evan Thomas lived out his life in a remote corner of Wales, but enjoyed wide local fame as a bone-setter. Richard, one of his five sons, continued the practice. Richard had in turn three sons and four daughters, all of whom practiced bone-setting to some extent. One of the daughters emigrated to the United States and settled in Waukesha, Wisconsin; she was known locally as a bone-setter. Evan Thomas (figure 1.1), the oldest son, was aggressive and successful enough to establish himself as a full-time practitioner of bone-setting in Liverpool, although his practice resulted in many conflicts with the local physicians. Coming to believe that the future of irregular practitioners like himself was bleak, he apprenticed all of his sons into the medical profession. The best known of the five was Hugh Owen Thomas.[5]

The Sweet family of Rhode Island is the best-known family of bone-setters to practice in the United States.[6] James Sweet, the founder, emigrated from Wales to Narragansett before the American

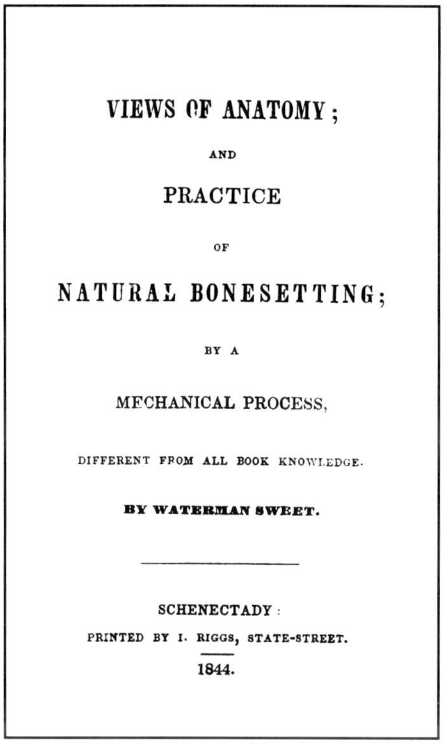

VIEWS OF ANATOMY;

AND

PRACTICE

OF

NATURAL BONESETTING;

BY A

MECHANICAL PROCESS,

DIFFERENT FROM ALL BOOK KNOWLEDGE.

BY WATERMAN SWEET.

SCHENECTADY:

PRINTED BY I. RIGGS, STATE-STREET.

1844.

Figure 1.2 Waterman Sweet's book on bone-setting, first published in 1844. The Sweet family is the best-known family of bone-setters in the United States.

Revolution, bringing his vocation with him. His son, Benoni, enjoyed a wide reputation as a bone-setter. Benoni's grandson, Job, was so widely known for his talents that Aaron Burr sent for him to care for his daughter, Theodosia, in New York City. Other members of the large family known to be bone-setters were Jonathan, William, John, Charles, and Samuel. For the most part they earned their living as farmers, mechanics, laborers, and fishermen throughout New England. Samuel's son Waterman Sweet was the most successful and widely traveled of the family. In 1844, he published a small book, *Views of Anatomy; and Practice of Bonesetting by a Mechanical Process Different from All Book Knowledge*[7] (figure 1.2). In this book, Sweet attributes his success to an innate gift, describes some of his manipulations, discusses the use of emollients, poultices, and other local applications, and concludes with an extensive collection of testimonials from satisfied patients.

Waterman Sweet's son left New England to practice bone-setting in the west, and we have this description of him from a doctor in Missouri:

> *I well remember Professor Frank H. Hamilton telling his class of a family by the name of Sweet, claiming to be "natural bone-setters," practicing in New England and New York; and quite recently, I have heard of a scion of the same stock with like inherited wonderful gifts working his racket in our near neighborhood. He is pictured as a little, gray old man, dressed in gray jeans, with a slouched black hat, and, as he industriously gums his plug of tobacco, he looks, for all the world, every inch of him a western farmer or drover. He says of himself: "I am a natural bone-setter. I belong to a family of bone-setters before me; my father, Waterman Sweet, practiced more than my grandfather—enough at least to make a comfortable living. I have a brother practicing the same in New York state, and a son who will make a bone-setter if he gives it attention; two other sons have not the natural gift. I can't tell why I succeed. It is very simple if only you know how. It requires a great deal of observation and practice and is done by manipulating the joint—no drugs, no medicine, and it generally requires but little time. It is a natural gift and it was so with my father and my grandfather. I make a speciality of dislocations and hip diseases. Sometimes women's and frequently children's hips are thrown out during childbirth. The joint is not put in place, the blood becomes clogged, ulcers appear, and they call that hip disease. I have operated successfully on such cases from one to twenty years standing."*[8]

Since they believe their talent to be innate, bone-setters have never concerned themselves with education beyond apprenticeship. Percivall Pott commented on this lack of education in 1773 in his book on the treatment of fractures:

> *No part of surgery is thought to be so easy to understand, as that which relates to fractures and dislocations. Even, the most inexpert, and least*

instructed practitioner, deems himself perfectly qualified to fulfill this part of the chirurgic act; and the majority even of these, are affronted by an offer of instruction, on a subject with which they think themselves already so well acquainted.

This is also the opinion of a considerable part of the people. They regard bone-setting (as it is called) as no matter of science; as a thing which the most ignorant farrier may with the utmost ease become soon and perfectly master of; nay, that he may receive it from his father and family, as a kind of heritage.

We all remember the great, though short-lived reputation of the late Mrs. Mapp. We all remember the absurdity and impracticality of her own promises and engagements were by no means equal to the expectations and credulity of those who ran after her, that is, of all ranks and degrees of people; from the lowest labourer or mechanic, up to those of the most exalted rank and station; several of whom not only did not hesitate to believe implicitly the most extravagant assertions of an ignorant illiberal drunken female savage, but even sollicited her company, and at least seemed to enjoy her conversation.[9]

Mrs. Mapp was the daughter of an English bone-setter and practiced herself at Epsom. She was widely known, both for her eccentricities and for the social status of some of her patients. "Crazy Sal," as she was called, was immortalized by Hogarth in his print *The Arms of the Company of Undertakers*[10] (figure 1.3), where she shares top billing with two other famous quacks, "Spot" Ward and Chevalier Taylor.

For the most part, bone-setters were illiterate or, at best, badly educated, and lived in poor rural districts. Howard Marsh described a trial in which the court requested a bone-setter to articulate the tibia and fibula. He was unable to do so. Because they lacked formal education, bone-setters have left few accounts of their methods. What descriptions we have are almost entirely anecdotal.[11]

The extent to which incantations, charms, magic, and prayers entered into their practice has varied widely and does not concern us here. We shall deal primarily with their methods of treating fractures and dislocations, and secondarily with their methods of treating other injuries and diseases of joints.

Until Wilhelm Conrad Roentgen's discovery of the X ray, bone-setters and surgeons alike had to rely on the same methods for diagnosing fractures and dislocations. These methods were the patient's history of injury, pain and loss of function, physical findings of deformity, loss of normal motion, false motion, crepitus, visible bone fragments in a wound, swelling, and ecchymosis. Fracture healing was indicated by palpable nontender callus and loss of false motion. The success of the bone-setter thus depended on his powers of observation and the extent of his experience. To these factors the surgeon could add the combined experience of the past as set forth

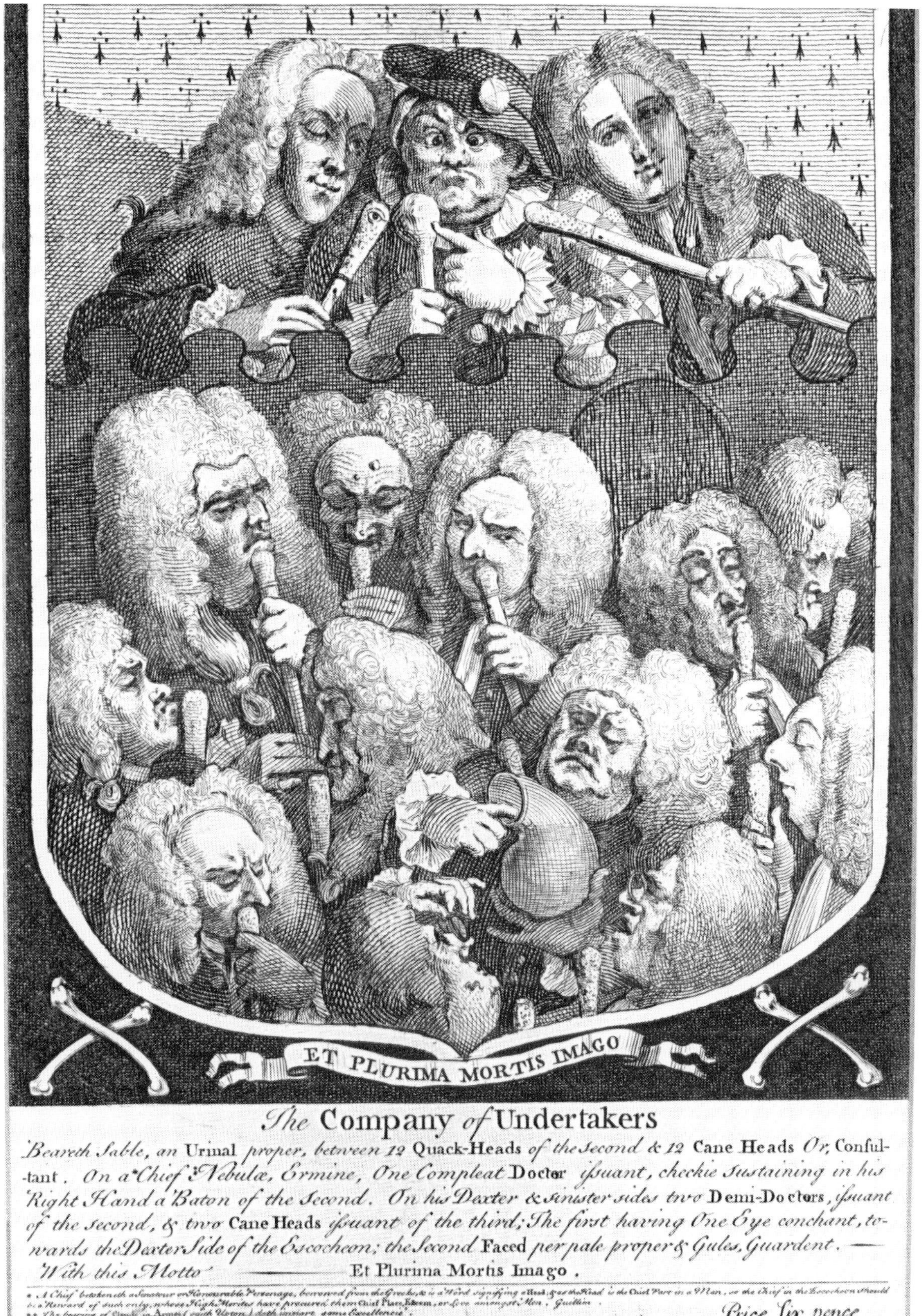
ET PLURIMA MORTIS IMAGO
The Company of Undertakers
Beareth Sable, an Urinal proper, between 12 Quack-Heads of the Second & 12 Cane Heads Or, Consul-
-tant. On a Chief Nebulæ, Ermine, One Compleat Doctor issuant, checkie Sustaining in his
Right Hand a Baton of the Second. On his Dexter & Sinister sides two Demi-Doctors, issuant
of the second, & two Cane Heads issuant of the third; The first having One Eye conchant, to-
wards the Dexter Side of the Escocheon; the Second Faced per pale proper & Gules, Guardent. —
With this Motto —— Et Plurima Mortis Imago.
Price Six pence

Figure 1.3 *The Arms of the Company of Undertakers* by William Hogarth. Mrs. Mapp, the eccentric Epsom bonesetter, also called "Crazy Sal," is the central figure at the top, pointing to the bone she is holding. The character to her left holding the cane containing an eye is the notorious itinerant quack oculist and author, Chevalier Taylor.

in the medical literature and, as time went on, an increasing knowledge of anatomy.

The actual treatment of the fracture or dislocation, particularly if it was several days or weeks old, was preceded by a period during which local applications were made to the affected area. These consisted of water, wine, and a wide variety of herbal or animal substances such as butter, linseed oil, and neat's-foot oil prepared as lotions, ointments, poultices and other embrocations. Their application was accompanied by rubbing and massage. These preliminaries were designed to reduce swelling and edema, promote muscle relaxation, and gain the confidence of the patient.

Diaphyseal fractures were aligned by manual traction by the bone-setter and his assistants. Dislocations and metaphyseal fractures were reduced by manipulation. This was carried out suddenly and unexpectedly after the patient's attention had been distracted. In his lecture "Cases that Bone-Setters Cure," James Paget describes, with a critical eye, the treatment of one of his patients:

> *I believe that, in the large majority of cases, bone-setters treat injuries of joints, of whatever kind, with wrenching and other movements of them. The proceeding was described to me lately by a gentleman who had a well marked fracture at the lower end of his radius. He had been to a distinguished bone-setter, who, with a glance at the wrist, said "You ha' put out your wrist tha's what you ha' done"; then violently stretched and moved the joint; then said: "Now you go and hold that under my pump" and after the cold douche, took his fee. The fracture, being none the better for this treatment, was, at a second visit a few days later, again, wrenched pumped upon and paid for. But this time, much pain and swelling followed; and the patient had the wisdom to call himself a fool, and to go to his usual medical attendant; who sent him to me.*[12]

After applying traction or manipulating the part, the bone-setter applied a dressing. Immediately before this, the skin may have been covered with a thick ointment that could be incorporated into the dressing. The bandage might also be applied with the addition of wax, bitumen, egg white, flour, or even mud to promote cohesion and rigidity. In addition to the bandages, the dressing might also include a splint. A wide variety of local materials were used for splints, the only limits being the availability of the material and the imagination of the practitioner.[13] Sometimes the bone-setter did not use splints, relying on the bandage to prevent displacement.

Of particular interest was the fact that fractures were reduced slowly over a period of days with repeated episodes of treatment, sometimes as often as twice a day. The bone-setter continued to treat the fracture until it did not displace spontaneously after the dressing was removed. Adjacent joints were seldom immobilized, and early passive and active motion was promoted by rubbing and massage.

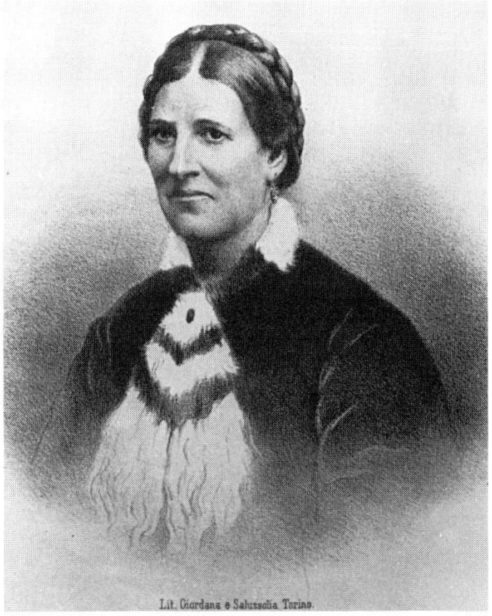

Figure 1.4 Regina Dal Cin, who began her "practice" as a bone-setter as a child of nine, eventually achieving notoriety in Italy for her treatment of congenital dislocations of the hip, which she claimed to reduce readily by manipulation. From *Brevi cenni sulle lussazioni e sulle loro riduzioni* (Torino: n.p., 1872).

This pattern of functional treatment has had its medical advocates throughout the centuries.

While it is fair to assume that many patients benefited from the ministrations of bone-setters, it is equally fair to assume that malunion and nonunion resulted in many fractures. R. L. Huckstep, writing from Kampala, Uganda, in 1961, had this to say:

> *The witch doctor, and local bone-setter, still flourish throughout the country, often with the help of illicit drugs such as penicillin and sulfonamides to add potency to the native brew. The late results of their ministrations alone, in the form of old dislocated joints and malunited fractures, would keep an orthopod busy for the rest of his life.*[14]

Harold B. Boyd's description of his encounter with an aged bone-setter in Kenya is an interesting vignette.[15] I have seen few patients whose fractures have been treated by bone-setters and all had bad results; but after all, consultants are not apt to see cases of successful treatment.

To discuss bone-setters without digressing from the treatment of fractures and dislocations into the treatment of other injuries and diseases of joints would be inappropriate, because it is in this area that bone-setters have had their greatest impact on their medical contemporaries.

William Cheselden in 1784 described the treatment of clubfeet by a bone-setter:

> *Children are sometimes born with their feet turned inwards, so that the bottom of the foot is upwards: in this case the bones of the tarsus, like the vertebrae of the back in crooked persons, are fashioned to the deformity. The first knowledge I had of a cure of this disease was from Mr. Presgrove, a professional bone-setter, then living in Westminster. I recommended the patient to him, not knowing how to cure him myself. His way was by holding the foot as near the natural posture as he could, and then rolling it up with straps of sticking plaster, which he repeated from time to time as he saw occasion, until the limb was restored to a natural position, but not without some imperfection, the bandage wasting the leg, and making the top of the foot swell and grow larger. After this, having another case of this kind under my care, I thought of a much better bandage, which I had learnt from Mr. Cowper, a bone-setter at Leicester, who set and cured a fracture of my own cubit when I was a boy at school. His way was, after putting the limb in proper position, to wrap it up in rags dipped in the whites of eggs, and a little wheat flour mixed; this drying, grew stiff, and kept the limb in a good posture.* [16]

Regina Dal Cin (figure 1.4) achieved notoriety in Italy for her treatment of congenital dislocations of the hip, which she claimed to reduce readily by manipulation.[17] Dal Cin's parents were innkeepers in modest circumstances. She began her "practice" as a child of nine when she treated a fracture in her mother's leg following a carriage accident.[18] We have a description of one of her clinics at the city hospital in Trieste in 1871:

No cases of reduction of the femur have been witnessed by me. Many cases of muscular rigidity of the upper and lower extremities, and more especially of the small articulations, have been either completely and instantaneously cured or partially ameliorated. No attempt has been made in cases of old dislocations with fistulas or scars. Signora Dal Cin is a wonderful manipulator. Her practice extends back nearly forty years, under the guidance of her mother and grandfather. She is about fifty-five years old, and an intelligent looking woman. Her activity, flexiblity, and sensibility of the tips of her fingers, and her habit of incessantly talking to the patient while operating, our correspondent thinks, are the qualities on which her success in manipulating rigid muscles depends.[19]

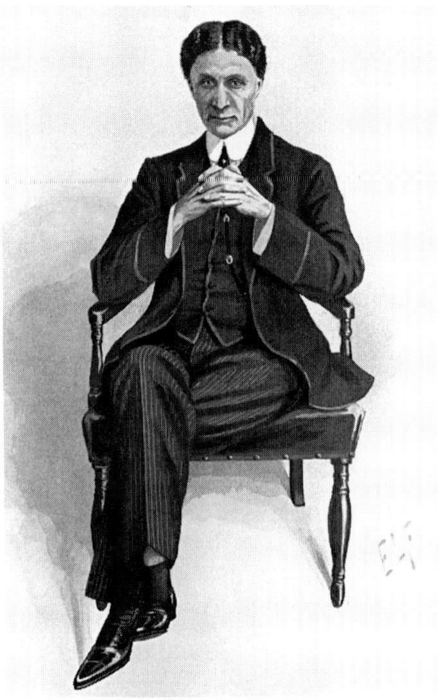

Figure 1.5 Sir Herbert Barker (1869–1950), bonesetting entrepreneur and member of the upper class, whose practice was filled with wealthy and famous patients. Barker was knighted in 1922 for his services to patients in World War I. This chromolithograph by Elf appeared in *Vanity Fair.*

The whole spectrum of injuries, such as sprains, subluxations, ligamentous and meniscal tears, and osteochondral fractures, as well as such conditions as osteoarthritis, rheumatoid arthritis, septic joints, and osteochondritis dissecans, have provided a fertile field for bone-setters. Richard Wiseman, writing in 1676, recognized this:

In several observations in this book I have had occasion to take notice of the inconvenience many people have fallen into through the wickedness of those who pretend to the reducing of luxated joints by the peculiar name of bonesetters: who (that they may not want imployment) do usually represent every bone dislocated they are called to look upon; though possibly it be but a ganglion, or other crude tumour or preternatural protuberance of some part of a joint. In which cases their rash extensions do frequently cause sad accidents. But their more gainful way is, by extending, and dressing up joints rather wrencht than dislocated: in which if they escape undetected, they must needs reap great credit, the patient recovering so soon the ease and use of them. Whereas if the joints happen really to be luxated, scarse one of them knoweth how to reduce them.[20]

There are conditions which can best be treated by programs of passive and assisted motion and manipulation rather than by rest and immobilization. The problem until recently has been how to distinguish between them. Bone-setters achieved their greatest success in patients with internal derangements of the knee and with joints such as "frozen" shoulders, which could be benefited substantially by manipulation and an active assisted range of motion exercises. Their greatest disasters, and there were many, occurred following the manipulation of septic and particularly tuberculous joints.

Bone-setting reached its zenith in the career of Sir Herbert A. Barker (figure 1.5), during the early part of this century. Barker's father was a lawyer; his mother, a distant relative of the family of George Washington. Orphaned at an early age, Barker attended a boarding school. Before continuing his education, he decided to visit Canada, and it was on this voyage that he discovered his "gift" for healing at age eighteen. In the absence of a ship's doctor, he apparently reduced a dislocation of the elbow of a passenger who had fallen during rough weather. Returning to England, he decided that instead of going on to university, he would accept the invitation of his mother's cousin, John Atkinson, to study bone-setting. John Atkinson was an established London bone-setter with a society practice. Atkinson and Barker were both descended from yeoman farmers who had practiced bone-setting in northern England for over two hundred years. As an entrepreneur and member of the upper class, Barker enjoyed a vogue that filled his office with wealthy and famous patients. During his lifetime, he fought a long battle as an irregular against the medical establishment. In this struggle he was largely successful, and he was knighted in 1922 because of his services to patients during World War I.[21]

In recent years, there has been some interest in China in assimilating some of the methods of splinting fractures used by the traditional bone-setters into the mainstream of medical practice.[22]

Notes

1. "Hawaiian Health," *MD* 3 (1959): 136–39.

2. Herodotus, *The Histories* (Edinburgh: Penguin, 1952), 132.

3. Joseph-François Malgaigne, *Surgery and Ambroise Paré*, trans. and ed. Wallace B. Hamby (Norman, Okla.: University of Oklahoma Press, 1965), 168–71.

4. E. H. Ackerknecht, "Primitive Surgery," *Am Anthro* 49 (1947): 25–45.

5. David LeVay, *The Life of Hugh Owen Thomas* (Edinburgh and London: E. & S. Livingstone, 1956).

6. A. Wilder, "The Sweet Family of Narragansett," *Med Trib* 9 (1895): 193–201.

7. Waterman Sweet, *Views of Anatomy; and Practice of Natural Bonesetting by a Mechanical Process Different from All Book Knowledge* (Schenectady, N.Y.: Riggs, 1844).

8. A. J. Steele, "The Osteopathic Fad," *Trans State MO Med Assoc*, 38th Session, May 21, 1895, 343–58.

9. Percivall Pott, *Some Few General Remarks on Fractures and Dislocations,* 2d ed. (London: Hawes, Clarke & Collins, 1773), 1–2.

10. N. B. Gwym, "An Interpretation of the Hogarth Print *The Arms of the Company of Undertakers*," *Bull Hist Med* 8 (1940): 115–27.

11. For fuller descriptions of the practice of bone-setting, see Ackerknecht, "Primitive Surgery"; G. M. Bennett, *The Art of the Bone-Setter* (London: Hutchinson, 1927); G. W. Harley, *Native African Medicine* (Cambridge, Mass.: Harvard, 1941); Wharton P. Hood, *On Bone-Setting (So Called)* (London: Macmillan, 1871); D. D. O. Oyebola, "Yoruba Traditional Bonesetters: The Practice of Orthopaedics," *J Trauma* 20 (1980): 312-22; Sweet, *Views of Anatomy*; and A. F. Whiting, "Leaves from a Hopi Doctor's Casebook," *Bull NY Acad Med* 47 (1971): 125–46.

12. James Paget, "Cases That Bone-Setters Cure," in Howard Marsh, ed., *Clinical Lectures and Essays* (New York: D. Appleton, 1895).

13. Ackerknecht, "Primitive Surgery," 84–100

14. R. L. Huckstep, letter to the author, Sept. 18, 1961.

15. Harold B. Boyd, "I Consulted with an African Witch Doctor," *Clin Orthop* 16 (1982): 14–15.

16. William Cheselden, *The Anatomy of the Human Body*, 12th ed. (London: Printed for J. F. & C. Rivington, J. Dodsley, T. Cadell, R. Baldwin, T. Lowndes, 1784).

17. "Regina Dal Cin," *G Accad Med Torino* 3 (1871): 871–80, 931–38.

18. Tomaso Lugli, letter to the author, June 1981.

19. A. Joannides, "Bone-setting on the Continent," *Lancet* 1 (1871): 734.

20. Richard Wiseman, *Of Wounds, Of Gun-Shot Wounds, Of Fractures and Luxations*, facsimile of books 5, 6, and 7 from *Severall Chirurgical Treatises*, first published in 1676 (Bath, England: Kingsmead, 1977), 478.

21. Herbert A. Barker, *Leaves from My Life* (London: Hutchinson, 1927).

22. See, for example, D. M. Amerasinghe and P. G. Veerasingham, "Early Weight Bearing in Tibial Shaft Fractures Protected by Wooden Splints," *Injury* 14 (1983): 405–14; Fang Hsien-Chih et al., "The Integration of Modern and Traditional Chinese Medicine in the Treatment of Fractures," *Chin Med J* 82 (1963): 493–504; and Shang T'ien-Yu and Ku Yun-Wu, "Fracture Treatment: Combination of Western and Traditional," *Indian Med J* 56 (1962): 7–8.

CHAPTER TWO

The Literature of Fractures

If thou examinest a man having a dislocation in his mandible, shouldst thou find his mouth open [and] his mouth can not close for him, thou shouldst put thy thumb[s] upon the ends of the two rami of the mandible in the inside of his mouth, [and] thy two claws [meaning two groups of fingers] under his chin, [and] thou shouldst cause them to fall back so that they rest in their places.

—*Edwin Smith Papyrus*[1]

THIS TRANSLATION OF Case 25 from the *Edwin Smith Papyrus* is the earliest description of a surgical procedure still being used for the reduction of a dislocation of the mandible. It represents a written tradition almost 5,000 years old. The earliest illustrated surgical manuscript that has been preserved contains a representation of this procedure[2] (figure 2.1). This manuscript and the illustrations were preserved in a tenth-century Byzantine copy of a commentary on the Hippocratic treatise *On Dislocations* by Apollonius of Kitium, a contemporary of Julius Caesar.

The difference between bone-setters, who passed on their "gift" and an oral tradition to their descendants, and the literate surgeon who is able to ingest, preserve, and transmit experience by means of the written word is enormous. Such a written record of medical experience was of course not possible without an available, relatively inexpensive material to write upon (papyrus), suitable inks and pens or brushes, and most important of all, a system of writing. From the beginning, we must recognize that progress in the treatment of fractures and dislocations, as in all aspects of medicine, has depended heavily on discoveries and improvements in unrelated areas of technology.

The *Edwin Smith Papyrus* is an incomplete copy of the earliest known treatise devoted to surgery; it was composed about 2,800-3,000 B.C.[3] Edwin Smith, an American Egyptologist who lived in Luxor from 1858 to 1876, purchased portions of the papyrus from an Egyptian dealer in antiquities (that is, a grave robber) in 1862. Because he knew the ancient Egyptian hieratic script, Smith was able to reconstruct the papyrus as it now survives. After his death, the papyrus was given to the New York Historical Society. Although Smith had begun a translation of the work, and many Egyptologists

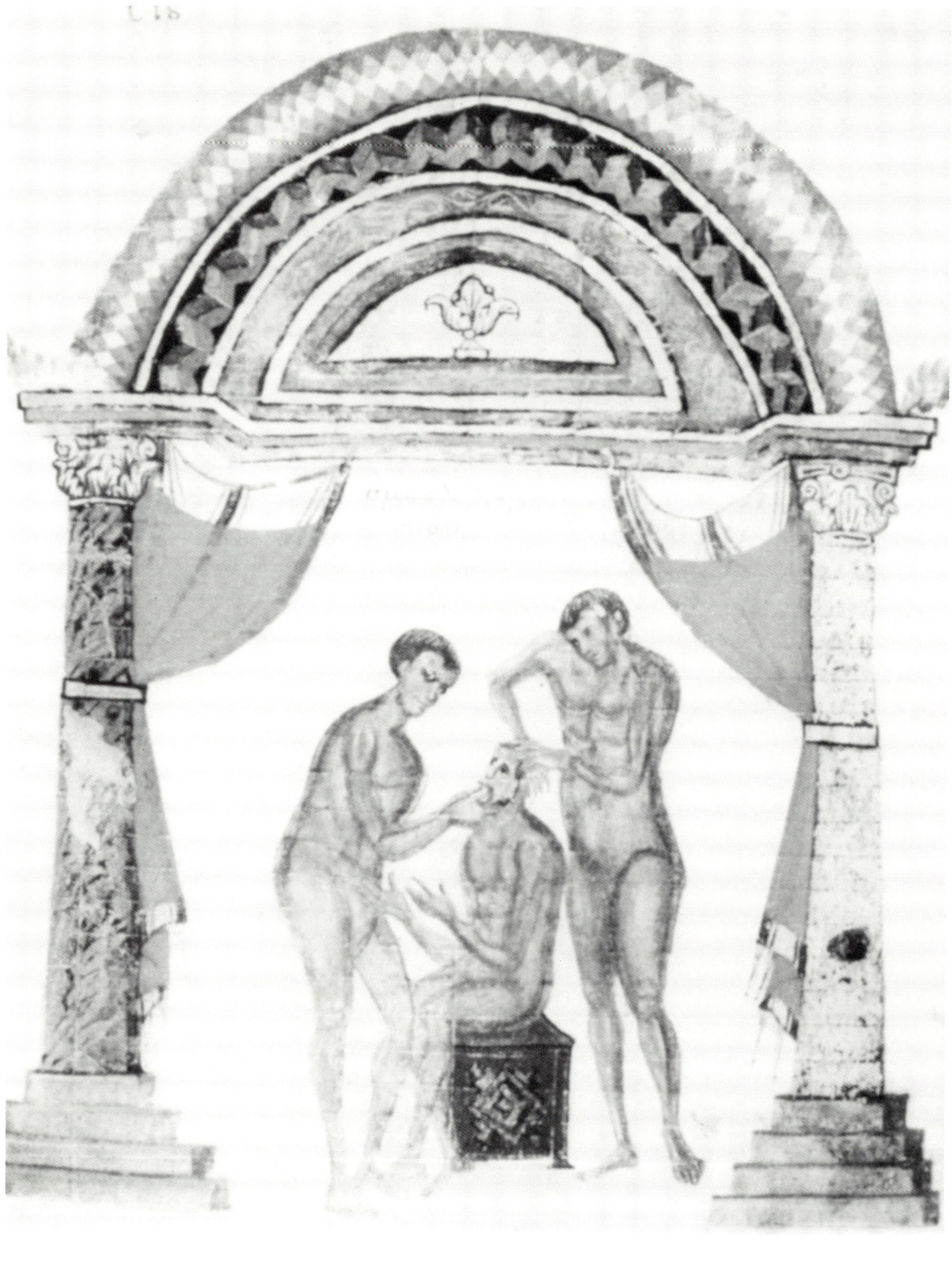

Figure 2.1 The reduction of a dislocation of the mandible, as shown in the oldest illustrated surgical text extant, a 10th century Byzantine manuscript. From Apollonius, *Commentario di Apollonio di Kition sul "Peri Arthron" di Ippocrate*, Codice Laurenziana LXXIV, 7 sec. IX (Firenze: Biblioteca Laurenziana, n.d.)

had some knowledge of its contents, it was not until James Breasted's translation of the papyrus in 1930 that surgeons became aware of what it contained.

The papyrus consists of a series of case reports of which only forty-eight are preserved, arranged in order from the head downward. This arrangement, *eis podas ec cephales, a capite ad calces* (from head to foot), did not change in medical literature for the next 4,500 years. The description of cases in the papyrus introduced, for the first time in any written language, words for *brain*, *fracture*, *open fracture*, and *comminuted fracture*. The closure of wounds by means of sutures and by strips of adhesive plaster was described for the first time. The observations of the effects of injuries of the brain and spinal cord, and the relationship between the pulse and the action of the heart hint at a fund of knowledge greater than is revealed in the fragments of the treatise that have survived. Each case is presented with a brief account of the history and physical findings. A prognosis is given: favorable, uncertain, or unfavorable. A plan of treatment is stated: can treat and cure; can treat and try to cure; cannot treat. The treatment is rational and chiefly surgical. In only one of the forty-eight cases is there a resort to magic.

It is particularly interesting to see how easily these short case summaries can be paraphrased into a problem-oriented record:

Case 31: *Data base: History of injury to neck with immediate loss of sensation in arms and legs. Exhibits priapism with dribbling, incontinence and abdominal distention.*

Problem: Dislocation of cervical vertebra.

Plan: An ailment not to be treated.

Case 37: *Data base: 1) Wound over upper arm and 2) fracture of the humerus.*

Plan: 1) If the wound does not connect with the fracture, the arm should be splinted and the wound dressed daily with grease, honey and lint.

2) If the wound connects with the fracture, that is, if it is an open fracture, this is an ailment not to be treated.[4]

Unfortunately, the number of cases of fractures and dislocations that have been preserved in the *Edwin Smith Papyrus* is too small to provide a substantial insight into ancient Egyptian methods of diagnosis and treatment. Like bone-setters, the Egyptian surgeons used local applications of honey and other substances and placed heavy emphasis on bandaging. Splints of wood padded with linen were used, and sometimes a roll of linen alone was used as a splint. Cartonnage, a bandage composed of layers of linen glued together and incorporating plaster, was also employed.

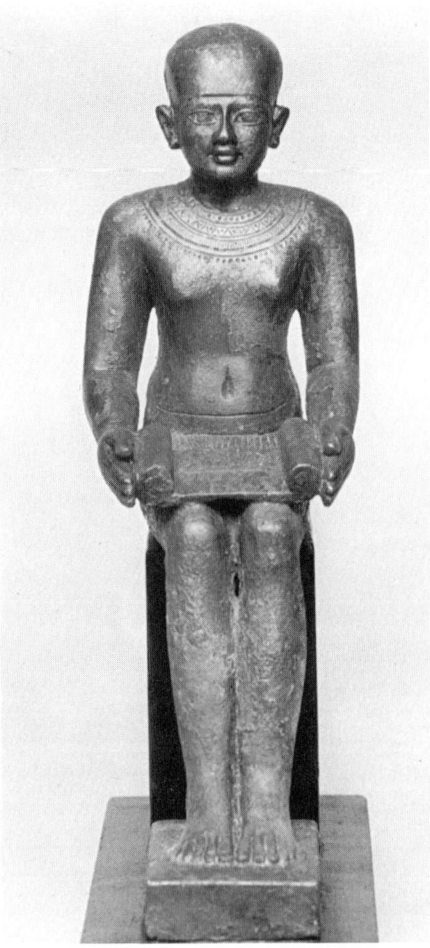

Figure 2.2 Imhotep: A bronze statuette of the early Ptolemaic period depicting this genius of many talents: administrator, architect, engineer, scholar, and physician, whom Osler called "the first physician to stand out clearly from the mists of antiquity."

The appearance of the first of the great surgical texts, the *Edwin Smith Papyrus*, literally at the beginning of recorded history, is astonishing. Its level of sophistication and its accuracy of observation illustrate the fund of knowledge that can be accumulated, preserved and communicated in a preliterate society. This should not be surprising when one considers that in the late Neolithic period the obliquity of the ecliptic and the precession of the equinoxes had already been noted.[5] This pool of information was the birthright of all the ancient writers and questions about the priority of discovery cannot now be answered: The authors were in many ways the conduits through which inherited information was transmitted.

The author of the *Edwin Smith Papyrus* is unknown. While Breasted speculated that Imhotep was the author, there is no direct evidence supporting this association. We can conclude only that if Imhotep was the author, its contents would ensure him of an imperishable reputation as a surgeon. Imhotep (figure 2.2) was a genius of many talents: administrator, architect, engineer, scholar, and physician.[6] As the chief minister of Zoser, founder of the Third Dynasty, Imhotep supervised the construction of the step pyramid at Saqqara (c. 2780 B.C.). He also had a wide reputation as a physician. William Osler considered him to be the "first figure of a physician to stand out clearly from the mist of antiquity."[7] As time passed, Imhotep became a legendary figure, eventually entering the pantheon of Egyptian healing deities.[8] The chief centers of worship of Imhotep were in Memphis and on the island of Philae.[9] The Greeks identified him with their own Asclepios, and he later became the Aesculapius of the Romans. While little is known about his medical knowledge, we can accept the importance of his contributions on the basis of his reputation among the Egyptians as the "first great man in Medicine."[10] To place Imhotep in time, one must consider that the era of Hippocrates (460–377 B.C.) falls almost exactly halfway between Imhotep and our own century (figure 2.3).

Hippocrates, the Asclepiad of Cos, was the great physician of the Golden Age of Greece (figure 2.4). Among his contemporaries were Pindar, Aeschylus, Sophocles, Euripides, Aristophanes, Pheidas, Praxiteles, Xenophon, Socrates, Plato, Herodotus, Thucydides and Pericles. While there is no doubt that Hippocrates practiced and taught at the school of Cos, the methods he used and the priciples he elucidated are unknown. No single word in medical literature can be attributed to him. However, his name gradually became associated with the collection of anonymous Greek medical manuscripts from the fourth and fifth centuries that was assembled in the great library at Alexandria.[11] While Henry Sigerist believed that the basic elements of the *Hippocratic Corpus* consisted of the remnants of the libraries of the medical schools of Cos and Cnidus,[12] they were instead probably gathered in a haphazard manner.[13] Hippocrates' name came to be fixed firmly to the collection by Celsus, who hailed Hippocrates as "the oldest medical writer" and by Galen who called

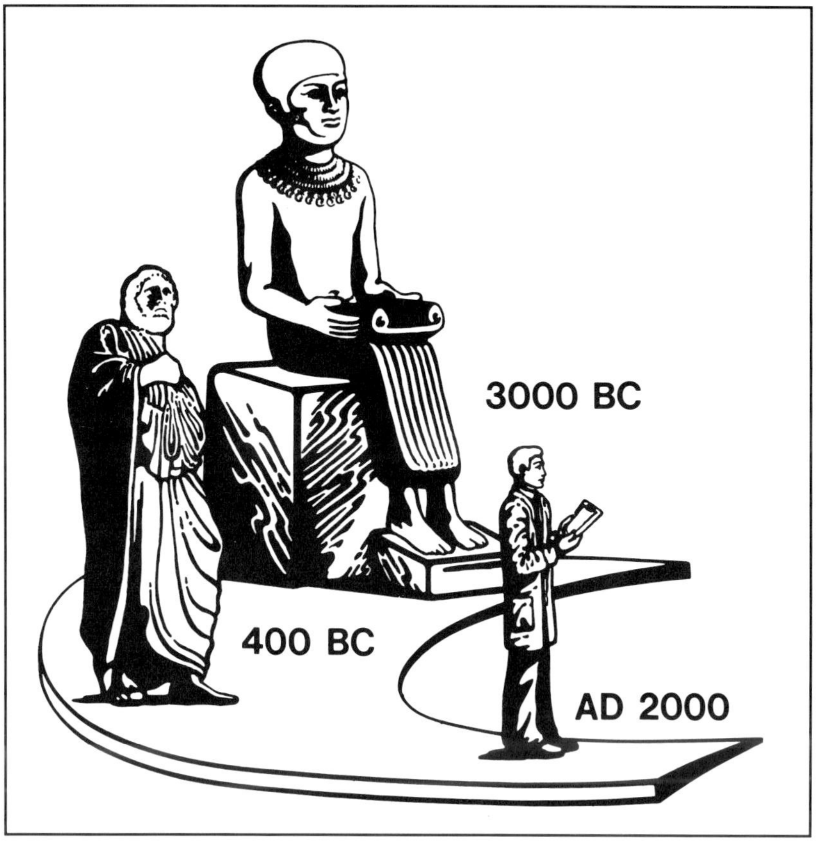

Figure 2.3 A drawing of Imhotep, Hippocrates and a surgeon of today, indicating that Hippocrates lived about half way between Imhotep's day and the industrial age.

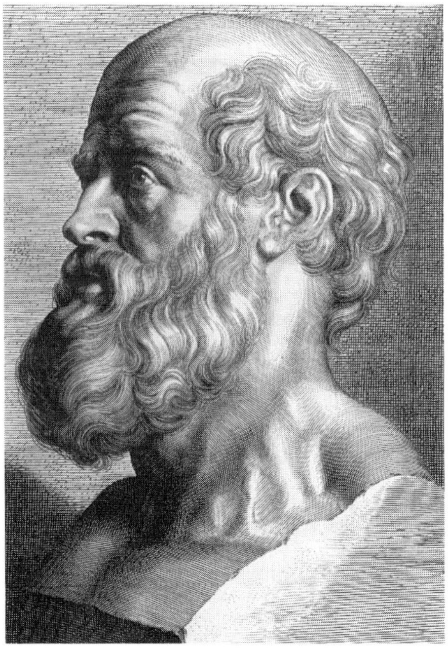

Figure 2.4 Hippocrates. Engraving by Paul Ponce (1603–1658) after a drawing by Peter Paul Rubens (1577–1640). (Antwerp [?], 1638.)

him "the father of medicine."[14] In speaking of Hippocrates, it is best to adopt the view of Fielding Garrison: "By Hippocrates, we mean that great mind behind the greater texts, which evince firsthand study of actual conditions rather than mere summation of past knowledge."[15]

The works of Hippocrates on the treatment of fractures can be examined conveniently in the English translation of Francis Adams.[16] They are four in number: *On Surgery*, *Mochlicus*, *On Fractures*, and *On Dislocations*. The methods and materials described by Hippocrates had been used for centuries before his birth and continued to be used for centuries after his death. Supplies generally available in an agrarian society were used to implement these methods.

The basic element in the armamentarium was the bandage. Perfected by the Egyptians as part of the art of embalming, bandages were applied to the living by physicians. They consisted of rolls of cloth, usually linen, of varying width and length. "Son of man, I have broken the arm of Pharaoh, King of Egypt; and lo, it shall not be bound up to be healed, to put a roller to bind it, to make it strong to hold the sword." Thus Ezekial in the course of a metaphor described a treatment in the seventh century B.C. (Ezek. 30:21).

Later, Hippocrates described six different ways of applying these roller bandages so that they conformed to the varying shapes and configurations of the trunk and extremities. Skill with the roller remained the hallmark of the accomplished surgeon. "It should be done quickly, without pain, with ease and with elegance; quickly by dispatching the work; without pain, by being readily done; with ease, by being prepared for everything; and with elegance, so that it may be agreeable to the sight"[17] (figure 2.5). Failure to apply the bandage properly resulted in sloughing of the skin and soft parts—complications with which Hippocrates was familiar.

Cerate was often used to stiffen the bandage. This was an ointment consisting of lard or oil mixed with wax, rosin, pitch, or similar ingredients to give a medicated preparation that was firm and did not melt upon contact with the skin. A thin layer was applied to the skin before application of the first bandage, and more cerate was rubbed into the bandages as they were wound in place. Rigidity and strength were obtained by increasing the number of layers or rolls of bandages. In closed fractures, the initial treatment consisted of the applicaton of bandages, the head of the first bandage being placed over the site of the fracture. The rollers were extended proximally and distally with decreasing pressure. The limb was not allowed to become dependent. The bandages were renewed daily with increasing compression as the swelling subsided. The reduction of the fracture was delayed until the seventh day after injury or until the swelling was minimal.

Wooden splints of a wide variety of shapes and sizes were used. Some of them were gutter splints. Small splints of sheet lead were used occasionally. The splints were not allowed to touch the bony prominences for fear of damage to the skin due to pressure. In cases of nasal fracture, linen rolls were inserted into the nostrils and pieces of leather were glued to the skin. This dressing was reinforced by mixtures of wheat flour and aromatic gums and resins such as manna or frankincense. Fractures of the mandible were treated by binding the teeth together with wire, linen thread, or horse hair.

Hippocrates relied heavily on mechanical aids to reduce displaced fractures and dislocation: "And all other mechanical contrivances should be either properly done, or not be had recourse to at all, for it is a disgraceful and awkward thing to use mechanical means in an unmechanical way."[18] Forcible extension was obtained by means of axles and levers, and by suspension in a wide variety of methods. The illustrations of these techniques described by Hippocrates have delighted surgeons and intrigued artists through the centuries. The position of choice for immobilizing fractures of the upper extremity was with the forearm in pronation and the elbow flexed to a right angle. In the lower extremity, the hip and knee were fixed in full extension. After reducing the fractures, the bandages were reapplied and reinforced by splints. These dressings were left undisturbed for twenty days.

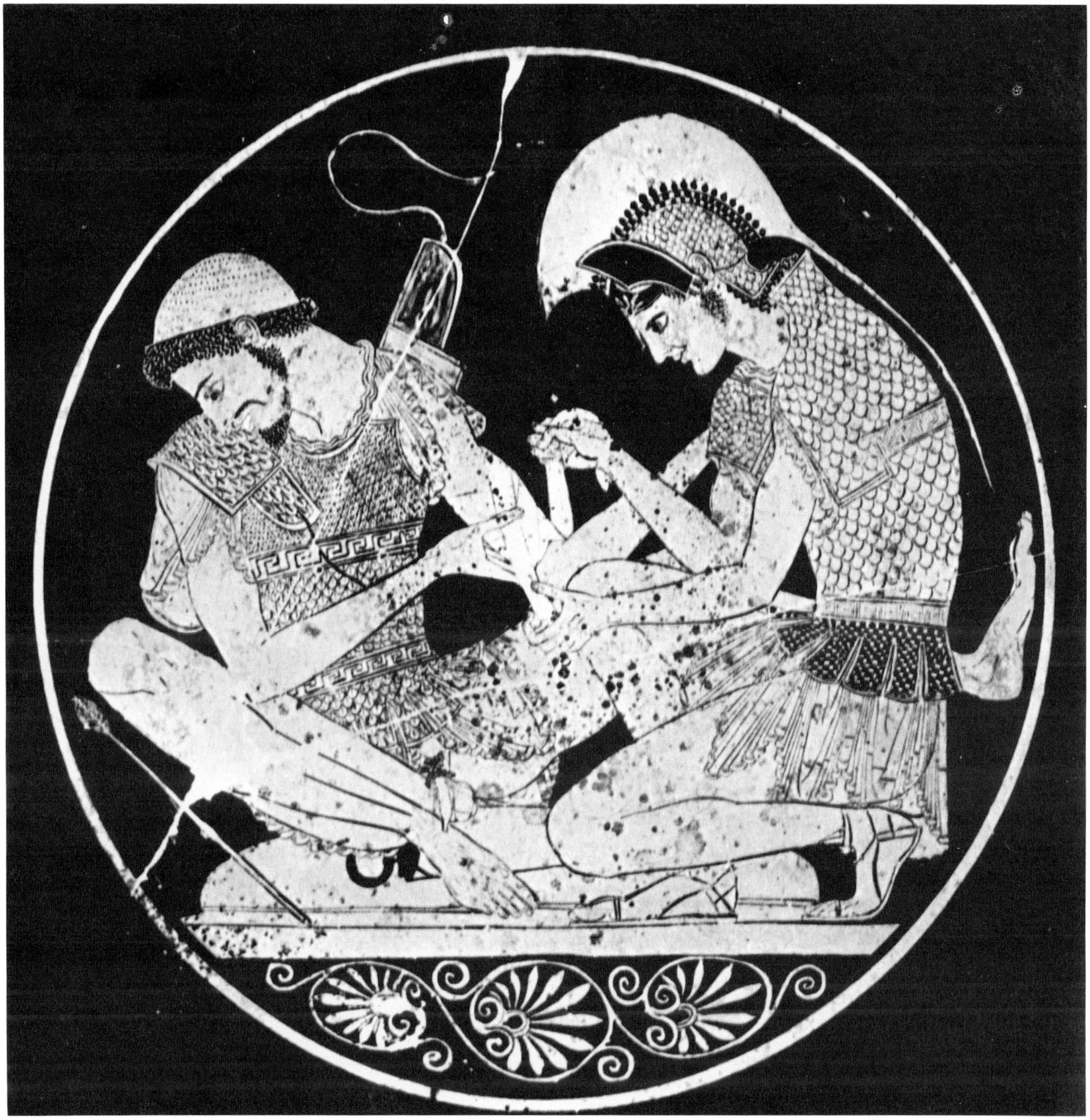

Figure 2.5 The Attic bowl of Sosias portrays Achilles applying a roller bandage to the arm of his friend Patrochlus during the Trojan War.

Hippocrates observed that cancellous bone healed more rapidly than cortical bone. He also knew that open fractures could heal: "But all bones get consolidated more slowly if not laid properly and if not kept steady in the same position, and in this case callus is more feeble."[19] Table 1 shows the estimates he gave of the average time for healing for various fractures, (based on good immobilization), although he admitted that they were not precise. While healing of fractures of the upper extremity with shortening was acceptable because it could be concealed, shortening of the lower extremity was not acceptable because the patient would limp after the fracture healed.

"In all dislocations, reduction is to be effected, if possible, immediately. . . ."[20] In keeping with this view, Hippocrates describes the method used by Imhotep for the reduction of dislocations of the mandible. Like Imhotep, he recognized that dislocations of the spine could be complicated by retention of urine and loss of sensation and motor function, eventually resulting in death. He distinguished acromioclavicular separations from dislocations of the shoulder, and he knew that in the former, in spite of the cosmetic deformity, function was unimpaired. Primary and recurrent dislocations of the shoulder were frequent. Hippocrates described four methods of reduction. For recurrent dislocations of the shoulder he advised perforation of the soft tissue of the anterior axillary fold in several places with a red hot wire. Following this, the arm was bound to the side for a long period to permit scars to form and to contract. The result was limitation of abduction and external rotation of the shoulder, the goal of many subsequent operations for this condition advocated today.

Table 1 *The Healing Time of Fractures, As Given by Hippocrates*

mandible	20 days
ribs	20
spine	speedily and easily
forearm	30
femur	50 days
tibia	40
ankle	40
foot	20

The Hippocratic works on surgery exhibit only a rudimentary understanding of human anatomy, though he was the first to mention individual muscles by name—for example, the masseter and temporalis muscles. Some of his best descriptions, particularly of the anatomy of the shoulder, are suspected of being later interpolations.[21] The foundations for the systematic study of anatomy were laid by Herophilus and Erasistratus in the great Alexandrian school of anatomy (300–250 B.C.). An example of this new knowledge can be found in the commentary on Hippocrates' *On Articulations*, written by Apollonius of Kitium in the first century B.C. This work contains a description of the *ligamentum teres* of the hip joint attributed to an earlier surgeon, Hegeter.[22]

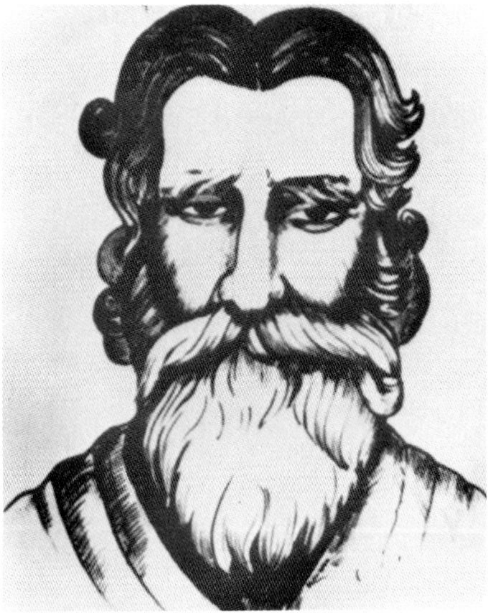

Figure 2.6 An idealized portrait of Suśruta, whose writings form the basis of our knowledge of surgery in ancient India. From P. K. Duraiswami and S. M. Tuli, "5,000 Years of Orthopaedics in India," *Clin Orthop* 75(1971): 269–80.

Ancient India also produced important medical works. Suśruta (figure 2.6) was said to be the son of the sage Visvamitra, a contemporary of Rama.[23] So vague is the chronology of the development of Indian medicine, however, that Suśruta can be dated only between the broad limits of 600 B.C. and A.D. 600.[24] Suśruta's name has become attached to a collection of manuscripts, the *Suśruta Samhita*, considered to be one of the greatest medical works of Sanskrit literature.[25] It is distinguished especially by its description of the practice of surgery in the Brahman period. Suśruta used drugs to allay pain and apprehension. Before reduction of a fracture or dislocation, formentations of bark, honey and clarified butter (*ghee*) were applied to the area of injury. Massage was used to decrease induration and swelling and to relax the muscles. After the fracture was reduced, a pulp of bark mixed with glue and flour was put on the limb and a splint of bark or wood was bound in place. Splints or narrow strips of bamboo tied together with string were used extensively. The dressings were removed and reapplied at frequent intervals. Suśruta also described the method of reducing a dislocation of the mandible used by Imhotep. Like Hippocrates, Suśruta used short iron levers to reduce open fractures.

A. Cornelius Celsus (25 B.C.–A.D. 50) was a Roman man of letters who compiled an encyclopedia consisting of books on agriculture, military arts, rhetoric, philosophy, law and medicine. Only the books on medicine have survived. After being lost for centuries, a copy of the manuscript was discovered in Milan in 1443. Its importance was recognized immediately, and it was one of the earliest medical books to be printed, being preceded only by the works of Albucasis (1471) and Avicenna (1476). *De medicina*, first printed in Florence by Nicolaus in 1478, was written in A.D. 30 and consists of eight books—four dealing with diseases treated by diet and regimen, and four dealing with diseases treated by drugs and surgery. It contains the first important history of medicine and the best account of Roman medical practice. Celsus quotes from the works of ninety-four ancient medical authors whose writings have survived only in fragments. Every medical student and physician is familiar with the four signs of inflammation given by Celsus: *rubor*, *tumor*, *calor*, and *dolor*.[26] Because of the style of his Latin, Renaissance scholars hailed Celsus as the medical Cicero, and he was considered, along with Hippocrates and Galen, as one of the greatest medical authorities of antiquity.

Although Celsus provided more accurate anatomical descriptions of the bones, he closely followed the principles laid down by Hippocrates for the treatment of fractures and dislocations. Celsus advised the use of local applications and bandages, changed at frequent intervals during the first week following injury. After the final reduction, often obtained with the help of mechanical devices, the fractured limb was placed in a suitably padded gutter splint. Celsus recognized the value of an intact fibula in the case of a fractured tibia. Celsus was not an innovator, perhaps because he was not a physician, and surgical practice did not suffer from the disappearance of his work for centuries. However, after its rediscovery and publication, Celsus' work did have an important effect on the vocabulary and prose style of the Renaissance medical writers.

Soranus (A.D. 98–138) was born in Ephesus, studied in Alexandria and practiced in Rome during the reigns of Trajan and Hadrian. His book *On Diseases of Women* was the best work on obstetrics, gynecology and pediatrics of antiquity.[27] For example, it contains an early description of rickets. He also wrote a small book, *De fracturam signia*, *(On the Signs of Fractures)*, which contains a classification of skull fractures. He was an expert on bandages, and some examples of his technique survived in the book *De fasciis liber* by Galen.[28]

Galen (A.D. 130-200) was born in Pergamon during the reign of Hadrian[29] (figure 2.7). Pergamon was then the capitol of the

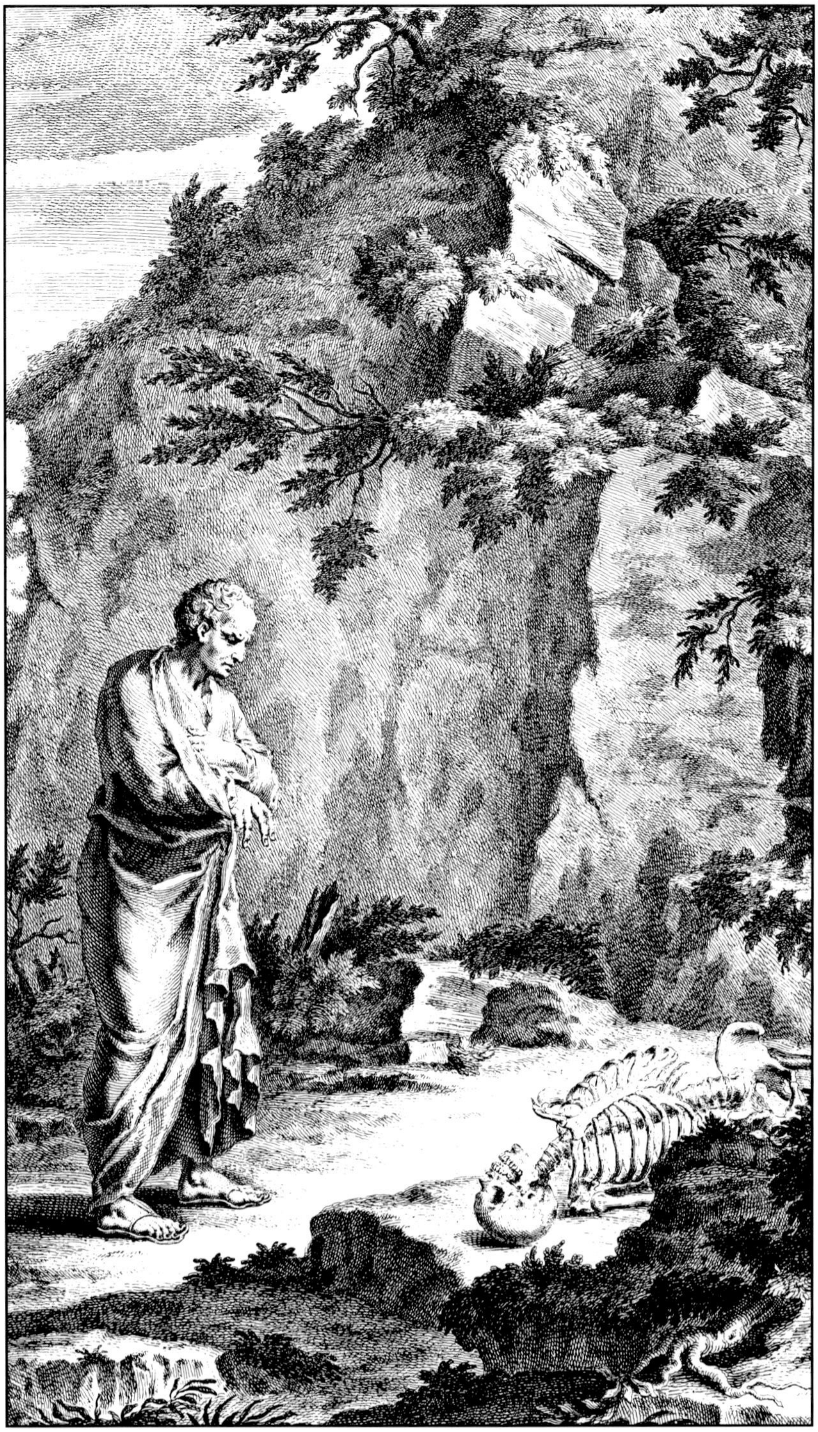

Figure 2.7 Galen looking at the bones of a robber. From William Cheselden, *Osteographia: or, The Anatomy of the Bones* (London: 1733), frontispiece.

province of Asia and a city distinguished for its wealth and culture. Galen received an excellent education and at the age of fifteen began the study of anatomy. He pursued his work first in Pergamon and later in Smyrna, Corinth and Alexandria. In Alexandria, he combined his study of anatomy with the study of medicine. He returned to Pergamon in 158 to assume the post of physician to the gladiators,

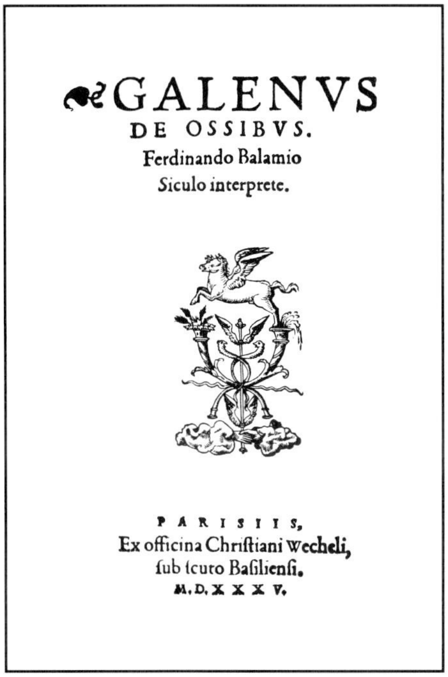
GALENVS
DE OSSIBVS.
Ferdinando Balamio
Siculo interprete.

PARISIIS,
Ex officina Chriſtiani Wecheli,
ſub ſcuto Baſilienſi.
M.D.XXXV.

Figure 2.8 Galen's book on bones, printed for the first time in 1535.

a position he held for three years. During this time he was responsible not only for the treatment of their wounds, injuries and illnesses, but also supervised their diet and conditioning. This practical experience perhaps qualifies him for the title "the father of sports medicine."[30]

In 161, Galen began medical practice in Rome. This attempt was cut short by controversy and opposition from established physicians, and he retreated to Pergamon. He returned to Rome when Marcus Aurelius became emperor to oversee the medical care of Marcus' son Commodus, then a child of eight. Galen was the court physician during the reigns of Marcus Aurelius and Commodus. During this period he enjoyed an immense practice at the center of the political and intellectual life of the Roman Empire. Following the death of Commodus in 192, Galen retired to a life of writing and meditation in Pergamon.

In his book *De ossibus ad tirones*, *(On Bones for Beginners*), Galen used an anatomical nomenclature that included the terms *skeleton*, *epiphysis*, *apophysis*, *trochanter*, *bregma*, *zygoma*, *mastoid*, *sphenoid*, *odontoid*, *thorax*, *phalanx*, *cuboid*, *carpus*, and *metacarpus*[31] (figure 2.8). While the terms he used may not have originated with him, they appear for the first time in this work. *De usu partium* (*On the Usefulness of Parts of the Body*), was written between 169 and 175 at the suggestion of his friend and patron, the ex-consul Flavius Botheus.[32] It was a major work and contained a collection of anatomical and physiological observations that illustrate the diversity of his interests and the untiring purpose with which he pursued them. It had a wide circulation among his contemporaries and affected medical thought for centuries. In his *De fasciis liber* (*Book on Bandages*), Galen described a wide variety made of wool, linen, and leather of various widths, lengths and patterns.[33] Of particular interest was his description of the spica. In Latin, *spica* means "ear of grain." When used as a surgical term, *spica* refers to a type of bandage in which the turns of the bandage cross one another in a pattern suggesting the head of wheat or barley (figures 2.9, 2.10). Galen refers to a shoulder spica, first described by Glaucis, a surgeon of the third century B.C.[34]

In addition to these works, Galen composed a series of commentaries on the Hippocratic books, *On Fractures* and *On Dislocations*.[35] His purpose was to clarify obscure points, to affirm truths, and to expose untruths. He explained the meaning of arcane Greek words and endeavored to answer the question: "What did Hippocrates mean when he said. . . ?" Galen included anatomical information in his commentaries and based some of his discussion on his own experience. By refurbishing and renewing these Hippocratic books, Galen perserved them in a useful form, extending their influence into the nineteenth century. However, he introduced no real changes or innovations of his own into the treatment of fractures.

Oribasius (325–403) was also born in Pergamon and educated in Alexandria. He became the court physician, friend and confidant of

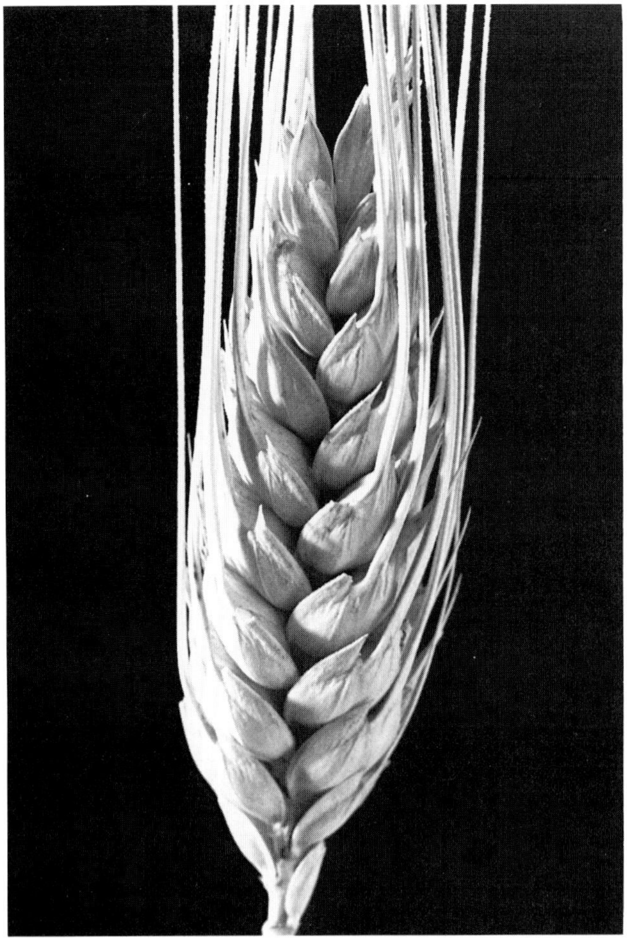

Figure 2.9 A spica, or ear, of grain.

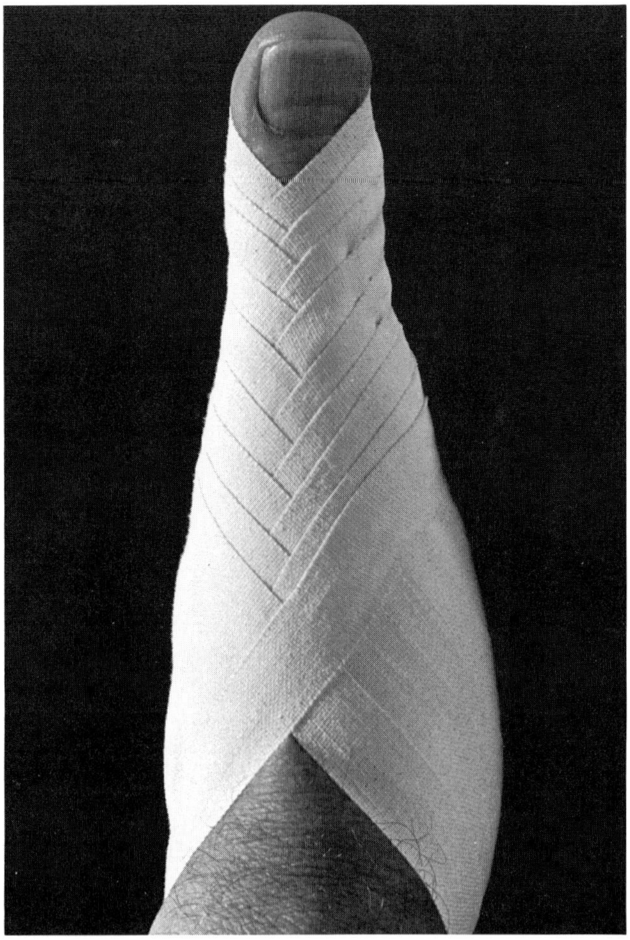

Figure 2.10 A thumb spica applied to demonstrate the pattern suggesting a spica of grain.

the Emperor Julian, a nephew of Constantine. Oribasius accompanied the emperor on his expedition against the Parthians and was present at the emperor's death, which was caused by a penetrating wound of the liver. Having lost his position in the change of regime, Oribasius spent the remainder of his long life compiling an encyclopedia of the medical knowledge of the Greeks and Romans. Seventy volumes were written, only sixteen of which have survived.[36] They were valuable because Oribasius gave his sources and quoted them accurately. Through this work, Oribasius preserved fragments from many authors that might otherwise have been lost. Toward the end of his life, Oribasius wrote a popular synopsis of his encyclopedia. The methods for the treatment of fractures and dislocations described by Oribasius were essentially those of Hippocrates and Galen.

Paul of Aegina (652–90) was the last of the Greek authors and compilers. His surviving work consists of seven books, the sixth of which deals with surgery and includes the treatment of fractures and dislocations.[37] The entire collection is valuable because it gives a rather complete summation of the methods of treatment used by the ancients. The nineteenth-century English translation by Francis Adams with its scholarly notes makes this material readily available. Paul included nothing new in his section on the treatment of fractures and dislocations, but he was a practical and experienced surgeon who did make original comments on lithotomy, trephination, tonsillectomy, paracentesis, and amputation of the breast.[38]

The great authors who wrote in Arabic provided the bridge over which the collected medical knowledge of the Greeks and Romans reached Western Europe. Their original contributions to the practice of surgery were limited because Islam prohibited the study of human anatomy. Although the encyclopedic medical works of Rhazes and Avicenna influenced medical education and practice for centuries, their treatment of fractures and dislocations was essentially that of Paul of Aegina. Only Albucasis (936–1013) broke new ground. The three surgical books of his collection, the *Altasrif*, are unusual because in addition to their restatement of Greek and Roman material, they contain interpolated anecdotes and case reports from his own practice.[39] Albucasis demonstrated his independence of thought by advocating that in patients with fractures of the shaft of the femur, the knee should be flexed completely. All other writers from Hippocrates to the time of Percivall Pott, with the exception of Fabricius de Aquapendente, advocated the treatment of fractures of the femur with the knee in full extension. Albucasis described a variety of plasters and poultices to be applied to the fractured limb:

> *This is a description of the plasters used for repair, applied to fracture, dislocation or sprain. Description of a common simple plaster for the repair of fractures, suited to most constitutions, particularly for women and children, because in it there predominates neither hot nor cold. Take mill dust, that is, the fine flour that sticks to the walls of a mill as the grindstone moves. Pound it as it is, without sieving, with egg white, to a medium consistency; then use.*
>
> *Description of another plaster for the repair of a fracture, luxation or dislocation: take ten drachms each of pulse, gum-mastic, acacia, elecampane, mughath, and sukk, five drachms each of myrrh, and aloes; twenty drachms of clay of Armenia or Asia Minor; all should be pounded fine and mixed with water of tamarisk, or with egg white if the patient be of a warm constitution; then use this plaster, which is excellent for uniting, quickly repairing broken bones, and suits most people because of its mildness.*[40]

These concoctions were applied to the broken limb following the reduction of the fracture, and the usual bandages and splints were then applied. After drying, some of these mixtures helped to provide more rigid fixation; others were favored for their emollient and healing properties. The use of these plasters and poultices contrasted sharply with the practice of the ancient authors since the dressings with which they were combined were left undisturbed for days and weeks rather than being changed and reapplied every few days.

The Church became the repository of knowledge following the fall of the Roman Empire in the West, preserving what little learning there was in Europe during a long and tumultuous period. Clerical orders became the only routes to literacy and education available to the ambitious. It is thus not surprising that clerics at all levels of the church hierarchy engaged in the practice of medicine. Women were not excluded from this work, and some like Hildegard of Bingen (1098–1179) were well known.[41] The foundation of a nursing order of women was a natural development. The Church also had an important role in the founding of hospitals. For example, l'Hôtel Dieu was founded in Paris in the seventh century by St. Landry, Bishop of Paris, and St. Bartholomew's Hospital in London was founded in 1123 by Rahere, the first prior of the Priory of Austin Canons in Smithfield. The Crusades saw the growth of orders such as the Knights Hospitalers, who were dedicated to the care of the sick and wounded.

The success of these clerical physicians was their undoing, however. They became more interested in their patients than in their preaching, more preoccupied with the things of this world than with those of the next—including fine clothes, servants, and fine wines, rich food, and other temptations of the flesh. These abuses of the religious life eventually led to drastic reform.

The Church's reform of medical practice was only a small part of a larger program that addressed all the abuses among the clergy.[42] It was instituted by a series of Church councils held between 1130 and 1147.* The reforms were expressed as canons, from the Greek word meaning a "rod," a "line," or a "ruler;" it carried a secondary meaning of "straightness," "fixity," or a "norm" or "standard." The term was used by early Christian theologians to define the Church's position in matters of faith and practice, dogma and discipline. Canons were thus designed to straighten out deviations from correct behavior and to keep wayward and rebellious clerics and parishioners in line. Some of these canons forbade clerics to practice or even to study medicine. The practice of surgery was in particular proscribed. The dictum *ecclesia abhorret a sanguine* was observed throughout Western Europe, though with a few notable exceptions. Among these were some of the most important surgeons of the period: Hugh of Lucca, Bruno, Theodoric, Arnold of Villanova, William of Salicet, Lanfranc, Henri de Mondeville and Guy de Chauliac. Two physicians even became popes, John XXI (reigned 1276–77) and Paul II (1464–71). In spite of these exceptions, surgery ceased to be part of the intellectual mainstream of medical life and thought. Rushing to

* The councils of Clermont (1130) and Rheims (1131), the Second Lateran Council (1139), the Councils of Montpellier (1162), Tours (1163), and Paris (1212), the Fourth Lateran Council (1215), and the Council of LeMans (1247).

fill the gap left by the departure of the educated clerical surgeon came the self-taught specialists and quacks, the bone-setters, the lithotomists, the oculists, and the herniotomists. Thus the Church reforms, precipitated by the lax spiritual discipline of clerical practitioners, forced surgery and surgeons into a decline that lasted almost five hundred years.

The *Surgery* of Theodoric (d. 1267) provides a good measure of the state of the practice of surgery in medieval Europe.[43] It draws from ancient Greek and Roman authors as well as from Arabic ones, especially Albucasis. Theodoric was his son and protege of Hugh of Lucca, who was physician to the Bolognese in Syria and in Egypt during the Crusades, and the *Surgery* is based substantially on Hugh's work.[44] Theodoric was also influenced by Bruno of Longoburg. These three surgeons promulgated the concept that wounds, properly cleansed, brought into apposition and carefully maintained in an undisturbed dry dressing could heal *per primum* without the formation of "laudable pus." Only Henri de Mondeville and Paracelsus supported this point of view until the work of Joseph Lister in the nineteenth century.

Theodoric stated his approach to the treatment of fractures very simply:

> *And the first objective is the true and correct reduction or realignment of the broken or separated bones. The second is the maintenance of the afore-mentioned state by proper binding. The third objective is to restore the intervening flesh to its proper place.*[45]

Theodoric believed that displaced fractures should be reduced as soon as possible because delay made the reduction more difficult. This was in contrast to the treatment of Hippocrates and Galen who advised waiting four to seven days. Following reduction, Theodoric described two approaches to maintaining position. The first, the method of Hugh of Lucca and derived from Arabic physicians, consisted in the application of bandages soaked in egg whites, the placement of suitable pads and cushions, and then the binding on of splints made of wood. This initial dressing was intended to remain undisturbed for two or three weeks if possible. The second was the method of Hippocrates and Galen, in which the dressings were changed and reapplied every three days. William of Salicet (1210–1277) was the leading surgeon at the medical school in Bologna. His book on surgery contained many original observations and included the first discussion of surgical anatomy.[46] In the section devoted to the treatment of fractures, he follows Theodoric and advocates the use of bandages soaked in egg white and other materials and changed at long intervals. He emphasized *sonitus ossi fracti* or crepitus as a diagnostic sign of fracture. Unfortunately, he did not follow Theodoric's ideas on the treatment of wounds. The teachings of

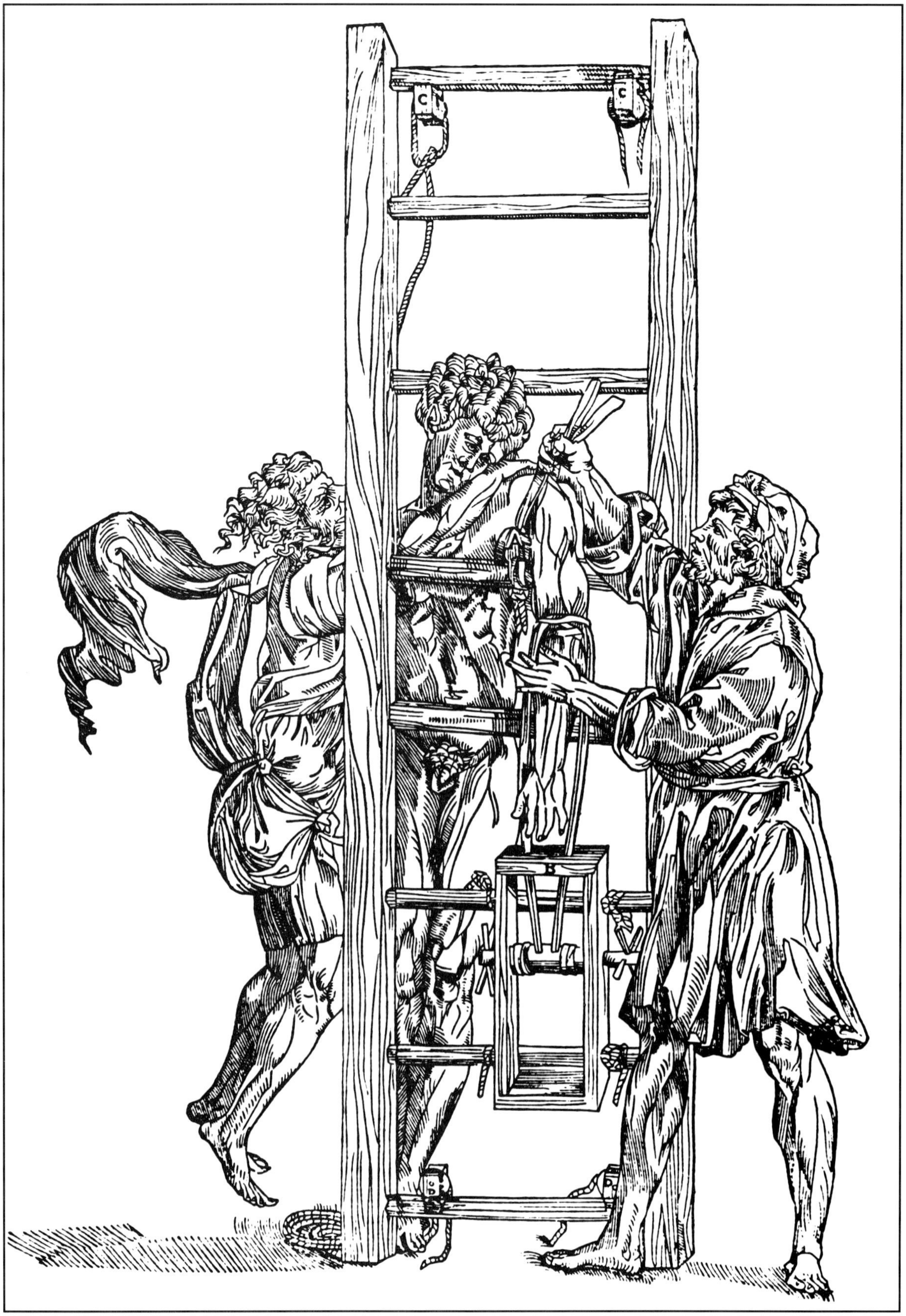

Figure 2.11 Woodcut, after drawings attributed to Francesco Primaticcio, showing the method of reducing a dislocation of the shoulder. From Guido Guidi, *Chirurgia è graeco in latinum conversa* (Paris: Gaultier, 1544). Guidi's magnificent book was printed in the residence of Benevenuto Cellini under the patronage of François I.

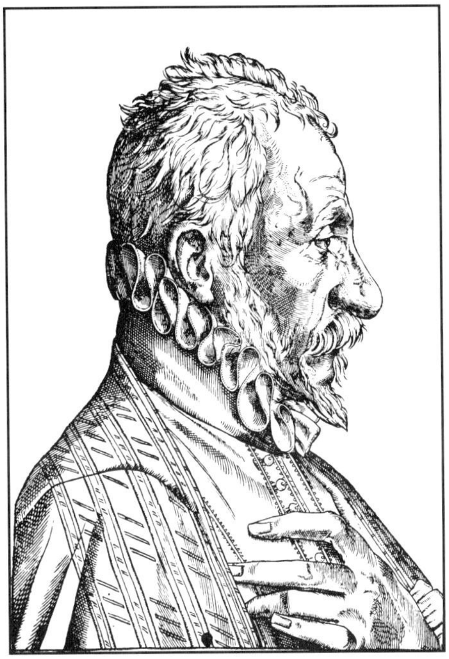

Figure 2.12 Ambroise Paré (1510–1590). Woodcut from the first edition of his collected writings, *Les Oeuvres de M. Ambroise Paré, conseiller, et premier chirurgien du Roy* (Paris: Gabriel Buon, 1575).

William of Salicet, along with all of the erudition of the Italian school of surgery, were carried to France by his student Lanfranc.[47]

Guy de Chauliac (d. 1368) was the last of the great cleric-surgeons. He was well educated, having studied in Paris, Montpellier, Bologna and Prague.[48] He collected an extensive library of medical books by ancient Arabic and contemporary authors. Interestingly, however, he had a very limited knowledge of the works of Hippocrates, and none at all of Celsus. Before being called to Avignon by Pope Clement VI, he had been an itinerant surgeon and and had thus traveled widely. He was in Avignon when the plague broke out in 1348 and described the disease, including his own case, in some detail. He remained in Avignon as the physician to succeeding popes, Innocent VI and Urban V.

La Grande Chirurgie of Guy de Chauliac, which appeared in 1363, contains descriptions of the methods of treating fractures in use at the end of the medieval period,[49] including both the ancient method of using frequent dressing changes and the methods of the Arabic authors, which incorporated stiffening materials into dressings that were changed at long intervals. In addition to using splints made of wood, he utilized other materials such as leather, horn and iron. Guy de Chauliac was also the first to describe the use of isometric traction to the leg applied by a weight attached to a cord and passing through a pulley.

The beginning of the modern era in medicine was marked by the publication of *De humani corporis Fabrica* of Vesalius in Basle in 1543. The following year, the *Chirurgia è graeco in latinum conversa* of Guido Guidi (Vidius) was published in Paris in a sumptuous folio edition under the patronage of François I.[50] In the *Chirurgia*, Guidi presented Latin translations of surgical sections from the works of Hippocrates, Galen and Oribasius, to which he added a commentary. Much of the material deals with the treatment of fractures and dislocations. The beauty of the book lies in its marvelous illustrations (figure 2.11) that were redrawn for Guidi, most likely by the Mannerist Francesco Primaticcio, but perhaps also with the participation of other Italian masters, from the earliest known illustrated surgical manuscript, *Commentario di Apollonio di Kition sul "Peri Arthron" di Ippocrate*.[51]

The great change that marked the emergence of medical literature from the medieval and the Renaissance periods into the modern era was the shift from the use of Greek, Latin and Arabic to the vernacular languages of the evolving European nations: Italian, French, Spanish, English and German.

Ambroise Paré (1510-1590) was a leader of the movement to publish in the vernacular (figure 2.12). Poorly educated and initially knowing little of either Greek or Latin, he slowly became an accomplished and prolific author whose books enjoyed wide circulation. His importance in the history of surgery has been delineated by Geoffrey Keynes:

Paré's contribution to surgery is usually summarized by mentioning his three important "discoveries"—the harmfulness of treating gunshot wounds with boiling oil, the use of the ligature in amputations, and podalic version in obstetrics—but in reality his contribution was far greater than this. He was, in fact, by virtue of his personality and his independent mind, the emancipator of surgery from the dead hand of dogma. There was no comparable practitioner, during his time, in England or in any other country, and his influence was felt in every part of Europe. He left in his collected "Works" a monument to his own skill and humanity which is unsurpassed in the history of surgery.[52]

A great deal of scholarly work has been concentrated on collecting and collating the works of Ambroise Paré, and because of their interest and importance a surprising amount of the material is available in English.[53] Paré had a thorough knowledge of the ancient, Arabic and medieval and Renaissance authors and quoted them frequently. However, he was not merely a plagiarist or a compiler. Paré himself liked to repeat that he had done no more wrong to an author he copied "than a candle which lights itself from another."[54] In fact, when Paré writes from his own experience, his style is more simple and direct than when he is summarizing the accounts of his predecessors.[55] His work on the treatment of fractures and dislocations is often original: an example is his description of a patient with an intracapsular fracture of the neck of the femur, the first such case to be described in medical literature. Of particular interest are his comments on separation of the proximal femoral epiphysis and his observations that the parts of bones near the joints "are bloodless and more difficult to cure."[56]

Sometimes fracture of the neck of the femur occurs at the hip joint, which I saw when called to treat a good woman. Seeing that the leg was shorter than the other, with a prominence the trochanter makes externally and below the joint of the ischium, I assumed this was the head of the bone, dislocated and not fractured. Then I pulled and set the bone, it seemed, in its socket, after which the two legs were equal in length and contour, and I dressed and treated it as a dislocation. Two days later I found her in great pain, the leg short again and the foot turned inward. I removed the bandages and found that the prominence had reappeared.

Then I tried again to replace the bone in its socket and I felt the bone crepitate. Then I found there was no joint cavity, so I knew this was a fracture and not a dislocation.

(Likewise, the epiphysis of the head of this bone sometimes separates and disjoins, so the Surgeon is deceived, thinking it a dislocation and not a disjunction of the epiphysis of this bone.)

Again I reduced the bone, applying splints on the compresses and made a bandage of two parts, crossing them at the joint and around the body like a St. Andrew's cross. The rest of the cure was made as described earlier; I put a hoop over the foot to keep pressure off the toes. I attached a rope to a frame over the middle of the bed, as one should always do in case of fractures of the thigh and leg, to let the patients raise themselves by their arms when they see to their affairs, and also to let them turn a little to lift the back and hips to relieve pressure on the parts, which when denied a long time, produces pain and a strange heat. On this can follow ulceration, most often of the rump, which produces pain, fever, and such great upset that death follows, if not well treated. More important than the fracture alone is that near the joints the parts are bloodless and more difficult to treat and harder to cure, because of the nerves, tendons, and common ligaments which carry the greatest complications. A fracture made in the middle of the bone is easier to treat and heals quicker.[57]

Paré's account of the treatment of fractures and dislocations is a good summary of the state of the art at the end of the sixteenth century.

One hundred years after Paré, an English surgeon, Richard Wiseman (d. 1676), published a treatise in English that contained a large number of observations from his own experience, including the first description of tuberculosis of the joints, "white swellings."[58] In the section devoted to skeletal injuries, he describes forty-two patients with fractures, twenty-eight of which were open fractures, as well as fifteen patients with dislocations. He advocated prompt amputation in cases of gunshot fractures.

Wiseman was a royalist during the English Civil War and thereafter spent twenty-three years in exile on the Continent before returning to England after the Restoration. Charles II promptly appointed Wiseman as one of his personal surgeons. During the Civil War and his years in exile, Wiseman gained extensive experience in the treatment of wounds in the various armies and navies in which he served. Unfortunately, he died in the year his *Severall Chirurgical Treatises* was published.

Joseph Guichard Duverney (1648-1730) was the first of the modern academic surgeons:[59] his teaching appointment was at the king's medical school, the Jardin du Roi, and his research was supported by the Académie des Sciences of Louis XIV. His surgical practice was in the public hospitals of Paris. Among his students of anatomy were members of the court, including the Dauphin, the king's heir. Duverney's book on the ear, published in 1683, was the first scientific monograph on the subject.[60] After his death at eighty-two, one of his students edited and published his manuscripts on bone diseases and fractures. Appearing twenty-one years after Duverney died, *Maladies des os* contains careful clinical observations supported by anatomical dissections. There are excellent descriptions of the gross pathology of rickets and osteoporosis. Included is the report of a case of an isolated fracture of the wing of the ilium—now called Duverney's fracture.

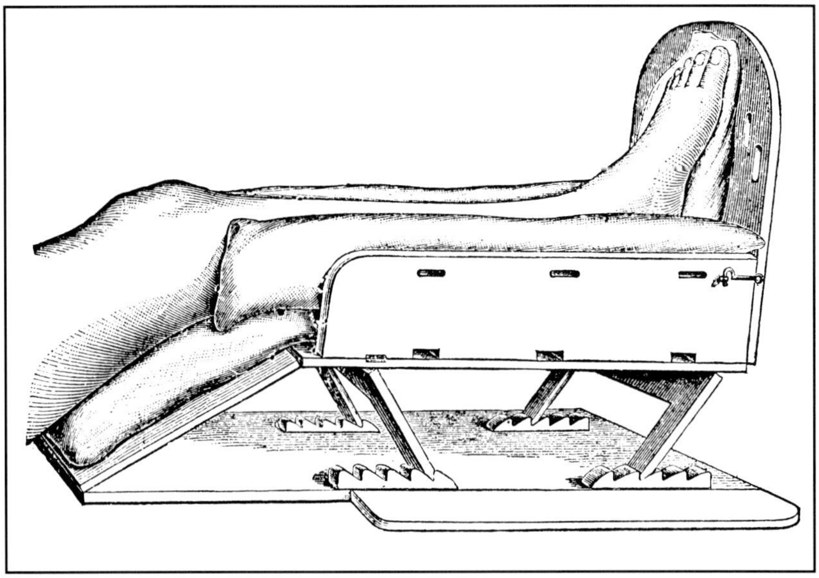

Figure 2.13 Jean-Louis Petit's apparatus for the treatment of fractures of the tibia. It was the prototype of many other models. From L. A. Stimson, *Treatise on Fractures and Dislocations* (Philadelphia: Henry C. Lea's Son, 1883), 1:571.

Jean-Louis Petit (1674–1750), the foremost surgeon in Paris during the first half of the eighteenth century, invented the screw tourniquet, was the first to open the mastoid for mastoiditis, and gave a good description of osteomalacia. His book, *L'art de guérir les maladies des os*, contained practical directions for the treatment of fractures and was printed in numerous editions (figure 2.13).

Lorenz Heister (1683–1758) was a well-traveled scholar, who gained practical experience in the wars between France and the United Provinces. In 1718, he published the first systematic textbook of surgery, *Chirurgie, in welcher alles, was zur Wund-Artzney gehöret, nach der neuesten und besten Art.*[61] He had intended to publish his work in Latin, but chose German instead so that his students could read it for themselves. The importance of Heister's work is apparent from the number of editions and translations that were printed: seven in German, three in Latin, and ten in English, as well as Spanish, French, Italian, and Dutch editions! In addition to discussing the usual treatment of fractures and dislocations, he also comments on the use of the tourniquet and of spinal braces.

William Cheselden (1688–1752) was born near Leicester and was the son of a well-to-do farmer. After attending a local school until he was fifteen, he was apprenticed for a period of seven years to James Ferne, a surgeon in London. During this time, he studied anatomy with William Cowper and assisted Ferne at St. Thomas Hospital. In December 1710, he finished his apprenticeship and became licensed to practice surgery. While waiting for his practice to develop, he began a series of lectures on anatomy. From this venture came his *Anatomy of the Human Body*, a textbook that went through thirteen editions, and his *Osteographia, or the Anatomy of the Bones*, which is

OSTEOGRAPHIA,

OR THE

ANATOMY

OF THE

BONES.

BY WILLIAM CHESELDEN

SURGEON TO HER MAJESTY;

F. R. S.

SURGEON TO S[T] THOMAS'S HOSPITAL,

AND MEMBER OF THE ROYAL ACADEMY OF SURGERY AT PARIS.

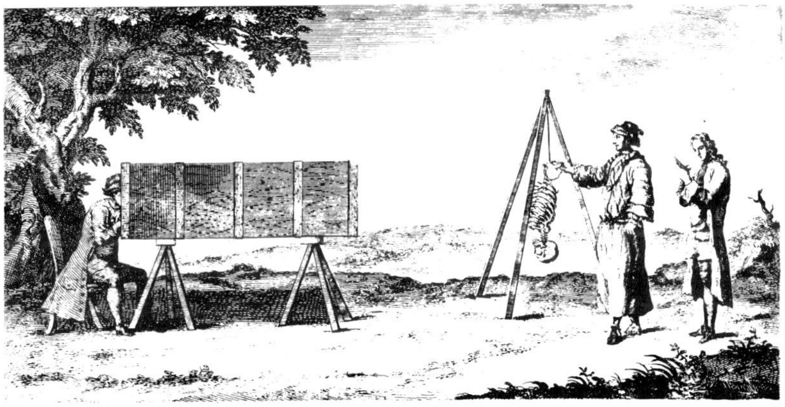

LONDON MDCCXXXIII.

Figure 2.14 The title page of Cheselden's *Osteographia*. The vignette shows Cheselden making a drawing under the camera obscura.

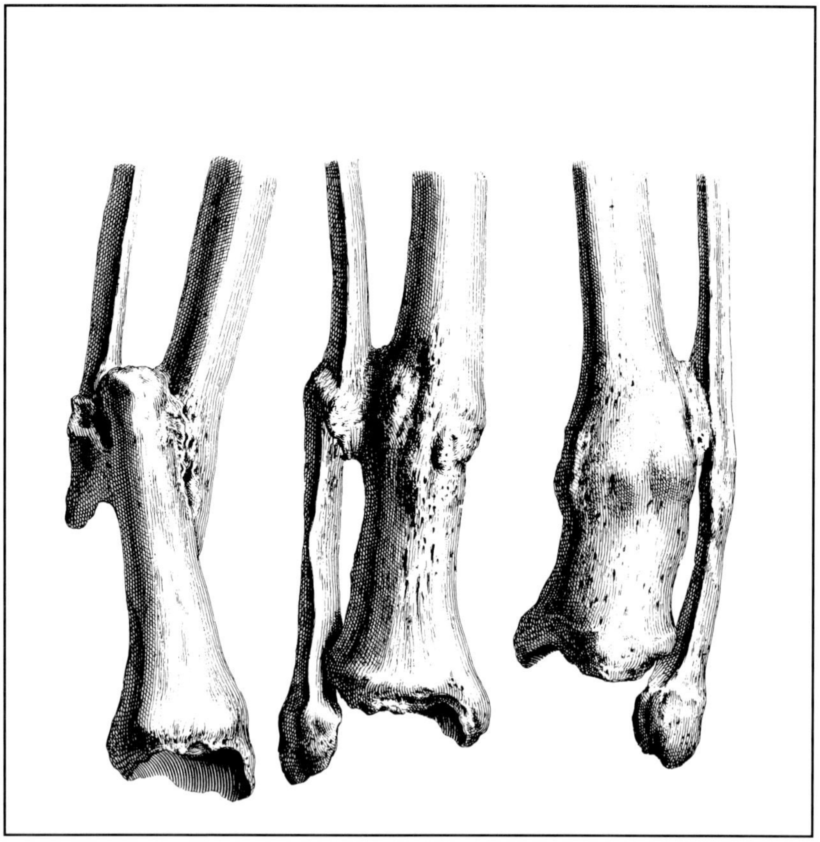

Figure 2.15 Engravings of healed fractures from Cheselden's *Osteographia*.

considered one of the great works of anatomy of the eighteenth century[62] (figure 2.14).

In addition to his explication of normal anatomy, Cheselden included some examples of diseased bones (figure 2.15). As a practitioner and teacher, Cheselden was England's leading surgeon until his death, counting among his pupils notable surgeons in their own right such as Samuel Sharp and John Hunter.

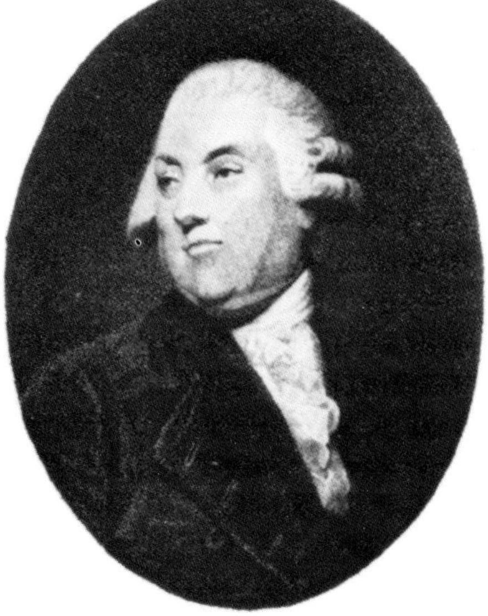

Figure 2.16 Percivall Pott (1714–1788). Engraving by Heath after Sir Joshua Reynolds.

Percivall Pott (1714–1788) succeeded Cheselden as the leading surgeon in London, a position he maintained until his retirement in 1787[63] (figure 2.16). At that time, he had been associated with St. Bartholomew's Hospital "as man and boy for half a century." Among his most enduring works is his small monograph of the treatment of fractures, *Some Few General Remarks on Fractures and Dislocations* (1765)[64] (figure 2.17). His *Remarks* logically develops the concept that the displacement of fracture fragments is due to the contraction of the muscles attached to them. To counteract or minimize these muscular forces, the limb should therefore be arranged in a position in which the muscles are in the greatest state of relaxation. In the lower extremity, this is with the hip and knee partially flexed (figure 2.18). Pott's concept has been accepted and is used today to explain many of the common patterns of displacement in fractures. When first propounded, however, the idea was opposed by physicians who adhered to a tradition going back to Hippocrates: that fractures of the femur and tibia should be treated with the hip and knee in full extension. Pott's own application of his concept, in which the patient lay on his side, was not practical, but it rapidly led to the use of the double-inclined plane (figure 2.19) invented by Robert Chessher (1750–1831), the first British orthopedist.[65]

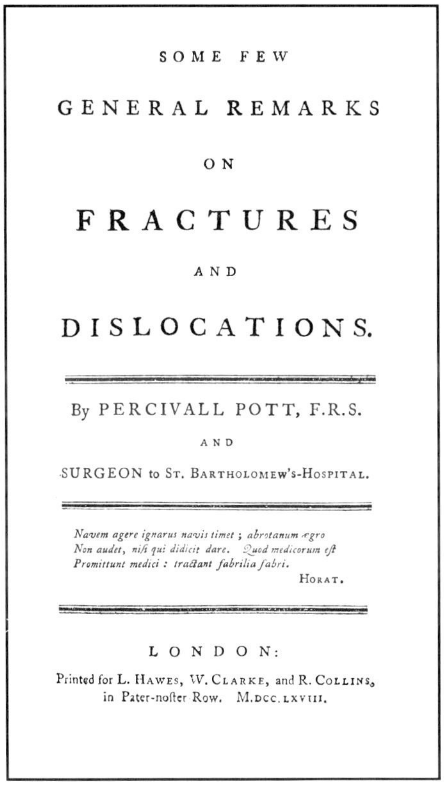
SOME FEW
GENERAL REMARKS
ON
FRACTURES
AND
DISLOCATIONS.

By PERCIVALL POTT, F.R.S.
AND
SURGEON to ST. BARTHOLOMEW'S-HOSPITAL.

Navem agere ignarus navis timet; abrotanum ægro
Non audet, nisi qui didicit dare. Quod medicorum est
Promittunt medici: tractant fabrilia fabri.
HORAT.

LONDON:
Printed for L. HAWES, W. CLARKE, and R. COLLINS,
in Pater-noster Row. M.DCC.LXVIII.

Figure 2.17 Successor to Cheselden, Pott argued that the displacement of fracture fragments is due to the contraction of the muscles attached to them.

In the *Remarks*, Pott describes what he believed to be the most frequent type of ankle fracture. The fracture of the fibula is well above the distal tibio-fibular syndesmosis, which appears to be intact in spite of rupture of the medial ligaments and displacement of the talus laterally. However, if such a fracture in fact occurs, it must be exceedingly rare. What then is a Pott's fracture? I believe that this term should be used as a generic term to include all fractures of the ankle caused by external rotation violence.

One of Percivall Pott's students from the United States was John Jones (1729–1791), who was born in Jamaica, Long Island[66] (figure 2.20). After a preparatory education in New York, he was sent to Philadelphia to study medicine with his cousin, Thomas Cadwalader. Four years of apprenticeship were followed by an extensive trip abroad during which he visited Paris, London and Edinburgh. It was during this trip that he first became acquainted with Pott, and the two formed a firm friendship. In New York Jones developed a large practice, participated as an army surgeon during the French and Indian War, and took an active part in forming the medical school at King's College in New York in 1767. Jones then became the college's first professor of surgery. The school collapsed during the turmoil of the Revolution, and when British forces occupied New York in 1776, Jones left for Philadelphia. As a medical officer in the Continental Army, his major contribution was a small manual "addressed to the surgeons of the army and navy of the United States, to whom it was intended to afford a knowledge of the improved practice of treating some of the most common surgical complaints; and thereby to lessen the unavoidable misfortunes attendant upon the struggle about to be made for the liberties and independence of this country."

The book, *Plain Concise Practical Remarks on the Treatment of Wounds and Fractures* (figure 2.21), was dedicated to his cousin and preceptor, Thomas Cadwalader. The preface reads in part:

> *The present calamitous situation of this once happy country, in a peculiar manner, demands the aid and assistance of every virtuous citizen; and though few men are possessed of those superior talents, which are requisite to heal such mighty evils as now threaten the whole body politic with ruin and desolation; yet every man has it in his power to contribute something toward so desireable an end and if he cannot cure the fatal disease of his unfortunate country, it will at least afford him*

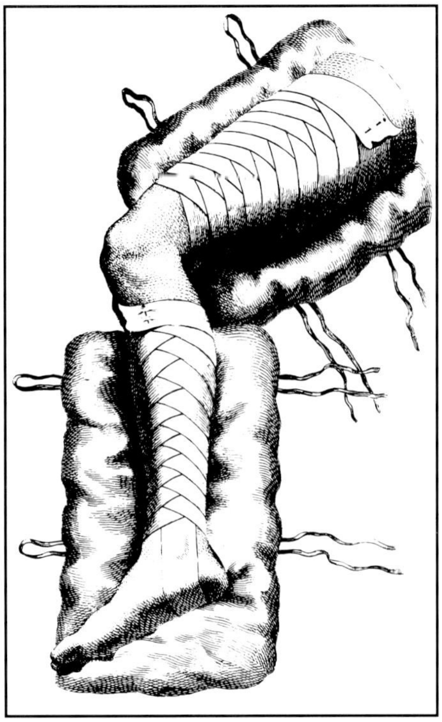

Figure 2.18 Pott's method of obtaining flexion of the hip and knee in the treatment of fractures of the shaft of the femur. From Pott, *Some Few General Remarks on Fractures and Dislocations* (London: Hawes, Clarke and Collins, 1767), facing p. 37.

some consolation to have poured a little balm into her bleeding wounds.[67]

This little volume has the distinction of being the first book on surgery and on the treatment of fractures to be written and published in the United States, and its appendix is the first American work on public health and hygiene. It is the progenitor of all subsequent surgical manuals written for use in the U.S. armed forces. The first edition was published in New York in 1775, and a second edition was published in Philadelphia in 1776. It summarized the best surgical opinions of the day in a simple and useful way and must have been of tremendous value to young army surgeons, many of them poorly educated and without access to contemporary medical literature. Jones enjoyed a fine career as a surgeon in Philadelphia after the revolution, where he was consulted by Benjamin Franklin and George Washington.

The chief surgeon of l'Hôtel Dieu in Paris at the end of the eighteenth century was Pierre Joseph Desault (1744–1795), whose students included Xavier Bichat, Guillaume Dupuytren, and Dominique Jean Larrey. Desault made many contributions to the treatment of fractures, particularly with his concepts of wound debridement. His lectures were collected and published by Bichat and appeared in English translation in the United States.[68] At the height of his clinical work, Desault founded, edited and published the *Journal de chirurgie*, the first periodical devoted entirely to surgery.

At the beginning of the nineteenth century, the importance of medical journals, as repositories for case reports, observations, clinical notes, descriptions of foreign travel, and reviews of books and lectures grew rapidly. They flourished in most lively medical communities as forums for discussion among local physicians. Most of them had small circulations and short lives. It was in such a provincial

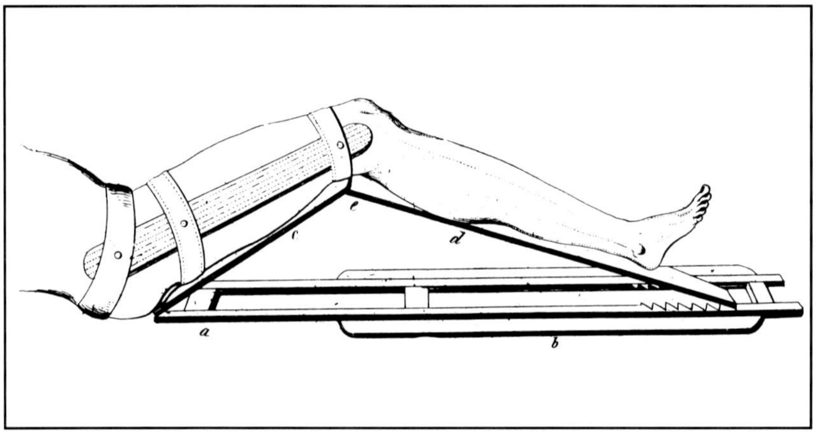

Figure 2.19 The double-inclined plane devised by Robert Chessher, (1750–1831), the first British orthopedist. From A. L. Richter, *40 Lithographirte Tafeln nebst Erklarung und Erlauterung derselben zu dem theoretich-pratischen Handbuch der Lehre von den Bruchen und Verrenkungen der Knochen* (Berlin: Enslin, 1828), Tafel XV, figure 3.

journal, the *Edinburgh Medical and Surgical Journal*, that Abraham Colles's (1773–1843) article "On the Fracture of the Carpal Extremity of the Radius" appeared in 1814[69] (figure 2.22). Although Colles's description was not the first nor the most accurate, his name has been firmly attached to this common fracture of the distal end of the radius.[70] Colles was a great teacher and enjoyed a long career as a professor of surgery in Dublin.

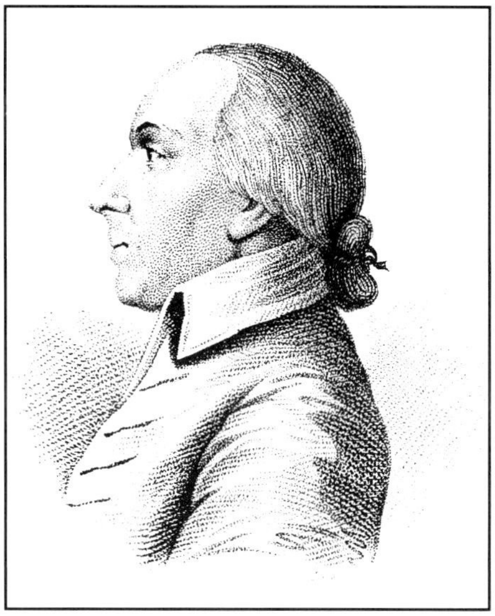

Figure 2.20 John Jones (1729–1791).

Similarly, the papers of John Rhea Barton (1794–1871) on bending fractures in children and his "Views and Treatment of an Important Injury of the Wrist" appeared in medical journals in the United States[71] (figure 2.23). The latter paper describes a fracture-dislocation of the radio-carpal joint, now called Barton's fracture.[72] These are only two examples of the many significant articles on the treatment of fractures and dislocations that began to appear in periodicals rather than in books.

A contemporary of Desault, Giovanni Battista Monteggia (1762–1815) held a similar position as chief surgeon of the Spedale Maggiori in Milan[73] (figure 2.24). His accomplishment, like Desault's, was unusual considering the disturbed political situation in Piedmont during his tenure. The second edition of Monteggia's *Istituzioni chirurgiche* (1813–16) is his major work and lasting monument.[74] This edition was the last in which he had an active part in preparing, but other editions appeared as late as 1837, twenty-two years after his death. In this systematic treatise, he calls not only upon his own observations but upon those of his predecessors and contemporaries. The volumes are thus replete with references to the works of Gerard van Swieten, Adolph Leopold Richter and Humboldt; to Duverney, Petit, Desault, Louis, Bichat, Abel Boyer, Larrey, Emile Littré, and François Chopart; to the Bells, Benjamin, Charles and John; Pott, John Brown, Samuel Sharp, and John Hunter. Especially interesting are his references to American authors such as Benjamin Rush, Nathan Smith, and Philip Syng Physick. In thus collecting and correlating this tremendous mass of foreign literature and making it available to his Italian colleagues, Monteggia made a major contribution to the development of surgery in Italy. Widely read by his own countrymen, his work received little attention elsewhere. For example, many have been surprised to find that one of the earliest descriptions of poliomyelitis came from him:

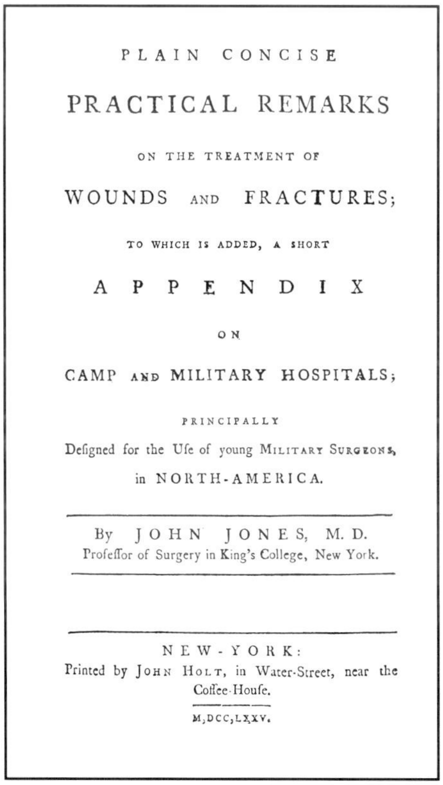

PLAIN CONCISE

PRACTICAL REMARKS

ON THE TREATMENT OF

WOUNDS AND FRACTURES;

TO WHICH IS ADDED, A SHORT

APPENDIX

ON

CAMP AND MILITARY HOSPITALS;

PRINCIPALLY

Defigned for the Ufe of young MILITARY SURGEONS, in NORTH-AMERICA.

By JOHN JONES, M. D.
Profeffor of Surgery in King's College, New York.

NEW-YORK:
Printed by JOHN HOLT, in Water-Street, near the Coffee-Houfe.

M,DCC,LXXV.

Figure 2.21 The first treatise on surgery and the work on the treatment of fractures published in the United States.

In this connection should be mentioned a certain kind of paralysis limited to one or other of the lower extremities which I have observed several times in practice but have not yet found in the literature. It occurs in children who are nursing, or not much later; it begins with two or three days of fever, after which one of these extremities is found quite paralyzed, immobile, flabby, hanging down, and no movement is made when the sole of the foot is tickled. The fever ceases very soon, but the member remains immobile and regains with time only an imperfect degree of strength. I knew such a person who even when adult remained dragging a weak leg, for it had not become cured by time.[75]

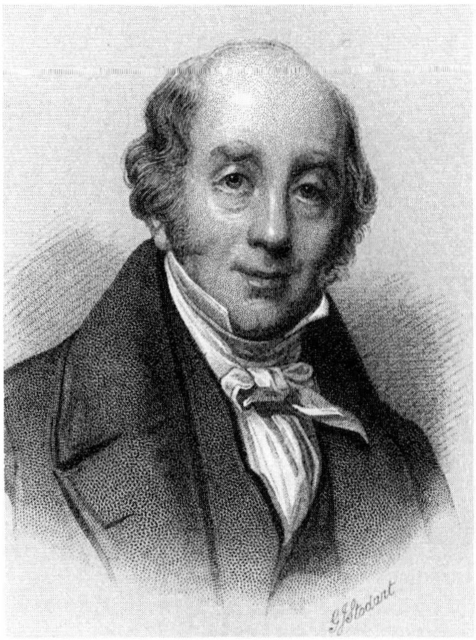

Figure 2.22 Abraham Colles (1773–1791), of Colles's fracture, engraved by G. J. Stodart.

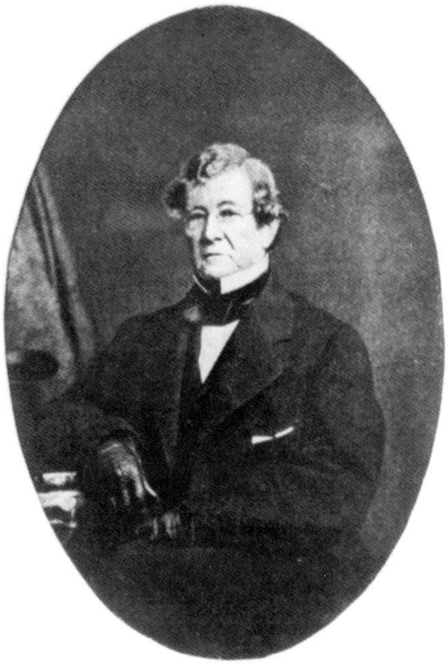

Figure 2.23 John Rhea Barton (1794–1871).

Only Michael Underwood (1789), Timothy Sheldrake (1806), and Johann Christian Gottfried Joerg (1810) preceded Monteggia in the description of poliomyelitis, and there is no question that this was an original observation on his part.[76]

Monteggia described the signs and symptoms accompanying a dislocation of the tendon of the long head of the biceps. Although this lesion had been noted by anatomists, he was the first to diagnose the clinical syndrome. And here also Monteggia described the case of a young woman who presented, after a fall on her outstretched arm, a fracture of the ulna at the junction of the proximal and middle thirds. The associated dislocation of the radial head was not noted until a month later!

In 1823, Joseph Wattmann (1789–1866), an Austrian surgeon, published a small book, *Descriptio Nexus Sceleti ad Luxationem Demonstrationem Pathologicam et Therapeuticam Inservientis*, describing a teaching manikin for the instruction of students in the maneuvers to be used in reducing dislocations.[77] It consisted of a human skeleton articulated by elastic straps. The joints were enveloped in a loose wrap (figure 2.25). The instructor could then produce a dislocation, ask the student to diagnose the type and require him to reduce it using the precribed maneuver. Wattmann was a professor of surgery at the University of Vienna from 1825 to 1848. A bold and versatile surgeon, he made important contributions to the understanding and treatment of air embolism complicating operations on the neck.

Adolph Leopold Richter (1798–1876) was a Prussian military surgeon. He was responsible for the reorganization of the Prussian Army medical service and bringing it to a high level of efficiency. One of his major works was the *Theoretisch-praktisches Handbuch der Lehre von den Bruchen und Verrenk ungen der Knochen* published in 1828.[78] It is accompanied by a valuable atlas illustrating all of the various types of dressings, splints and apparatus used in the treatment of fractures at that time.

Among John Hunter's students from the United States were Philip Syng Physick (1768–1837) (figure 2.26) and John Syng Dorsey (1783–1818), Physick's nephew. Physick was a talented surgeon who became the first professor of surgery at the University of Pennsylvania. Because of his many contributions, including his use of a seton in the treatment of ununited fractures, he has been called "the father of American surgery."[79] Physick's modification of Desault's long splint for the treatment of fractures of the shaft of the femur delayed wide use of the double inclined plane and the flexed position for the treatment of femoral shaft fractures in the United States for some time.

Physick did not publish his surgical lectures, but Dorsey, his nephew and closest associate, used much of this material in his *Elements of Surgery for the Use of Students*[80] (figure 2.27). This was the first systematic surgical textbook published in the United States and was even adopted for this purpose at the University of Edinburgh. Dorsey's premature death at age thirty-five from typhus was a significant loss.

William Gibson (1788–1868), a contemporary and colleague of Physick and Dorsey, modified and improved Physick's long splint, and his surgical lectures contain a great deal of information on methods of treating fractures in vogue at the time.[81] Samuel D. Gross (1805–1884), another Philadelphian who was to become the foremost surgeon of his generation in the United States, published

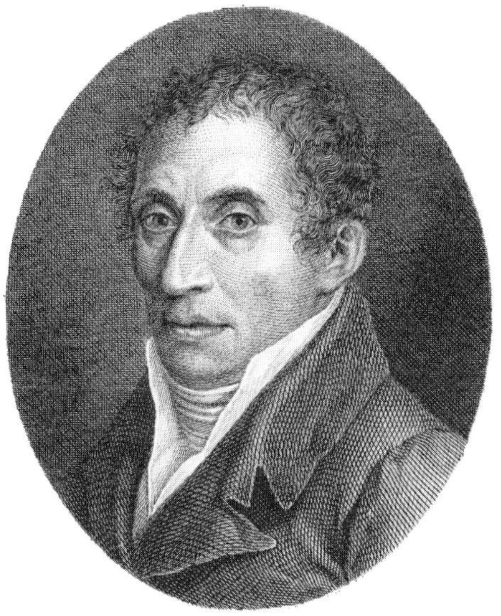

Figure 2.24 Giovanni Battista Monteggia (1762–1815), the first to diagnose the clinical syndrome of the dislocation of the tendon of the long head of the biceps. From F. E. Acerbi, *Della vita di Giambatista Monteggia* (Milan: Dova, 1816), frontispiece.

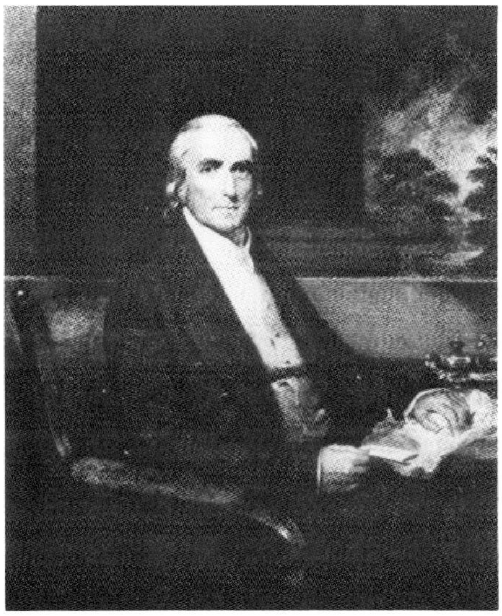

Figure 2.26 Philip Syng Physick (1768–1837) who has been called "the father of American surgery." From G. F. Sheldon and R. G. Sheldon, "Philip Syng Physick (1768–1837), The Father of American Surgery," *Bull Amer Coll Surg*, May 1979.

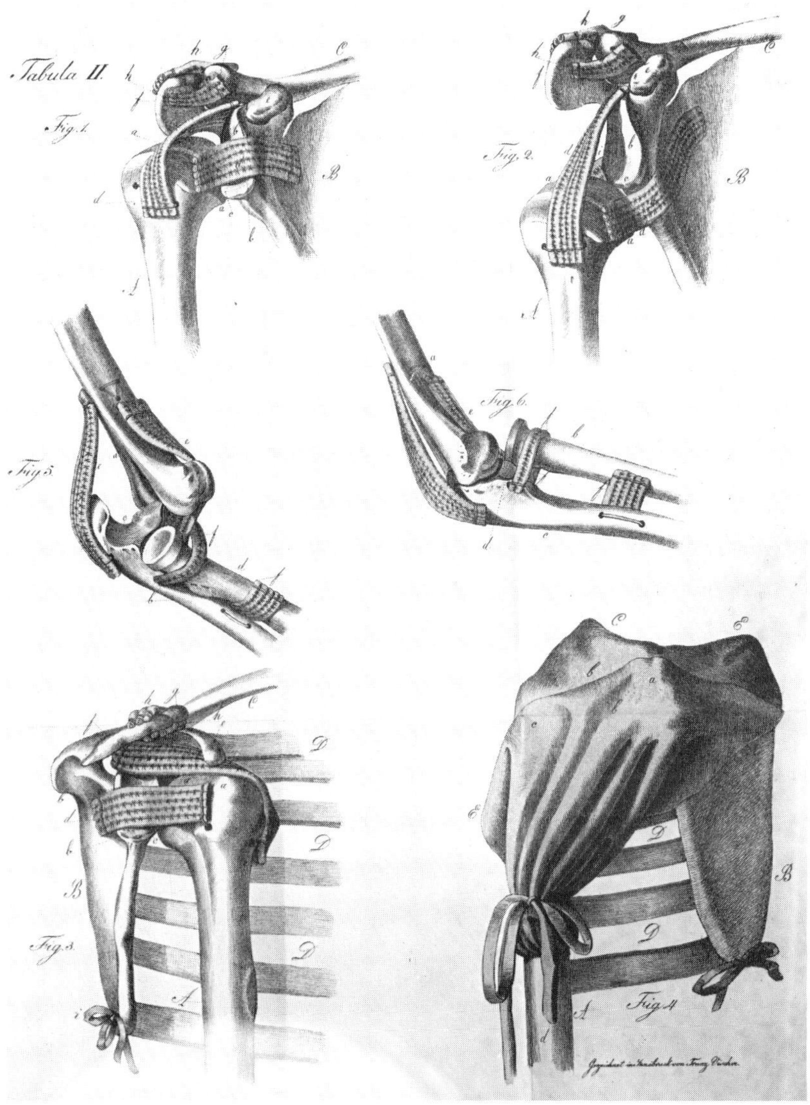

Figure 2.25 Details of the manikin devised by Joseph Wattmann (1789–1866) for the teaching of maneuvers for the reduction of dislocations. From Wattmann, *Descriptio Nexus Sceleti ad Luxationem Demonstrationem Pathologicam et Therapeuticam Inservientis* (Innsbruck, 1823), Tabula II.

a significant book at the young age of twenty-five, *The Anatomy, Physiology, and Diseases of the Bones and Joints*, which also dealt with the treatment of fractures.[82] This was Gross's first surgical text and the first textbook on orthopedics published in the United States.

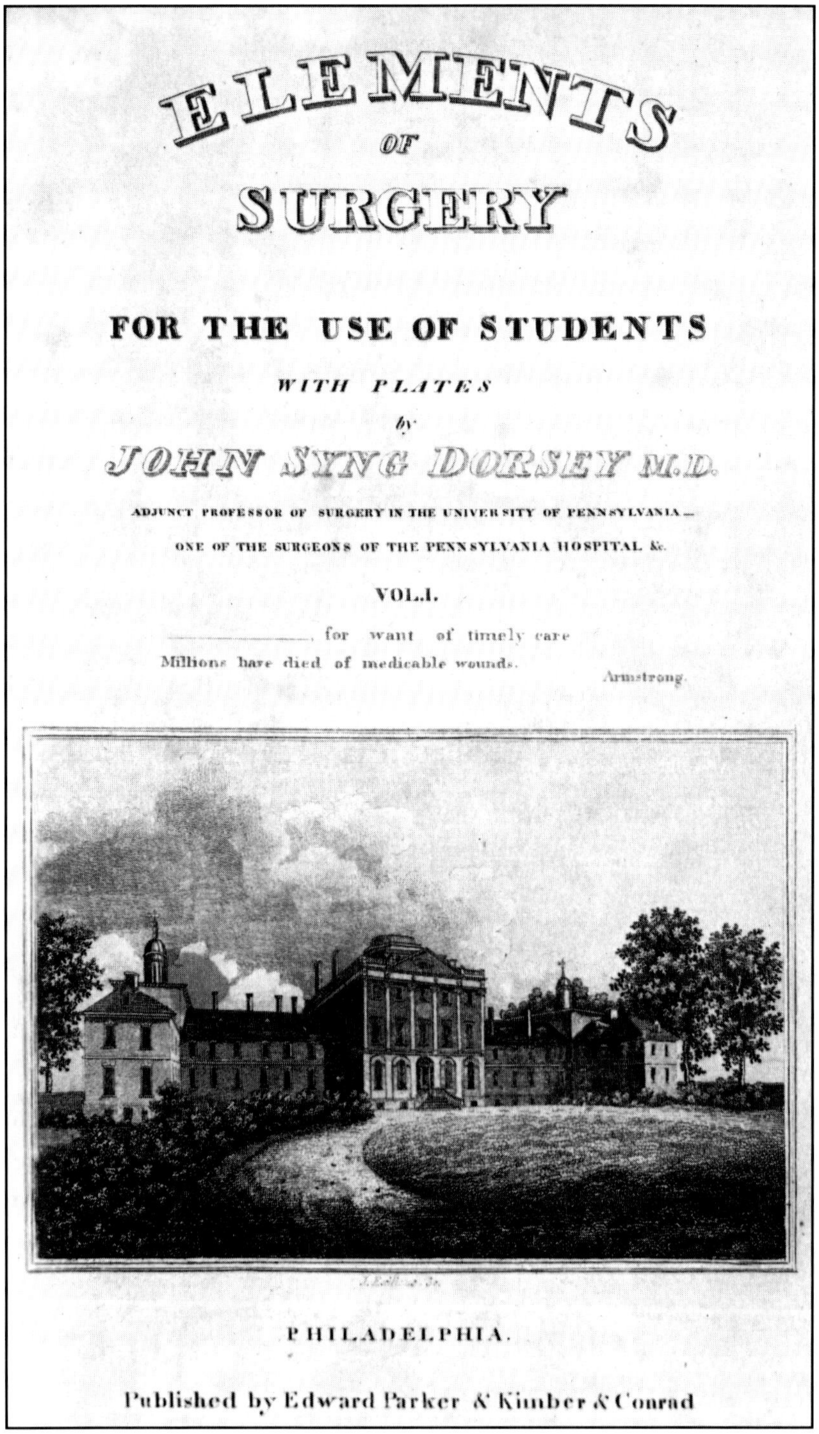

ELEMENTS

OF

SURGERY

FOR THE USE OF STUDENTS

WITH PLATES

by

JOHN SYNG DORSEY M.D.

ADJUNCT PROFESSOR OF SURGERY IN THE UNIVERSITY OF PENNSYLVANIA —

ONE OF THE SURGEONS OF THE PENNSYLVANIA HOSPITAL &c.

VOL. I.

——————, for want of timely care
Millions have died of medicable wounds.

Armstrong.

PHILADELPHIA.

Published by Edward Parker & Kimber & Conrad

Figure 2.27 The first systematic textbook on surgery written by an American. John Syng Dorsey included much previously unpublished material by his uncle, Philip Syng Physick, who never published his surgical lectures.

The French school of surgery excelled during the early decades of the nineteenth century under the leadership of Guillaume Dupuytren (1777–1835).[83] One of Dupuytren's contemporaries has left us a series of delightful sketches of the leading medical personalities of his day (figure 2.28). Before discussing Dupuytren, he prefaces his remarks: "If I could have avoided speaking of M. Dupuytren, it would have been a great relief to me, for I find myself in a very uncomfortable embarrassment. I am almost sure to leave all parties dissatisfied."[84] About no other surgeon have so violently differing opinions been expressed by associates and perpetuated by biographers. Many of his detractors are remembered today only because of their vitrolic epigrams directed against him. Perhaps the most widely known of these is that Dupuytren was the greatest of surgeons and the meanest of men. To understand the depth of this feeling today, one need only know that Dupuytren was deferred from the draft during the wars of Napoleon on the plea from the Faculty of Medicine that his services were essential, and that while the titles of most of his associates stemmed from the Emperor Napoleon, he was made a baron by Louis XVIII after the restoration of the monarchy.

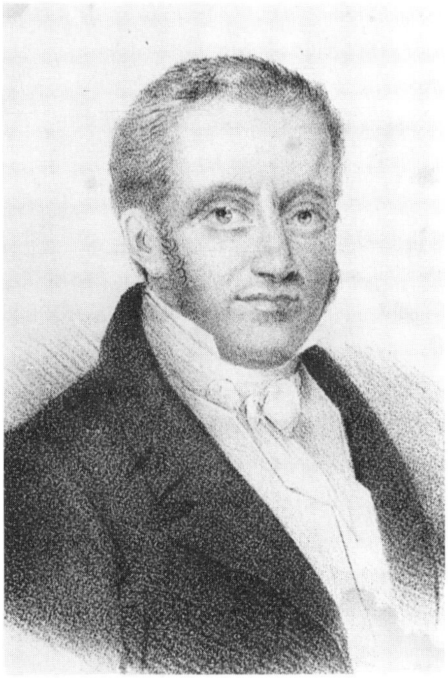

Figure 2.28 Guillaume Dupuytren (1777–1835), sometimes called "the greatest of surgeons and the meanest of men." His name has been applied as an eponym to at least twelve diseases, including *Dupuytren's contracture.*

Dupuytren was born in Pierre-Buffière, a small town in central France just south of Limoges. His father was an attorney of limited means and only because of the interest of a cavalry officer stationed in the town was Dupuytren able to go to Paris for his education. The grinding poverty and privation of his student years cast the shadows of avariciousness and parsimony over his later life. With absolute faith in his own ability, Dupuytren made work his religion. In a fiercely competitive system, he rose in twenty years from the position of prosector of anatomy to become chief surgeon of l'Hôtel Dieu. Born in poverty, he was at age fifty-three able to offer the deposed Charles X one million francs from his personal fortune. "Had not Monsieur Dupuytren been compelled to trim his student's lamp with oil from the dissecting room, he never would have succeeded in becoming Monsieur le Baron Dupuytren."[85]

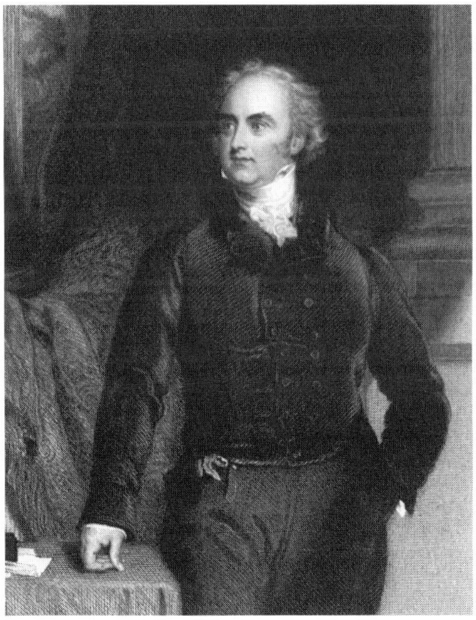

Figure 2.29 Astley Cooper (1768–1845).

As one Frenchman has aptly put it: "Modesty is not a defect of French character." Dupuytren's era was the high water mark of French surgery, and Paris was the center of the medical world. Amid a galaxy of brilliant minds, Dupuytren would not acknowledge a superior, but reigned alone, coldly critical of all of those about him. He had no friends among his medical colleagues. He was devoted to the care of his patients and never shirked his responsibilities to the inmates of l'Hôtel Dieu. Of the many crimes of which he was accused, no one ever suggested that he put his private interest above that of the meanest of his patients. His funeral cortege was interrupted as it made its way to the cemetery by crowds of workmen who took the coffin on their shoulders and bore it part of the distance. Among them was the coachman upon whom Dupuytren had performed the first successful resection of the mandible for a tumor many years before. These people were his friends.

Dupuytren's name has been applied as an eponym to at least twelve diseases, operations, and instruments, the most widely used term being, of course, *Dupuytren's contracture.*[86] Only rarely is reference made to Dupuytren's fracture. The description of this injury is not found in a brief case report of a single patient, but rather, consists of a long and learned treatise.[87] It contains a thorough review of the history of the treatment of ankle fractures, and of the normal anatomy and function of the ankle joint. Of special interest is the description of experimental fractures produced in cadavers to elucidate the mechanism of injury. The discussion of the history, signs, symptoms and complications is comprehensive. To all of this is added a description of a new method of treating these fractures with a report of the use of the method on 207 patients with the injury. Dupuytren's fracture has been defined by J. Grant Bonnin, a critical commentator on ankle injuries, as "a fracture of the fibula above the syndesmosis, but below the center of the fibula, with partial diastasis."[88]

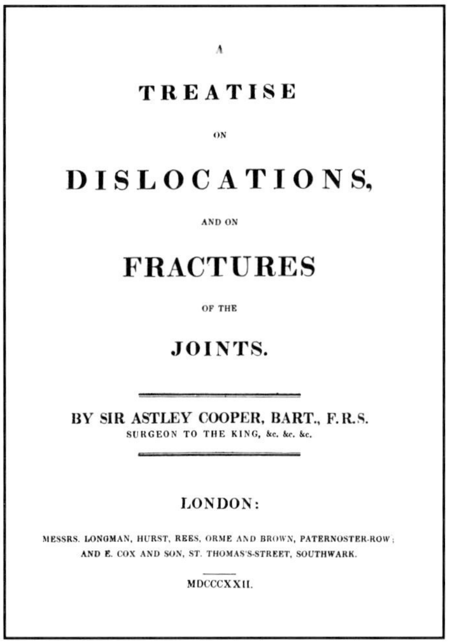
A
TREATISE
ON
DISLOCATIONS,
AND ON
FRACTURES
OF THE
JOINTS.

BY SIR ASTLEY COOPER, BART., F.R.S.
SURGEON TO THE KING, &c. &c. &c.

LONDON:
MESSRS. LONGMAN, HURST, REES, ORME AND BROWN, PATERNOSTER-ROW;
AND E. COX AND SON, ST. THOMAS'S-STREET, SOUTHWARK.
MDCCCXXII.

Figure 2.30 First edition of Cooper's *Treatise on Dislocations and on Fractures of the Joints* (1822).

Dupuytren's interest in fractures was not confined to those about the ankle. L'Hôtel Dieu received a continuing stream of patients injured in the streets of Paris. Dupuytren recognized the value of good emergency medical care and deplored the zeal of the uninformed bystander whose ministrations so frequently complicated a simple injury. An intensely practical man, he designated the first floor of the hospital for the reception of patients with fractures to avoid having to move them up and down the narrow stairways. He was a strong advocate of Percivall Pott's innovations and used the semi-flexed position in treating fractures of the lower extremity, contrary to the methods of treating them in extension that were well established in France. Dupuytren taught that the common injuries about the wrist were not dislocations, as Desault had argued, but were instead fractures of the distal radius.[89] His *Leçons orales* contains many comments on fractures in children and on pathological fractures. The problem of nonunion led him to study fracture healing. He was the first to differentiate between the provisional callus, which forms quickly, and the definitive callus, which produces the final union of the fracture.

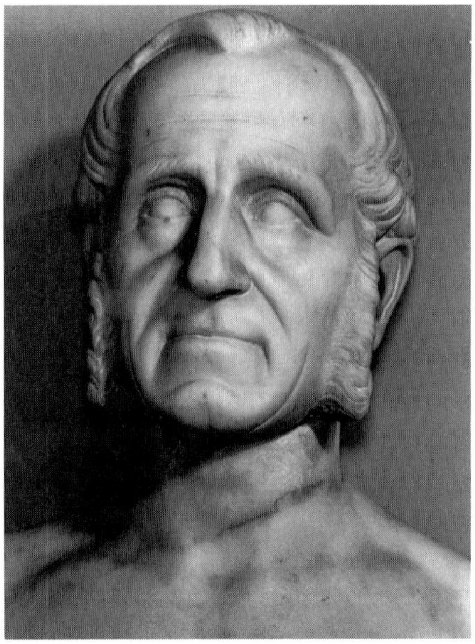

Figure 2.31 Bust of Robert William Smith (1807–1873), author of the first important work on fractures by an Irishman, in the Royal College of Surgeons, Dublin.

Another student of John Hunter, Astley Cooper (1768–1845) began to study medicine at Guy's Hospital at the age of sixteen[90] (figure 2.29). After seven years of study, he was made demonstrator of anatomy at St. Thomas Hospital and began to lecture on surgical subjects. In 1792, he took his bride to Paris, where he attended lectures by Desault and Chopart and heard the speeches of Danton, Marat and Robespierre. His experiences in Paris made him a staunch conservative for the rest of his life. Like Hunter, Cooper made the study of human anatomy a major part of his work in spite of his extensive surgical practice. His *Treatise on Dislocations and on Fractures of the Joints* (figure 2.30) first appeared in 1822 and went through numerous editions.[91] Cooper discussed not only anatomical and clinical problems in patients with fractures, but also, in the spirit of John Hunter, some animal experiments on the healing of fractures. The scope of Cooper's book, however, was limited. A more complete text was supplied by Joseph Amesbury (1795–1864) in 1831. His *Practical Remarks on the Nature and Treatment of Fractures of the Trunk and Extremities* strongly advocated the use of the double-inclined plane in the treatment of fractures of the shaft of the femur.

The great tradition of the Irish school of surgery, which reached its zenith with Abraham Colles, was maintained by Robert William Smith (1807–1873) (figure 2.31).[92] *A Treatise on Fractures in the Vicinity of Joints and on Certain Forms of Accidental and Congenital Dislocations*, in which the description of Smith's fracture appears, was the first important work on fractures by an Irish author.[93] In his initial chapter, "On the Diagnosis and Pathology of Fractures of the Neck of the Femur," Smith disagreed with Cooper as to the relative amount of shortening that accompanied intra- and extracapsular fractures, and showed that extracapsular fractures were initially shorter. In patients with old, ununited intracapsular fractures, however, he found large amounts of shortening and attributed Cooper's error to the fact that he based his opinion on the measurement of such cases. Because modern physicians' knowledge of these fractures is based primarily on radiographic characteristics, Smith's detailed reports of their pathological appearance as demonstrated by extensive dissection can still be read with profit. The introduction of statistical data into medical literature is a feature of this work; one table lists Smith's own experience with 28 extracapsular, 28 intracapsular and 4 impacted fractures of the hip, while another presents an analysis of 140 specimens of hip fractures in various Dublin museums.

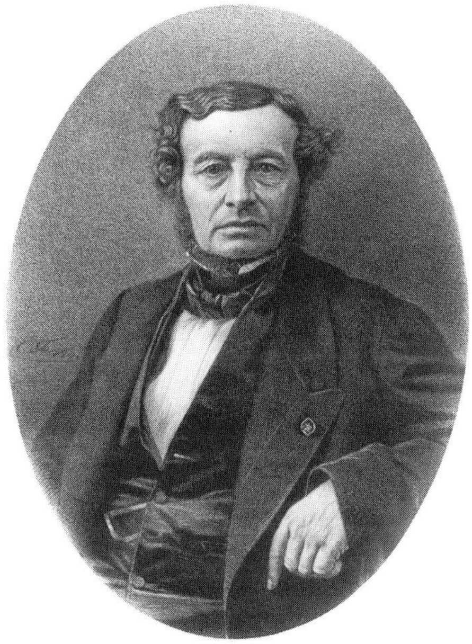

Figure 2.32 Joseph-François Malgaigne (1806–1865) included in his pioneering study a statistical analysis of 2,328 patients with fractures seen at l'Hôtel Dieu over an eleven-year period. Only 30 of the 2,328 patients were found to have more than one fracture, an indication that the forces producing injuries one hundred years ago were of a lesser magnitude than those encountered today.

In the chapter "On Fractures of the Bones of the Forearm in the Vicinity of the Wrist Joint," Smith corrected Colles's original description by placing the site of the fracture more distally. "The situation of the fracture is not so high as Mr. Colles states it to be; I have never seen it more than an inch above the carpal end of the bone; in the majority of cases it is not so much."[94] It was Smith who firmly attached Colles's eponym to the fracture that Colles described. In the same chapter Smith describes the fracture of the wrist with which his name is associated.

Smith was primarily a surgical pathologist. He was one of the founders of the Pathological Society of Dublin and performed the autopsy on Abraham Colles. In his magnificent *Treatise on the Pathology, Diagnosis and Treatment of Neuroma*, he anticipated Friedrich Daniel von Recklinghausen's description of neurofibromatosis by thirty-three years.[95] He was also an accomplished linguist, and his knowledge of the ancient medical writers was encyclopedic. His book on fractures points out a passage in Dupuytren's *Leçons orales* in which Dupuytren had been misquoted by his transcribers, an error which was corrected in later editions. Smith's references to foreign writers exceed in scope those of most British authors of the day, and because of his cosmopolitan interests, Smith became an ordinary, corresponding, or honorary member of many medical societies at home and abroad.

The midpoint of the nineteenth century was marked by the publication of three comprehensive textbooks on the treatment of fractures and dislocations. These works are modern in every respect, with broad discussions of the etiology, pathogenesis, treatment, complications, and prognosis of injuries, accompanied by a thorough review of the literature. The first was the *Traité des fractures et des luxations* (two volumes and an atlas), published in 1847 by Joseph-François Malgaigne (1806–1865) (figure 2.32).[96]

> *The character which I have mainly sought to give this work is that of reality. In a historical point of view, I have aimed at presenting a resume of all the doctrines and ideas maintained from the earliest times to our day, having recourse as much as possible to the original works. As to my teachings, I have asserted nothing unsupported by facts, drawn either from my own experience or from that of others. Where clinical observation was insufficient, I have sought substitutes for it in experiments upon dead bodies, or upon the lower animals; but above all, I have tried to clear up a great many mooted points by throwing upon them the light of pathological anatomy; and this is the object of my atlas.*[97]

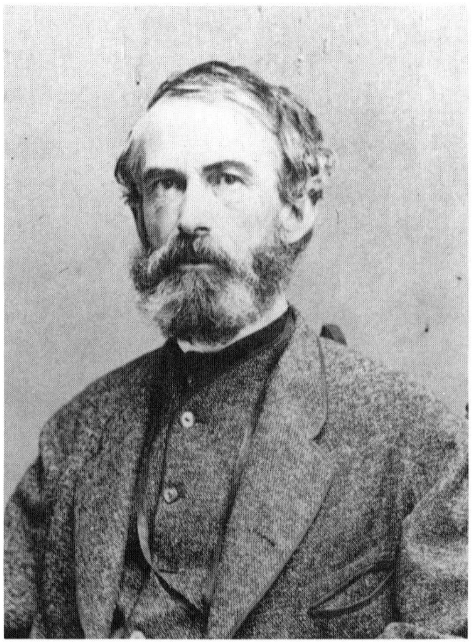

Figure 2.33 Frank Hastings Hamilton (1813–1886), author of the first complete book on the treatment of fractures and dislocations in English.

The opening statistical analysis of 2,328 patients with fractures seen at l'Hôtel Dieu over an eleven-year period is unique. The patients are classified according to age and sex, the time of year the fracture occurred and the bone fractured. It is interesting that only 30 of the 2,328 patients were found to have more than one fracture, an indication that the forces producing injuries one hundred years ago were of a lesser magnitude than those encountered today. The principles on which Malgaigne's treatment was based were those handed down in a great tradition through Paré, Petit, Desault, Boyer and Dupuytren. However, Malgaigne was not afraid to break with this tradition when his own observations and experiences showed his masters to be in error. He advocated the use of the semi-flexed position in treating fractures of the lower extremities described by Pott, in opposition to the methods of Desault, Larrey, Bichat, Jules Germain Cloquet and others. He proved his point by a series of ingenious experiments on animals and fresh cadavers, in which he showed that when the quadriceps and hamstring tendons are cut simultaneously with the knee partially flexed, the tendons retract equal distances, demonstrating that in this position the opposing muscles are equally balanced. Such was not the case when the tendons were sectioned with the knee fully extended.

Little escaped Malgaigne's observant eye or his inquiring mind. He described a patient with an ischemic contracture of the forearm due to a dressing too tightly applied thirty-four years before Richard Volkmann. He investigated the gas produced in gas gangrene by collecting a quantity of it, found that it burned with a blue flame, and identified it as carburetted hydrogen. He was imaginative in his approach to technical problems, such as maintaining the fragments of a displaced transverse patellar fracture in apposition. In the first volume of his book, Malgaigne described the double vertical fracture of the pelvis which bears his eponym.[98]

Malgaigne was the son of a poor rural practitioner and gained his medical education with difficulty. However, he was well versed in Latin and Greek and had worked as a secretary. This experience helped him in his work as an editor and medical historian. As an editor, he fought for the freedom to print critical articles and established this principle in a court of law.[99] His edition of the works of Ambroise Paré, with its historical introduction dealing with the progress of surgery from the sixth to the sixteenth century, established him as a great medical historian.[100] His monograph on the history of the treatment of fractures is still valuable.[101]

The second major text, *A Practical Treatise on Fractures and Dislocations*, was the first complete book on the treatment of fractures and dislocations in English. It was published in the United States in 1860 by Frank Hastings Hamilton (1813–1886) (figure 2.33).[102] Hamilton's work grew out of a collection of data on the results of the treatment of fractures assembled in an effort to provide physicians with information to use in defending malpractice actions.[103] Patients in the United States in the nineteenth century were as litigious as they are today, and most of the cases involved the results of the treatment of fractures and dislocations.[104] The *Boston Medical and Surgical Journal* on January 9, 1879, carried the following note:

> *As it is now, the unfortunate patient tries to retrieve his bad luck by levying upon the hard working surgeon without risking or staking anything for the chance of testing what may prove to be no case at all . . . .The suit depletes the surgeon's pocket and ruins his reputation. To pay is ruinous, to defend is ruinous, and to live in constant dread is ruinous . . . . The plaintiff carries around a lame leg with the surgeon's money to support it, and the surgeon carries around a lame reputation with nothing to support it.*[105]

It is interesting to note that four years before his election to the presidency, Abraham Lincoln successfully defended two physicians sued by a patient because his fractured leg had healed with some shortening.[106] Reports on the results of the treatment of fractures were limited, vague and anecdotal, and they provided no information on what result could be anticipated in an "average case." This is why Hamilton's publication of statistical tables that detailed the end results in a large group of patients with a wide variety of fractures was so important. These tables served as a standard against which an

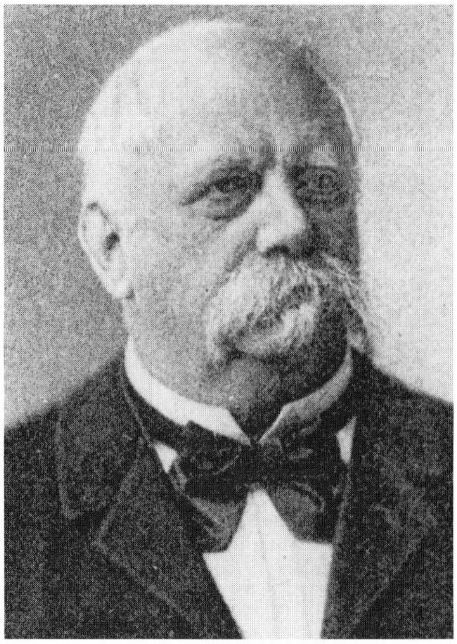

Figure 2.34 Ernst Julius Gurlt (1825–1899), most often remembered today for his mammoth history of surgery, although his work on fractures is unsurpassed as a source of obscure and arcane information. Frontispiece from *Arch klin Chir* 100(1913).

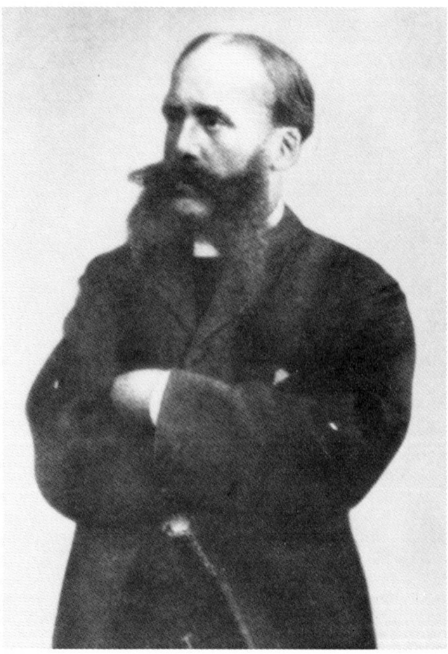

Figure 2.35 Richard Volkmann (1830–1889), of Volkmann's ischemic contracture. From H. Killian and G. Kramer, *Meister der Chirurgie und die Chirurgenschulen im Deutschen Raum* (Stuttgart: Georg Thieme, 1951), figure 31.

individual case could be compared and "had an incalculable influence on the results of suits for malpractice."[107] Originally published piecemeal in the *Transactions of the American Medical Association*, they were collected and published in a single volume in 1855.[108]

Frank Hastings Hamilton was born in Vermont. He began to study medicine as a preceptee, attended the College of Physicians and Surgeons of Fairfield, New York, and finally received the degree of Doctor of Medicine from the University of Pennsylvania. After entering practice, he taught in medical schools in Fairfield and Geneva, New York. After an extended trip to Europe, during which he visited the major clinics and hospitals, he became professor of surgery at the medical school in Buffalo. An early advocate of the use of ether anesthesia, Hamilton had a varied surgical practice. In 1854, he performed the first crossleg pedicle flap. In 1859, he followed his colleague Austin Flint to the Long Island College of Medicine and a short time later his book *A Practical Treatise on Fractures and Dislocations* appeared. After a period of distinguished service in the Medical Corps of the Union Army, Hamilton became professor of surgery at Bellevue Hospital. An indication of his reputation is apparent from the fact that he was called as a consultant after President Garfield had been shot.

The third major nineteenth-century work on the treatment of fractures and dislocations was the *Handbuch der Lehre von den Knochenbruchen* published in 1862 by Ernst Julius Gurlt (1825–1899).[109] Gurlt (figure 2.34) was educated in Berlin and had traveled in Austria, France and Great Britain, visiting surgical clinics. He was an assistant to Bernhard von Langenbeck, the leading German surgeon of the period, and later became a professor of surgery at Berlin. Like Malgaigne he had an interest in the history of medicine, and his monumental three-volume history of surgery covering the period from antiquity to the Renaissance is still a standard reference.[110] Gurlt's handbook on the treatment of fractures presents an exhaustive and detailed view of the literature on the subject. As a source for obscure and arcane information, he is unsurpassed.

One of Lister's first disciples in Germany was Richard Volkmann (1830–1889) who became a vigorous proponent of the antiseptic system[111] (figure 2.35). Volkmann wrote extensively on the treatment of fractures and is best remembered for his paper *Die ischamischen Muskellahmungen und Kontrakturen*, in which he describes what we now call Volkmann's ischemic contracture.[112] Using the pseudonym Leander, Volkmann later became well known as a poet and popular writer. His *Traumereien an Franzosischen Kaminen (Dreams by French Firesides)* went through thirty-one editions and was translated into five languages.[113]

At l'Hôpital de la Charité in Paris, the chief surgeon, Léon Gosselin (1815–1887), was accustomed to lecturing extensively on the treatment of fractures.[114] One of his students from the United

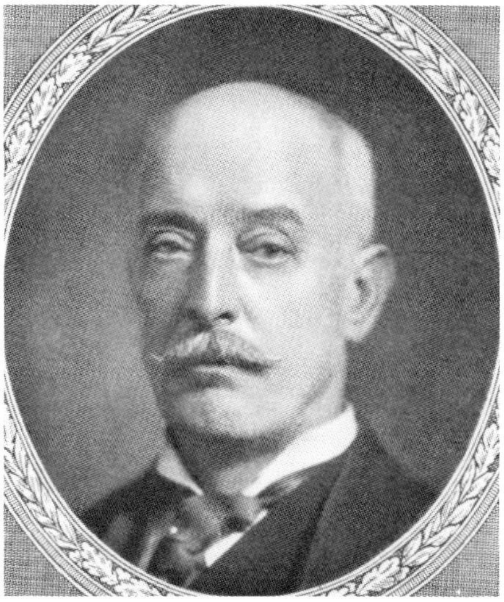

Figure 2.36 Lewis Atterbury Stimson (1844–1917). From *SGO* 44(1927): 571.

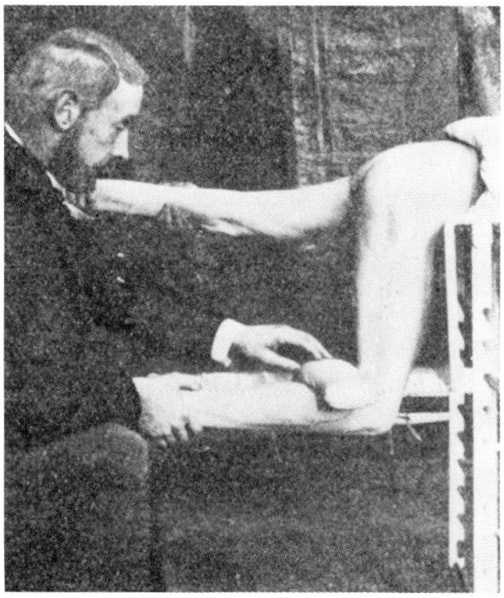

Figure 2.37 Stimson's maneuver for the reduction of a posterior dislocation of the hip. From Stimson, *A Practical Treatise on Fractures and Dislocations* (New York: Lea Brothers, 1905), p. 735.

States was impressed by this material and translated a portion of it into English.[115] Lewis Atterbury Stimson (1844–1917) was born in Patterson, New Jersey[116] (figure 2.36). His family was of old colonial stock, and his father was a successful stockbroker who counted Jay Gould and Jim Fisk among his acquaintances. Stimson graduated from Yale University in 1863, just in time to see action in the final period of the Civil War. After the war he married and went to work as a broker on Wall Street. In the next few years he became interested in the study of medicine, an interest perhaps stimulated by the chronic illness of his wife, who was a diabetic. In 1871, he took his family to Paris to seek treatment for his wife and to begin his medical education. While in Paris, he studied with Louis Pasteur, Auguste Nélaton, and Gosselin. Returning to the United States, he obtained his medical degree from Bellevue Hospital Medical College in 1875. At his graduation he was awarded the Wood Prize for an essay entitled "Bacteria and Their Influence upon the Origin and Development of Septic Complications of Wounds."[117] The following year he performed the first public operation in the United States demonstrating Lister's antiseptic technique; he went on to become an important influence on the introduction of antiseptic and aseptic techniques into American operating rooms. After the death of his beloved wife in 1876, Stimson devoted his life to his medical work. He made contributions to the technique of abdominal surgery and popularized the use of plaster of paris splints for the treatment of fractures. He described a method for the reduction of posterior dislocations of the hip (figure 2.37). Because of these contributions, Stimson became an influential figure on the New York surgical scene—for example, he played an important role in the development of Cornell University Medical College. Stimson's *Treatise on Fractures and Dislocations* was a thorough and well-documented exposition of the material, and it went through numerous editions.[118] In keeping with the progressive attitude of its author, those editions appearing after 1900 included sections on the importance and use of X rays.

The son of a bone-setter from Liverpool, who practiced general medicine and surgery in that community throughout his professional career, exercised an enormous influence on the treatment of fractures in spite of the fact that he never held an appointment as a professor, never headed a large clinic, never published a major textbook and was never held in great esteem by contemporary surgeons. Hugh Owen Thomas (1834–1891) was born in Wales[119] (figure 2.38). After a preceptorship with an uncle who was a physician, Thomas attended medical school in Edinburgh at the time James Syme was the professor of surgery and Joseph Lister was a house officer. From Edinburgh Thomas went to University College, London, for further medical training; his education also included a visit to major clinics in Europe. Thomas was a well-educated, talented eccentric who practiced in a highly individualistic way. His surgical practice became more and more specialized over time, eventually dealing primarily

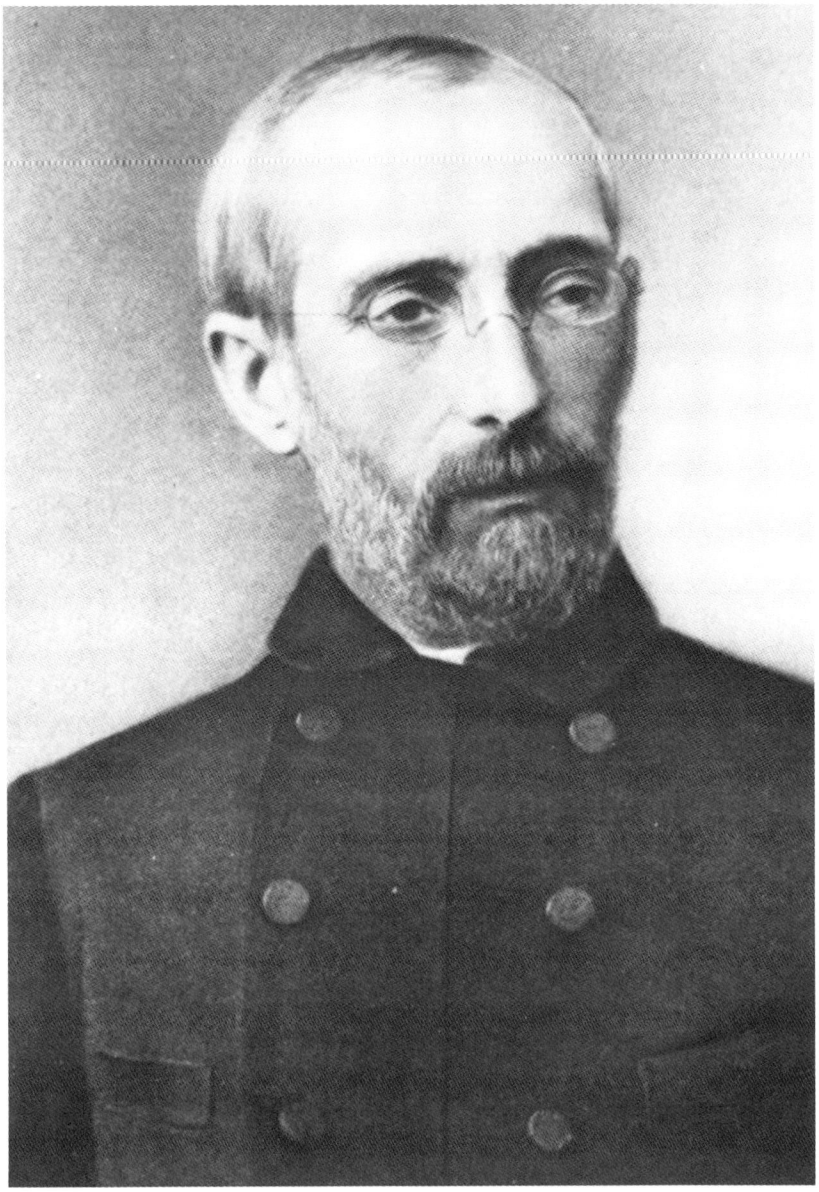

Figure 2.38 Hugh Owen Thomas (1834–1891) exerted an enormous influence on the treatment of fractures in spite of the fact that he never held an appointment as a professor, headed a large clinic, nor published a major textbook. He was also not held in great esteem by contemporary surgeons. From S. L. Koch and M. L. Mason, "Purposeful Splinting Following Hand Injuries," *SGO* 68(1939): 1–16.

with the treatment of bone and joint tuberculosis, deformities and skeletal injuries. He was the first to design a satisfactory ischial weight-bearing splint which, although primarily intended for the treatment of tuberculosis of the knee, he also used for the treatment of fractures of the shaft of the femur.[120] He was a great advocate of the practice of percussion and damming in the treatment of ununited fractures. He applied throughout his practice the same principle of "rest, absolute, uninterrupted and prolonged," which he used in the treatment of conditions ranging from tuberculous joints to fractures. However, *rest* meant many things to Thomas. In his small book *The Principles of the Treatment of Fractures and Dislocations*, published in 1886, he states:

Rest, as commonly interpreted, does not strictly express the meaning, I would, in a surgical sense, attach to this term; all modes of fixation or enforced immobility of a diseased part cannot be classed under the term. In surgical rest, the fixation or enforced immobility must be attained, by restraints applied to parts healthy, which tolerate them without harm, and at the same time, control the site of the lesion. Is confinement in plaster of Paris rest? We are told it is not: but is a little 'sustained pressure'. In fact, the instances in which immobility has led to degeneration of structures are not examples of rest. Confining a lesion in plaster of Paris, or by compressing bandages, is not rest, but the opposite of it, and a method of starving and injuring a diseased part, which is already below the normal standard of vitality.[121]

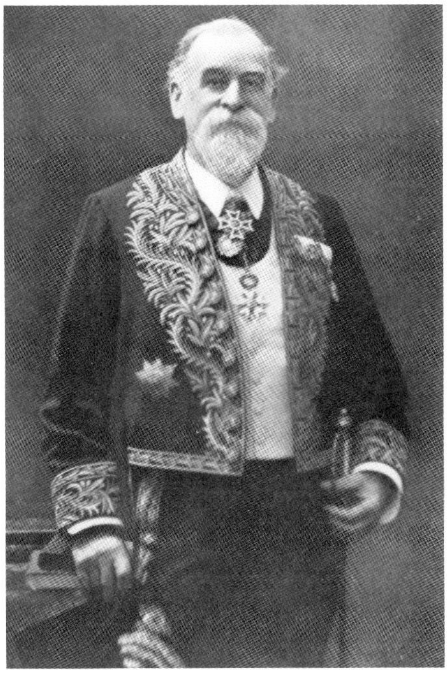

Figure 2.39 Just Lucas-Championnière (1843–1913) opposed the principles of treatment of fractures by rest espoused by Hugh Owen Thomas. From James B. Mennell, *The Treatment of Fractures by Mobilisation and Massage* (London: Macmillan, 1911), frontispiece.

This obscure and polemical style limited his circle of readers and his influence on his associates. However, Thomas's reputation was enhanced and his principles widely dispersed through the work of his nephew Robert Jones, who joined him in practice in 1878.

The concept of the treatment of fractures by rest espoused by Thomas was challenged by Lucas-Championnière, who taught that fractures, particularly those involving joints, were best treated through a program of mobilization and massage. Just Lucas-Championnière (1843–1913) was born in northern France and educated in Paris (figure 2.39). After a brief visit to Lister's clinic in Glasgow, he returned, excited by what he had seen, to introduce the antiseptic system of surgery in France. In 1876 he published the first authoritative book on the subject, *Chirurgie antiseptique*.[122] He also became well known for his work on hernia and neolithic trephination.[123]

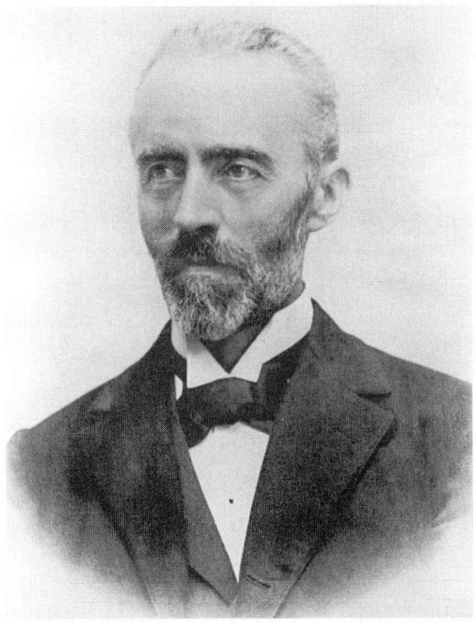

Figure 2.40 Theodor Kocher (1841–1917), of Kocher's fracture of the capitellum of the humerus.

In the foreword to a book by his English disciple James B. Mennell (1880-1957), Lucas-Championnière outlined his basic principles for the treatment of fractures:

Absolute immobilisation of the bony fragments does not provide the most favorable conditions for healing. A certain amount of movement of the fracture fragments provides the best conditions for repair. A certain amount of mobilisation and massage provide the best conditions for healing of the limb. Mobilisation and massage, in acting upon pain and muscle spasm, play an important role in healing that nothing else can replace. A large number of deformities caused by muscle contractions, disappear spontaneously with the cessation of the contractions after massage and mobilisation. The suppression of pain by massage and movement is an essential element in the treatment of fractures. The constriction and immobilisation of splints and dressings are bound to be detrimental to the healing of the injured limb. The restoration of

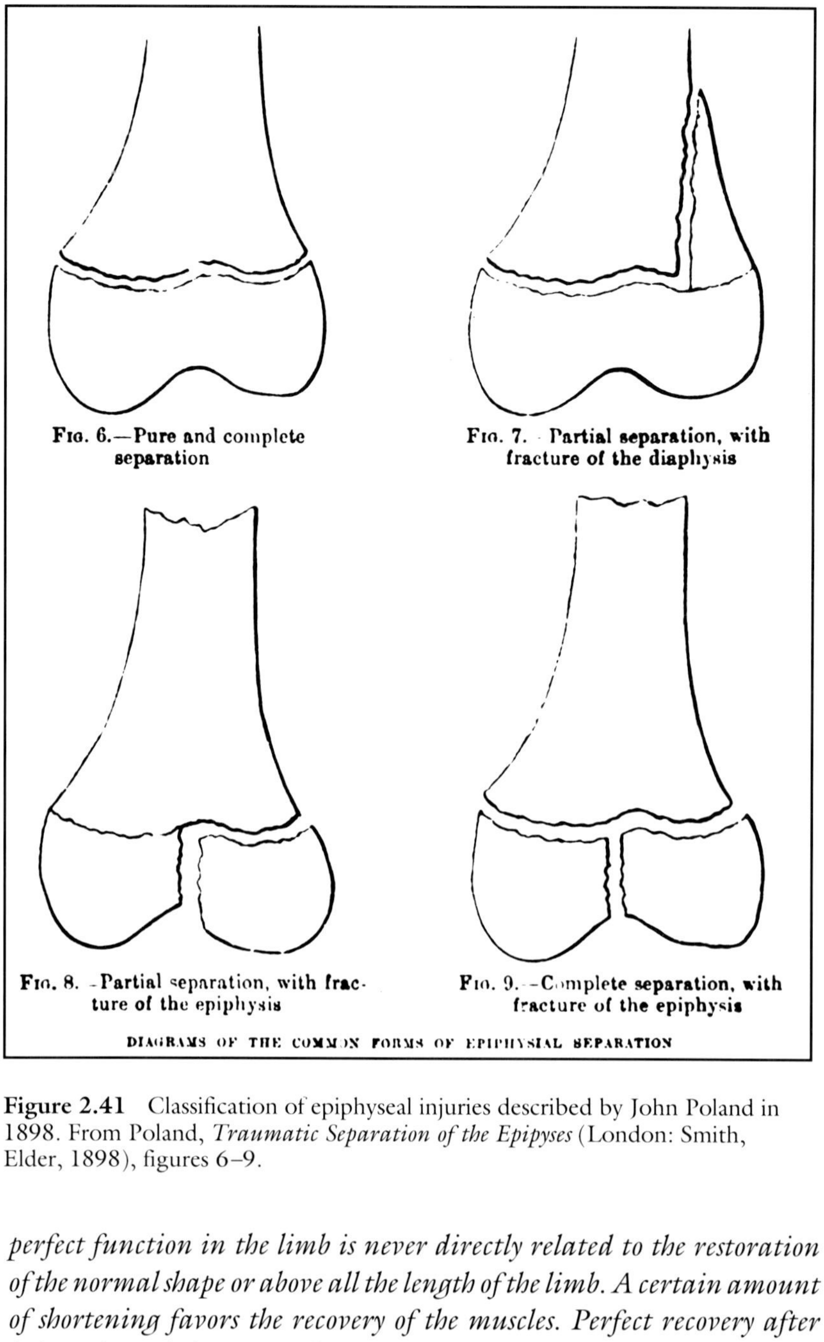

Figure 2.41 Classification of epiphyseal injuries described by John Poland in 1898. From Poland, *Traumatic Separation of the Epipyses* (London: Smith, Elder, 1898), figures 6–9.

perfect function in the limb is never directly related to the restoration of the normal shape or above all the length of the limb. A certain amount of shortening favors the recovery of the muscles. Perfect recovery after injury depends less upon the accurate restoration of form than on the rapid return of movement which promotes the life of the joints, tendons, muscles, nerves and vessels of the limb. Deprivation of movement for a short period of time, especially after injuries of the joints, will result in lesions which can never be restored.[124]

In practice, *massage* meant "to rub it gently, as if . . . stroking a cat," the slow and rhythmical repetition of a single movement, "little more than a caress." Mobilization for Lucas-Championnière consisted of active assisted exercise within the limits of pain. Treatment was carried out several times daily and was time-consuming and expensive. Mennell cautioned: "Never be afraid of rubbing too

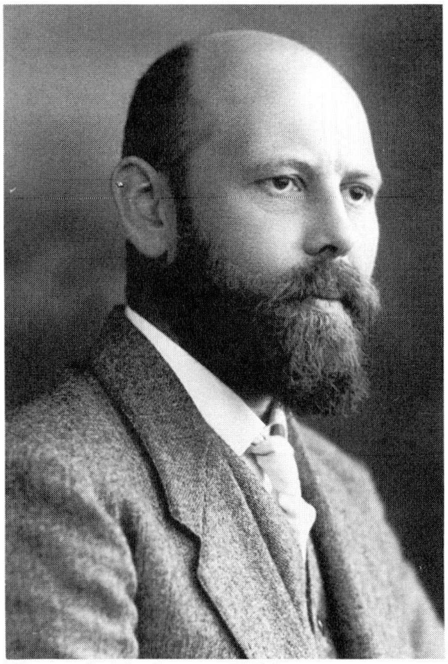

Figure 2.42 Lorenz Böhler (1885–1973) at thirty-eight years of age.

gently or of giving too small a dose of mobilization: always fear that massage is too heavy and movement too great."[125]

While his book *Le massage et la mobilisation dans le traitement des fractures*, like that of Thomas, did not have an immediate impact on the practice of treating fractures, Lucas-Championnière's had a subtle and persisting influence.[126] Programs of immediate mobilization of the joints and soft tissues—that is, continuous passive motion—in patients whose fractures have been reduced anatomically and rigidly fixed internally closely resemble those that Lucas-Championnière described, and it is in such treatment programs that the opposing concepts of "rest" and "movement" have been finally reconciled.

Until the end of the nineteenth century, all of our knowledge of fractures was gained by taking a history, performing a careful physical examination and, when the chance offered, carrying out an anatomical dissection. Such clinical and pathological correlations are illustrated nicely by the works of Theodor Kocher and John Poland, which were prepared just before the turn of the century.

Theodor Kocher (1841–1917) was a graduate of the University of Bern and had traveled extensively in many parts of Europe visiting surgical clinics[127] (figure 2.40). It was during a visit to Theodor Billroth's clinic in Vienna in 1870 that he was able to demonstrate successfully his "rotation-elevation" maneuver for the reduction of an anterior dislocation of the shoulder. Kocher's accomplishments as a surgeon and a teacher spanned forty-five years and eventually earned him a Nobel Prize. In 1896 he published his book *Beiträge zur Kenntniss einiger Praktisch wichtiger Fracturformen*, which is a careful description of the types of fractures occurring in the humerus and the hip.[128] It contains the description of the fracture of the capitellum of the humerus known as Kocher's fracture.

The monograph *Traumatic Separation of the Epiphysis*, published in 1898 by John Poland (1855–1937), was a substantial work, containing an exhaustive review of the literature on the subject as well as a system of classification for epiphyseal injuries (figure 2.41), which is remarkably current when compared to the classification in use today.[129] John Poland was educated and later worked at Guy's Hospital, where his uncle, Alfred Poland was on the surgical staff. John Poland was also on the surgical staff of the Royal National Orthopaedic Hospital and the City Orthopaedic Hospital.

A major French work on the treatment of fractures that appeared early in the century was written by Jean Tanton (1875–1918), a professor at the French military medical school Val-de-Grace. His work was published as a part of a surgical encyclopedia edited by A. LeDentu and Pierre Delbet.[130]

Lorenz Böhler (1885–1973) was born in the Vorarlberg region of Austria[131] (figure 2.42). While he was a medical student at the University of Vienna, his surgical teachers, Anton von Eiselsberg and Julius Hochenegg, opened the first wards in Europe specifically set

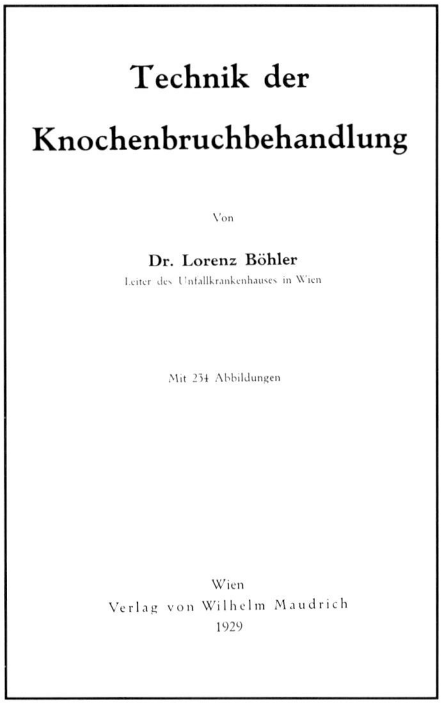

Technik der Knochenbruchbehandlung

Von

Dr. Lorenz Böhler
Leiter des Unfallkrankenhauses in Wien

Mit 234 Abbildungen

Wien
Verlag von Wilhelm Maudrich
1929

Figure 2.43 First edition of Böhler's highly influential and innovative textbook.

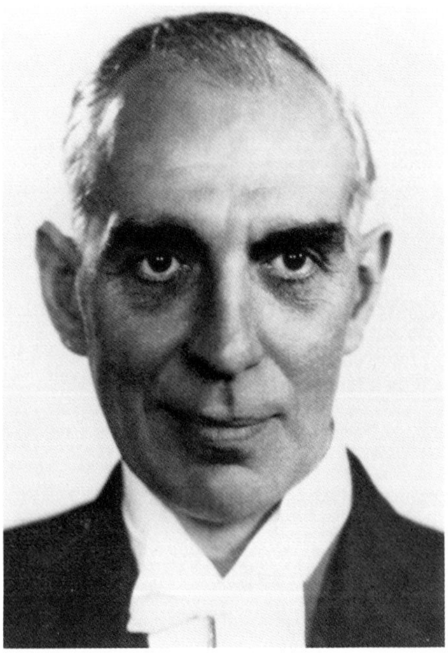

Figure 2.44 Reginald Watson-Jones (1902–1972). From his obituary, *J Bone Joint Surg* 54B(1972): 569–75.

aside for injured patients.[132] Following graduation, Böhler did his military service and then in 1914 traveled to the United States, where he remained for some months as a visitor at the Mayo Clinic. The organization and operation of this then unique clinic impressed him greatly. His experience in the treatment of casualties in World War I enhanced his clinical skills and developed his administrative abilility. He was able to organize an army hospital that specialized in the treatment of fractures and joint injuries and demonstrated that this specialized unit provided superior care. In 1917, Böhler first became aware of the magnitude of the problem of industrial injuries and began to plan a hospital for the care of the injured workers. Immediately after World War I, he had no opportunity to pursue his ideas, but in 1925 he was appointed director and chief surgeon of the Unfallkrankenhaus, or Accident Hospital, in Vienna, which was established and supported by a group of industrial insurance companies. It was to this hospital that Böhler was to give his enthusiastic leadership for the next thirty years.

His book *Technik der Knochenbruch-Behandlung*, appeared in 1929 (figure 2.43). It appeared in a modest first edition that grew as it passed through a number of editions in eight languages, becoming one of the most important and influential textbooks on the treatment of fractures and dislocations to be published in this century. Böhler's book presented the material in a systematic fashion and included careful follow-up and end result studies. Although he generally advocated a nonoperative approach, Böhler quickly recognized the value of intramedullary nailing for the internal fixation of long-bone fractures. Böhler was an influential teacher as well as an organizational genius: his students assumed the leadership of important accident hospitals, his clinic was filled with visitors from abroad, and his ideas spread throughout the world through his travels, lectures and books. Ernest W. Hey-Groves, in his preface to the fourth English edition of Böhler's textbook, published in 1935, commented:

> *A visit to Dr. Böhler's clinic in Vienna and the translation of his book have been to me a great pleasure and education. The fundamental principles which he has demonstrated, and to which I give my wholehearted support, are the necessity for unity of control, loyal and efficient team work, accurate knowledge of the after-results, and meticulous attention to detail. He has, moreover, demonstrated that the proper treatment of fractures is not only a scientific problem or philanthropic duty, but also a business proposition. In other words, it pays to treat fractures well!*[133]

At the end of World War II, Vienna was in ruins and the Unfallkrankenhaus, a wreck. Because of his hard work and indomitable spirit, Böhler's hospital survived the war and grew. In a new physical plant dedicated to his memory, Unfallkrankenhous Lorenz Böhler, his work is carried on today under the direction of his son, Jorg Böhler.

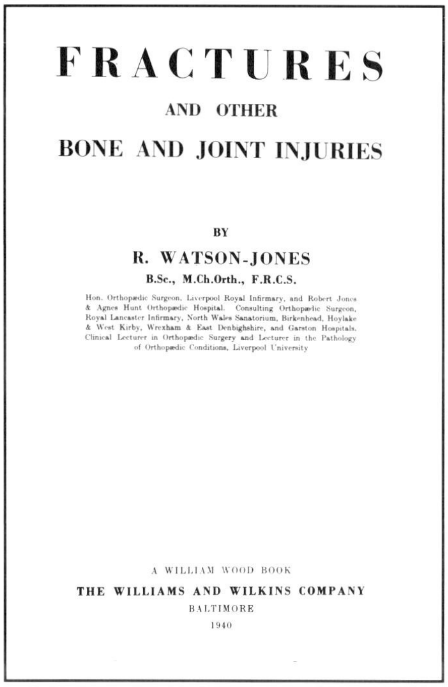
FRACTURES

AND OTHER

BONE AND JOINT INJURIES

BY

R. WATSON-JONES

B.Sc., M.Ch.Orth., F.R.C.S.

Hon. Orthopædic Surgeon, Liverpool Royal Infirmary, and Robert Jones & Agnes Hunt Orthopædic Hospital. Consulting Orthopædic Surgeon, Royal Lancaster Infirmary, North Wales Sanatorium, Birkenhead, Hoylake & West Kirby, Wrexham & East Denbighshire, and Garston Hospitals. Clinical Lecturer in Orthopædic Surgery and Lecturer in the Pathology of Orthopædic Conditions, Liverpool University

A WILLIAM WOOD BOOK

THE WILLIAMS AND WILKINS COMPANY

BALTIMORE

1940

Figure 2.45 Watson-Jones's book was dedicated to Hugh Owen Thomas and Robert Jones.

Reginald Watson-Jones (1902–1972) was a protege of Robert Jones who was appointed to the Liverpool Royal Infirmary in 1926 (figure 2.44). The growth of his fracture clinic there resulted in the institution of a course of lectures on the treatment of fractures. His textbook *Fractures and Other Bone and Joint Injuries* was a natural outgrowth of these lectures[134] (figure 2.45). The first edition appeared in 1940; it was quickly followed by a second in 1941 and a third in 1943. The latter editions were enriched by the material on war casualties that he gathered in his role as senior orthopedic consultant to the Royal Air Force. The book was used extensively throughout the English-speaking world and was especially popular in the United States. As a rule, the methods of treatment he advocated were conservative and nonoperative. In dedicating his book to Hugh Owen Thomas and Robert Jones, he expressed the belief that the book represented their philosophy of treatment. However, John Charnley (1911–1982) (figure 2.46) captured most accurately the spirit of Thomas and Jones in his small monograph *The Closed Treatment of Common Fractures* (figure 2.47).[135] If Charnley had done nothing more, this little volume would suffice to ensure his reputation, containing as it does the essence of the nonoperative approach to the treatment of fractures. His work demonstrates the essential sophistication of a simple approach and points out the importance of giving attention to seemingly minor details.

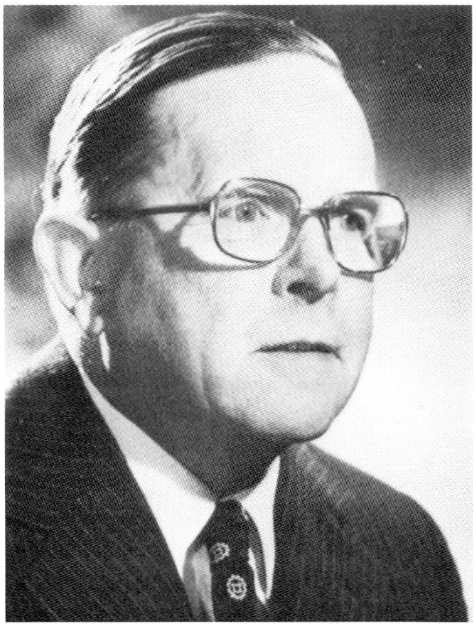

Figure 2.46 John Charnley (1911–1982). From his obituary, *J Bone Joint Surg* 65B(1983): 84–86.

For forty years following its first meeting in 1881, the American Surgical Association provided an important forum for the discussion of the treatment of fractures. Stimulated by the visit of Arbuthnot Lane to the United States in 1909, the Association included in its program in 1912 a symposium on the treatment of fractures in which twenty-eight speakers participated. Because of the conflicting opinions of the discussants, the Association appointed a Committee on Fractures whose members were, for the most part, distinguished senior fellows whose views were rooted firmly in the nineteenth century. The reports of this committee were published in 1922.[136] The organization of the American College of Surgeons in 1913 provided another platform for discussing the treatment of fractures, a subject which became of consuming interest because of the experiences of World War I. In 1922 the American College of Surgeons established a Fracture Committee consisting of forty-four surgeons with a special interest in the subject. This group was made up of a younger generation of surgeons; only three participants had participated in the symposium of 1912—William L. Estes, Jr., John B. Walker, and Charles L. Scudder (see table 2). The importance of this committee is apparent from the fact that, with only one exception, it included the author of every important textbook on the treatment of fractures published in the United States during the next fifty years.

*Table 2 The Committee on Fractures of the American College of Surgeons, 1922**

Frederic W. Bancroft, New York, Chairman
Robert H. Kennedy, New York, Secretary

Peter A. Bendixen, Davenport	Walter Estell Lee, Philadelphia
Willis C. Campbell, Memphis	George A. Leland, Jr., Boston
Isidore Cohn, New Orleans	Paul B. Magnuson, Chicago
H. Earle Conwell, Birmingham	Henry C. Marble, Boston
Salvador Cordoba, Caracas	Clay Ray Murray, New York
Frederic J. Cotton, Boston	Lloyd Noland, Birmingham
Bowman C. Corwell, Chicago	Hubley R. Owen, Philadelphia
William R. Cubbins, Chicago	Edwin W. Ryerson, Chicago
William Darrach, New York	Charles L. Scudder, Boston
Frank D. Dickson, Kansas City	W. O'Neill Sherman, Pittsburgh
Eldridge L. Eliason, Philadel.	Ernest A. Sommer, Portland
William L. Estes, Jr., Bethlehem	Kellogg Speed, Chicago
W. Edward Gallie, Toronto	Frederic J. Tees, Montreal
Fraser B. Gurd, Montreal	Jorge del Toro, Puerto Rico
Donald Guthries, Sayre	J. Huber Wagner, Pittsburgh
George W. Hawley, Bridgeport	John B. Walker, New York
Melvin Henderson, Rochester	Roscoe C. Webb, Minneapolis
William L. Keller, Washington	George E. Wilson, Toronto
Norman T. Kirk, Washington	John C. Wilson, Los Angeles
Samuel L. Leadbetter, Jr., Boston	Philip D. Wilson, New York

Ex-officio: Franklin H.Martin, Director-General

*From Franklin H. Martin, *Fifty Years of Medicine and Surgery*, (Chicago: Surgical Publishing Company, 1934), 350.

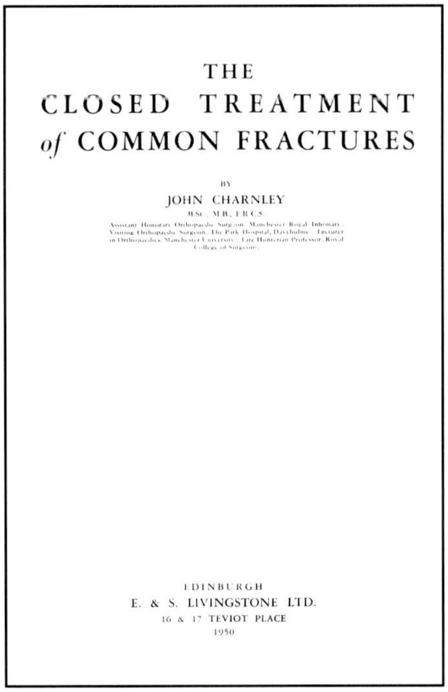
THE
CLOSED TREATMENT
of COMMON FRACTURES

BY
JOHN CHARNLEY
B.Sc., M.B., F.R.C.S.
Assistant Honorary Orthopaedic Surgeon, Manchester Royal Infirmary; Visiting Orthopaedic Surgeon, The Park Hospital, Davyhulme; Lecturer in Orthopaedics, Manchester University; Late Hunterian Professor, Royal College of Surgeons.

EDINBURGH
E. & S. LIVINGSTONE LTD.
16 & 17 TEVIOT PLACE
1950

Figure 2.47 A classic exposition of the nonoperative approach.

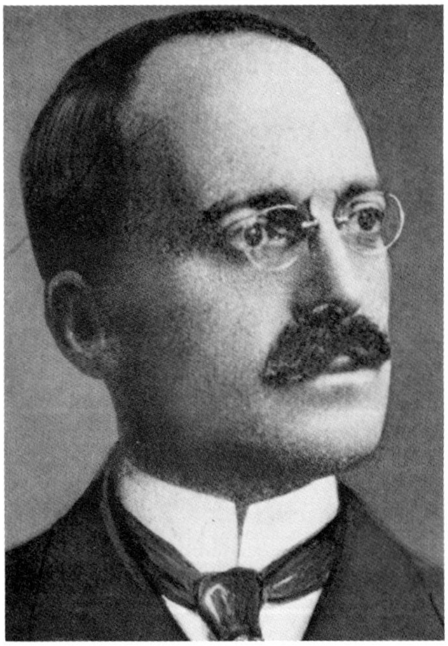

Figure 2.48 Charles Locke Scudder (1860–1949). From his obituary, *Trans Am Surg Assoc* 68(1950): 569–70.

Since its inception, the Fracture Committee has remained an active and important arm of the American College of Surgeons and is now known as the Committee on Trauma. The first product of the committee was an "Outline of the Treatment of Fractures," a syllabus adopted at a conference held in Boston in April 1922.[137] The surgeon most responsible for the establishment, organization and continuity of the committee was Charles Scudder (1860–1949).

Charles L. Scudder (figure 2.48) received undergraduate degrees from Yale before obtaining his medical degree from Harvard in 1888.[138] He began his work at Massachusetts General Hospital as a surgical extern and continued his service there in various capacities for fifty-six years, remaining active in the surgical outpatient clinic until 1943. His published papers reflect interests in urology, neurosurgery, gynecology, and abdominal and orthopedic surgery. His major interest, however, was in the treatment of fractures and dislocations. His book *The Treatment of Fractures* first appeared in 1900 and went through eleven editions, the last appearing in 1938.[139] The initial edition was produced with the assistance of his colleague Frederic J. Cotton, who supplied most of the drawings and references to the literature. The first paragraph of the preface predicted rapid progress in the treatment of fractures in the twentieth century:

The general employment of anesthesia in the examination and the initial treatment of fractures, especially of those near or involving joints has made diagnosis more accurate and treatment more intelligent. The application of the Roentgen ray to the diagnosis of fracture of bone has already contributed much toward an accurate interpretation of the physical signs of fracture. The greater certainty in diagnosis has suggested more direct and simpler methods of treatment. Antisepsis has opened to operative surgery a very profitable field in the treatment of fractures. The final results after the open incision of closed fractures emphasize the fact that anesthesia, antisepsis and the Roentgen ray are making the knowledge of fractures more exact, and their treatment less complicated. The attention of the student is diverted from theories and apparatus to the actual conditions that exist in the fractured bone, and he is encouraged to determine for himself how to meet the conditions found in each individual case of fracture.[140]

Scudder's book ended with three short chapters: "The Employment of Plaster of Paris," "The Ambulatory Treatment of Fractures," and "The Roentgen Ray and Its Relation to Fractures." The last chapter, written by his colleague E. A. Codman, a pioneer in the radiology of bone, considered some of the technical factors causing distortion on X rays and included a warning of the danger of exposure to X rays. The importance given to the subject is clear from the fact that the entire chapter occupies 13 pages in a volume containing 433.

Frederic J. Cotton (1869–1938) published his own book, *Dislocations and Joint Fractures*, in 1910. It was illustrated profusely by the author, who was also a talented artist. In the introduction Cotton also speaks of a new vista in the treatment of fractures:

We are fortunate today not only in having the x-ray as an accessory method of diagnosis, but in having, as a result of this diagnostic method and of a vast array of observations made directly at operation, a material for deductions not accessible to a previous generation. Wisdom did not begin with this generation, but we have had an unusual opportunity to learn.[141]

The establishment of the Fractures Service at Massachusetts General Hospital by Scudder in 1917 provided continuity in the collection of clinical material, which he used in preparing later editions of his book as well as a continuing series of monographs that might well be entitled "How We Treat Fractures at the MGH." The first of these, *Fractures and Dislocations: Immediate Management, After Care and Convalescent Treatment with Special Reference to the Conservation and Restoration of Function*, was compiled by Phillip D. Wilson and William Cochrane; Cochrane was appointed to fill the first chair of orthopedic surgery at the University of Edinburgh.[142] A second edition appeared in 1928 and was very popular.[143] In 1938 appeared *Experience in the Management of Fractures and Dislocations* by the Staff of the Fracture Service of the Massachusetts General

Hospital, Boston, under the general editorship of Phillip D. Wilson; it was based on an analysis of 4,390 cases.[144] The statistical presentation is impressive, as is the list of distinguished surgeons who contributed chapters. The series continued with the publication in 1958 of *Fractures and Other Injuries by Members of the Fracture Clinic of the Harvard Medical School*, edited by Edwin F. Cave.[145]

Several surgeons in New York contributed to medical journals regularly and significantly influenced the treatment of fractures through their participation in the organizational and educational activities of the Committee on Trauma. Among them were William Darrach (1876–1948), Clay Ray Murray (1890–1947), Frederic W. Bancroft (1880–1963), Robert Kennedy (1887–1978) and Preston Wade (1901–1982). It was Murray who said, "Hypothetically, the ideal treatment for any fractures would be to 'wish' the fragments into place, hold them there by 'moral suasion' and send the patient on about his business while the fracture heals."[146]

In Chicago, the Cook County Hospital nurtured an important fracture service begun by William Cubbins (1874–1959). Kellogg Speed (1879–1955), the head of this service from 1912 to 1933, gathered material for his book *A Text-Book of Fractures and Dislocations*, which went through four editions.[147] Speed was a star athlete in college and is remembered for his outgoing, aggressive personality. He was known for his aphorisms dealing with the care of the injured, the most notable of which was, "Splint 'em where they lie!" Another important textbook, *Management of Fractures, Dislocations and Sprains*, by J. Albert Key (1890–1955) of St. Louis and H. Earle Conwell (1893–1973) of Birmingham, first appeared in 1934 and went through six editions.

Notes

1. James H. Breasted, *The Edwin Smith Papyrus* (Chicago: University of Chicago Press, 1930), 304.
2. Apollonius, *Commentario di Apollonio di Kition sul "Peri Arthron" di Ippocrate*, Codice Laurenziana LXXIV 7, sec IX (Firenze: Biblioteca Laurenziana, n.d.).
3. Breasted, *Edwin Smith Papyrus.*
4. Lawrence Weed, *Medical Records, Medical Education and Patient Care: The Problem-oriented Record as a Basic Tool* (Cleveland: Case Western Reserve University Press, 1969).
5. G. de Santillana and H. von Dechend, *Hamlet's Mill: An Essay on Myth and the Frame of Time* (Boston: Gambit, 1969).
6. J. B. Hurry, *Imhotep, the Vizier and Physician of King Zoser* (Milford: Oxford University Press, 1926).
7. William Osler, *The Evolution of Modern Medicine* (New Haven: Yale University Press, 1921).
8. Kurt Sethe, *Imhotep, der Asklepios der Aegypter* (Leipzig: J. C. Hinrichs, 1902).
9. Henry E. Sigerist, *A History of Medicine* (New York: Oxford University Press, 1951), 1:289.
10. George Sarton, *A History of Science* (New York: W. W. Norton, 1970), 1:44.

11. Fielding H. Garrison, *An Introduction to the History of Medicine*, (Philadelphia & London: W. B. Saunders Co., 1929).

12. Sigerist, *History of Medicine.*

13. Wesley D. Smith, *The Hippocratic Tradition* (Ithaca, N.Y.: Cornell University Press, 1979).

14. Celsus, *De medicina*, with an English translation by W. G. Spencer (Cambridge, Mass.: Harvard University Press, 1960).

15. Garrison, *Introduction*, 93.

16. Hippocrates, *The Genuine Works of Hippocrates*, trans. Francis Adams (Baltimore: Williams & Wilkins, 1939).

17. Ibid., 159.

18. Ibid., 193.

19. Ibid., 187.

20. Ibid., 267.

21. Charles Singer, *A Short History of Anatomy from the Greeks to Harvey* (New York: Dover, 1957), 22-23.

22. Ibid., 33.

23. G. Mukhopadhyaya, *The Surgical Instruments of the Hindus* (New Delhi: R. K. Naahar, 1977); Udaya B. S. Prakash, "Suśruta of Ancient India," *SGO* 146(1978): 263-72.

24. P. K. Duraiswami and S. M. Tuli, "5000 Years of Orthopaedics in India," *Clin Orthop* 75(1971): 269-80.

25. Suśruta, *An English Translation of the Suśruta Samhita*, Based on the Original Sanskrit Text, edited and published by K. K. L. Bhishagratna (Calcutta: Wilkins Press, 1907).

26. Celsus, *De medicina*, (Edinburgi: Maclachlan et Stewart, 1831), 112.

27. Garrison, *Introduction*, 93.

28. Galen, *De fasciis liber*, in G. Guidi, *Chirurgia è graeco in latinum conversa* (Paris: Petrus Galterius, 1544).

29. George Sarton, *Galen of Pergamon* (Lawrence, Kan.: University of Kansas Press, 1954).

30. George A. Snook, "The Father of Sports Medicine," *Am J Sports Med* 6(1978): 128-31.

31. Galen, *De ossibus* (Paris: Christiani Wecheli, 1535); Singer, "Galen's Elementary Course on the Bones," *Proc Roy Soc Med* 45(1952): 767-76.

32. Galen, *De usu partium* (*On the Usefulness of the Parts of the Body*), trans. with an introduction and commentary by M. T. May (Ithaca, N.Y.: Cornell University Press, 1968).

33. Galen, *De fasciis.*

34. Ernest J. Gurlt, *Geschichte der Chirurgie und Ihrer Ausubung* (Berlin: A. Hirschwald, 1898), 1:311.

35. Guidi, *Chirurgia è graeco in latinum conversa* (Paris: Gaultier, 1544).

36. Oribasius, *Oeuvres d'Oribase, texte grec, en grande partie inédit traduit pour la première fois en français par les Drs. Bussemaker et Daremberg* (Paris: Imp. Nationale, 1851-76).

37. Paulus Aegineta, *The Seven Books of Paulus Aegineta*, translated from the Greek with a commentary and notes by Francis Adams (London: The Sydenham Society, 1844-47).

38. L. M. Zimmerman and Ilza Veith, *Great Ideas in the History of Surgery* (Baltimore: Williams and Wilkins, 1961), 74-75.

39. Albucasis, *On Surgery and Instruments*, Arabic text with English translation and commentary by M.S. Spink and G.L. Lewis (Berkeley and Los Angeles: University of California Press, 1973).

40. Ibid., 690.

41. Singer, "The Visions of Hildegard of Bingen" in *From Magic to Sciences: Essays on the Scientific Twilight* (New York: Dover, 1958).

42. For further discussion of the Church reforms, see A. Castiglioni, *A History of Medicine*, trans. and edited by E. B. Krumbaar, 2d ed. (New York: Knopf, 1958);

Paul Delaunay, *La Médicine et l'Eglise* (Paris: Editions Hippocrate, 1948); Paul Diepgen, "Über den Einfluss der autoritativen Theologie auf die Medicin den Mittelalters," *Abh Geistes Social Klasse Jahrgang* 1(1958): 1-20; P. Hughs, *The Church in Crisis: A History of the General Councils* (New York: Hanover House, 1961); H. J. Schroeder, *Disciplinary Decrees of the General Councils, Text, Translation and Commentary* (St. Louis: Herder, 1937); R. Somerville, *Pope Alexander III and the Council of Tours* (Berkeley and Los Angeles: University of California Press, 1977).

43. Theodoric, *The Surgery of Theodoric*, trans. Eldridge Campbell and James Colton (New York: Appleton Century Crofts, 1955-60).

44. Gurlt, *Geschichte der Chirurgie*, 1:740-41.

45. Theodoric, *Surgery*, 1:160.

46. Guillaume de Salicet, *Chirurgie de Guillaume de Salicet achevée en 1275, traduction et commentaire par Paul Pifteau* (Toulouse: Saint-Cyprien, 1898); R. A. Leonardo, *History of Surgery* (New York: Froben Press, 1943), 111.

47. Gurlt, *Geschichte der Chirurgie*, 765.

48. Guy de Chauliac, *La grande chirurgie de Guy de Chauliac composée en l'an 1363, revue et collationnée sur les manuscrits et imprimes latins et français par E. Niçaise* (Paris: Germer Baillière, 1890).

49. De Chauliac, *La grande chirurgie*, 353-69.

50. Guidi, *Chirurgia è graeco.*

51. Apollonius, *Commentario.*

52. Ambroise Paré, *The Apologie and Treatise of Ambroise Paré*, ed. Geoffrey Keynes (London: Falcon, 1951), xx-xxi.

53. See, for example, Paré, *The Case Reports and Autopsy Records of Ambroise Paré*, ed. Wallace B. Hamby, translated from *Oeuvres complètes d'Ambroise Paré*, ed. J.-F. Malgaigne (Springfield, Ill.: Charles C Thomas, 1960); *Surgery and Ambroise Paré*, trans. and ed. Wallace B. Hamby (Norman, Okla.: University of Oklahoma Press, 1965); *Ten Books of Surgery with the Magazine of the Instruments Necessary for It*, trans. R. W. Linker and Nathan Womack (Athens, Ga.: University of Georgia Press, 1969); and *The Apologie and Treatise of Ambroise Paré*, ed. Keynes.

54. Paré, *Oeuvres complètes d'Ambroise Paré revues et collationnées sur toutes les éditions par J.-F. Malgaigne* (Paris: Baillière, 1840), 1:337.

55. Janet Doe, *A Bibliography of the Works of Ambroise Paré* (Chicago: University of Chicago Press, 1937), xiii-xx.

56. Paré, *Case Reports*, 80-81.

57. Ibid., 81.

58. Richard Wiseman, *Severall Chirurgical Treatises* (London: R. Royston, 1676); id., "Of Wounds," "Of Gunshot Wounds," "Of Fractures and Luxations," a facsimile of Books 5, 6 and 7 from *Severall Chirurgical Treatises*, ed. John Kirkup (Bath: Kingsmead, 1977).

59. Leonard F. Peltier, "Joseph Guichard Duverney (1648-1730)," *Clin Orthop* 187(1984): 308-11.

60. Joseph Guichard Duverney, *Traité de l'organe de l'ouie* (Paris, 1683).

61. Lorenz Heister, *Chirurgie, in welcher alles, was zur Wund-Artzney gehöret, nach der neuesten und besten Art* (Nuremburg: J. Hoffmann, 1718).

62. William Cheselden, *The Anatomy of the Human Body* (London: N. Cliff and D. Jackson, 1713), and *Osteographia, or the Anatomy of the Bones* (London, 1733); see also K. F. Russell, "The *Osteographia* of William Cheselden," *Bull Hist Med* 28(1954): 32-49.

63. Peltier, "Eponymic Fractures: Percival Pott and Pott's Fracture," *Surgery* 52(1962): 280-86.

64. Percivall Pott, *Some Few General Remarks on Fractures and Dislocations* (London: L. Hawes, W. Clarke, and R. Collins, 1765).

65. R. T. Austin, "Robert Chessher of Hinckley (1750-1831)," Leicestershire County Council Libraries and Information Service, 1981.

66. Peltier, "John Jones: An Extraordinary American," *Surgery* 59(1959): 631-35.; id., "John Jones: An Extraordinary American," *Bull Am Coll Surg* (March 1978): 22-25.

67. John Jones, *Plain, Concise, Practical Remarks on the Treatment of Wounds and Fractures: To Which is Added an Appendix, On Camp and Military Hospitals* (New York: John Holt, 1775), 3.

68. Pierre-Joseph Desault, *Oeuvres chirurgicales; ou, Exposé de la doctrine et la pratique de P.-J. Desault par Xavier Bichat* (Paris: Méquignon, An IX (1801); id., *A Treatise on Fractures, Luxations and Other Affections of the Bones*, ed. Xavier Bichat, trans. Charles Caldwell (Philadelphia: Fry and Kammerer, 1805).

69. Abraham Colles, "On the Fracture of the Carpal Extremity of the Radius," *Edinb Med Surg J* 10(1814): 182-86.

70. Peltier, "Eponymic Fractures: Abraham Colles and Colles' Fracture," *Surgery* 35(1954): 322-28; id., "Fractures of the Distal End of the Radius: A Historical Review," *Clin Orthop* 187(1984): 18-22.

71. John Rhea Barton, "Remarks on Certain Injuries of the Bones in Children," *Am Med Rec* 4(1821): 9-20; id., "Views and Treatment of an Important Injury of the Wrist," *Med Exam* 1(1838): 365-68.

72. Peltier, "Eponymic Fractures: John Rhea Barton and Barton's Fracture," *Surgery* 34(1953): 960-70.

73. F. E. Acerbi, *Della vita di Giambatista Monteggia* (Milano: Dova, 1816); Franco Fusi, "Biografia di Giovanni Battista Monteggia," *Riv ortop trauma* 24(1956): 475-505; Peltier, "Giovanni Battista Monteggia and Monteggia's Fracture," *Surgery* 42(1957): 585-91.

74. G. B. Monteggia, *Istituzioni chirurgiche*, 2d ed. (Milano: Maspero, 1813–16).

75. Morris Fishbein and Ella Salmonsen, eds., *Bibliography of Infantile Paralysis 1789-1949*, 2d ed. (Philadelphia: J. B. Lippincott, 1951), 3.

76. Ibid.

77. Joseph Wattmann, *Descriptio Nexus Sceleti ad Luxationem Demonstrationem Pathologicam et Therapeuticam Inservientis* (Innsbruck, 1823).

78. A. L. Richter, *Theoretisch-praktisches Handbuch der Lehre von den Bruchen und Verrenk ungen der Knochen* (Berlin: Enslin, 1828).

79. G. F. Sheldon and R. G. Shelden, "Philip Syng Physick (1768-1837), The Father of American Surgery," *Bull Am Coll Surg* (May 1979): 16-27.

80. John Syng Dorsey, *Elements of Surgery for the Use of Students* (Philadelphia: Parker, and Kimber & Conrad, 1813).

81. William Gibson, "Reflexions on the Treatment of Fractures of the Thigh with an Account of a New Apparatus," *Phila J Med Phys Sci* 6(Feb. 1822): 217-38; id., *The Institutes and Practice of Surgery* (Philadelphia: Parker, 1824).

82. Samuel D. Gross, *The Anatomy, Physiology, and Diseases of the Bones and Joints* (Philadelphia: John Gregg, 1830).

83. Peltier, "Eponymic Fractures: Guillaume Dupuytren and Dupuytren's Fracture," *Surgery* 43(1958): 868-74.

84. J. L. H. Peisse, *Sketches of the Character and Writings of Eminent Living Surgeons and Physicians of Paris*, translated from the French by Elisha Bartlett. (Boston: Carter, Hendee & Babcock, 1831), 1.

85. Peltier, "Dupuytren's Fracture," 870.

86. Ibid.

87. Guillaume Dupuytren, "Mémoire sur la fracture de l'extrémité inférieure du péroné, les luxations et les accidents qui en sont la suite," in *Annuaire méd-chir hôp Paris* (Paris: Crochard, 1819).

88. J. Grant Bonnin, *Injuries to the Ankle* (London: Heineman, 1950), 165-66.

89. Peltier, "Fractures of the Distal End of the Radius," *Clin Orthop*, 1984, 18-22.

90. R. C. Brock, *The Life and Work of Astley Cooper* (Edinburgh: E. & S. Livingstone, 1952); Bransby B. Cooper, *The Life of Sir Astley Cooper, Bart.* (London: J. W. Parker, 1843).

91. Astley Cooper, *A Treatise on Dislocations and on Fractures of the Joints* (London: Longman, Hurst, Rees, Orme & Brown, 1822).

92. Peltier, "Eponymic Fractures: Robert William Smith and Smith's Fracture," *Surgery* 45(1959): 1035-45.

93. Robert W. Smith, *A Treatise on Fractures in the Vicinity of Joints and on Certain Forms of Accidental and Congenital Dislocations* (Dublin: Hodges & Smith, 1847).

94. Ibid., 132.

95. Smith, *A Treatise on the Pathology, Diagnosis and Treatment of Neuroma* (Dublin: Hodges & Smith, 1849).

96. Malgaigne, *Traité des fractures et des luxations* (Paris: J. B. Baillière, 1847); id., *A Treatise on Fractures, translated from the French with notes and additions by John Packard* (Philadelphia: J. B. Lippincott Co., 1859), 9-10; see also Peltier, "Eponymic Fractures: Joseph-François Malgaigne and Malgaigne's Fracture," *Surgery* 44(1958): 777-84.

97. Malgaigne, *Treatise on Fractures*, vi.

98. Peltier, "Malgaigne's Fracture," 777-84.

99. Peltier, "Guerin vs. Malgaigne: A Precedent for the Free Criticism of Scientific Papers," *J Orthop Res* 1(1983): 115-18.

100. Paré, *Oeuvres complètes.*

101. Malgaigne, *Recherches historiques et pratiques sur les appareils employées dans le traitement des fractures en général depuis Hippocrate jusqu'à nos jours* (Paris: H. Cousin, 1841).

102. Frank Hastings Hamilton, *A Practical Treatise on Fractures and Dislocations* (Philadelphia: Blanchard and Lea, 1860); J. D. MacCallum, and D. J. Adams, "Frank H. Hamilton," *Surgery* 33(1953): 468-76.

103. Hamilton, *Deformities after Fractures* (Philadelphia: T. K. & P. G. Collins, 1855).

104. F. L. Kozelka, "Legal Medicine in the United States," *Ciba Symposium* 1(1951): 1305-12; D. J. McCollum, "Letter: Century Old Complaint re: Malpractice," *N Eng J Med* 294(1956): 59.

105. McCollum, "Letter," 59.

106. Clark Heath, "Letter: How Abraham Lincoln Dealt with a Malpractice Suit," *N Eng J Med* 295(1976): 735-36.

107. Kozelka, "Legal Medicine," 1305-12.

108. Hamilton, *Deformities.*

109. Gurlt, *Handbuch der Lehre von den Knochenbruchen* (Hamm: G. Grote, 1862).

110. Gurlt, *Geschichte der Chirurgie* (Hildesheim: George Olms, 1964), 3 vols.

111. "Richard Volkmann (1830-1889), Proponent of Listerism in Germany," *JAMA* 198(1966): 780-81.

112. Richard Volkmann, "Die ischamischen Muskellahmungen und Kontrakturen," *Zentralbl Chir* 8(1881): 801-3.

113. J. S. Gravenstein, "Richard Volkmann-Leander," *SGO* 115(1962): 776-78.

114. Léon Gosselin, *Clinique chirurgicale de l'Hôpital de la Charité* (Paris: J. B. Baillière et Fils, 1876).

115. Gosselin, *Clinical Lectures on Surgery Delivered at the Hospital of La Charité*, trans. Lewis A. Stimson (Philadelphia: Henry C. Lea, 1878).

116. J. M. Hitzrot, "Lewis A. Stimson," *SGO* 44(1927): 571-73; Eric Larabee, *The Benevolent and Necessary Institution: The New York Hospital (1771-1971)*, (Garden City, N.J.: Doubleday, 1971), 277-88.

117. Stimson, *Bacteria and Their Influence upon the Origin and Development of Septic Complications of Wounds* (New York: D. Appleton and Co., 1875).

118. Stimson, *A Treatise on Fractures and Dislocations* (Philadelphia: Henry C. Lea's Son & Co., 1883).

119. David LeVay, *The Life of Hugh Owen Thomas* (Edinburgh and London: E. & S. Livingstone, 1956).

120. H. O. Thomas, *Diseases of the Hip, Knee, and Ankle Joints* (Liverpool: T. Dobb, 1875), 98-100.

121. Thomas, *The Principles of the Treatment of Fractures and Dislocations, Part IV* (London: H. K. Lewis, 1886), 21.

122. Just Lucas-Championnière, *Chirurgie antiseptique* (Paris: J. B. Baillière, 1876).

123. Lucas-Championnière, *Cure radicale des hernies* (Paris: Delahaye et Lecrosnier, 1887); id., *Trépanation néolithique, trépanation pré-Columbienne, trépanation des Kabyles, trépanation traditionelle* (Paris: G. Steinheil, 1912).

124. James B. Mennell, *The Treatment of Fractures by Mobilisation and Massage, with an introduction by Dr. J. Lucas-Championnière* (London: Macmillan, 1911), 3-4.

125. Mennell, *Treatment of Fractures*, 24.

126. Lucas-Championnière, *Le massage et la mobilisation dans le traitement des fractures* (Paris: Rueff, 1895).

127. E. Bonjour, *Theodor Kocher* (Bern: Paul Haupt, 1950); P. S. McGreevy and F. A. Miller, "Biography of Theodor Kocher," *Surgery* 65(1969): 990-99.

128. Theodor Kocher, *Beiträge zur Kenntniss einiger Praktisch wichtiger Fracturformen* (Basel and Leipzig: Carl Sallmann, 1896).

129. John Poland, *Traumatic Separation of the Epiphyses* (London: Smith, Elder, 1898); Robert B. Salter and W. R. Harris, "Injuries of the Epiphyseal Plate," *J Bone Joint Surg* 45A(1963): 587-622.

130. Jean Tanton, "Fractures du membre inférieur," Part IV of *Nouveau traité de chirurgie*, eds. A. LeDentu and P. Delbet (Paris: J. B. Baillière et Fils, 1915).

131. Friedrich Lorenz, *Lorenz Böhler: Der Vater der Unfallchirurgie* (Wien: W. Maudrich, 1955).

132. H. Spangler and P. Galle, "70 Jahre Unfallchirurgie an den Wiener Kliniken," *Wien klin Wschr* 13(1981): 423-28.

133. E. W. Hey-Groves, trans., Preface to the Fourth English Edition of L. Böhler, *The Treatment of Fractures*, (Baltimore: William Wood, 1935), 2.

134. Reginald Watson-Jones, *Fractures and Other Bone and Joint Injuries* (Baltimore: Williams and Wilkins, 1940).

135. John Charnley, *The Closed Treatment of Common Fractures* (Edinburgh: E. & S. Livingstone, 1950); "John Charnley," obituary, *J Bone Joint Surg* 65B(1983): 84-86.

136. American Surgical Association, *Treatment of Fractures: Reports of the Committee on Fractures of the American Surgical Association for 1913, 1914, 1915, 1916, 1917, 1918, 1921* (New York: American Surgical Association, 1922).

137. "Outline of the Treatment of Fractures," *AMA Arch Surg* 6(1923): 172-94.

138. Robert H. Kennedy, "Charles Locke Scudder," in *Profiles in Trauma*, ed. G. J. Curry, I. Cohn and F. V. Wade (Springfield, Ill.: Charles C Thomas, 1969), 189-94; "Charles L. Scudder," Obituary, *Trans Am Surg Assoc* 68(1950): 569-70.

139. Charles L. Scudder, *The Treatment of Fractures*, assisted by Frederic J. Cotton (Philadelphia: W. B. Saunders, 1900).

140. Ibid, 9.

141. Frederic J. Cotton, *Dislocations and Joint Fractures* (Philadelphia: W. B. Saunders, 1910), 17.

142. P. D. Wilson and W. Cochrane, *Fractures and Dislocations* (Philadelphia: J. B. Lippincott, 1925).

143. Wilson and Cochrane, *Fractures and Dislocations*, 2d ed. (Philadelphia: J. B. Lippincott, 1928).

144. Wilson, *Experience in the Management of Fractures and Dislocations* (Philadelphia: J. B. Lippincott, 1925).

145. Edwin F. Cave, ed., *Fractures and Other Injuries by Members of the Fracture Clinic of the Harvard Medical School*, (Chicago: Yearbook Publishers, 1958).

146. Clay Ray Murray in Harrison L. McLaughlin, *Trauma* (Philadelphia: W. B. Saunders, 1959).

147. Kellogg Speed, *A Text-Book of Fractures and Dislocations* (Philadelphia: Lea & Febiger, 1916).

CHAPTER THREE

Occlusive Dressings, Plaster of Paris, and the Ambulatory Treatment of Fractures

AT THE BEGINNING of the nineteenth century, the increasing population in the cities caused by the industrial revolution, the massive casualties of the Napoleonic Wars, and the shortage of trained surgeons emphasized the need for new methods of treating fractures. Ideally, these methods would be simple, inexpensive, require little special equipment, provide effective immobilization and require little, if any, adjustment during the weeks following their application. At this time, patients with fractures of the lower extremities—and often of the upper extremities as well—were treated in bed with restriction of all activity for many weeks until the fractures united. It was the practice of surgeons to dress wounds and fractures at frequent intervals. The bandages, pads, and splints were removed, the fractures manipulated, and the dressings reapplied. These dressing changes were difficult for patients and time-consuming for the surgeons; they also required large quantities of supplies. The continuing attendance of the surgeon and the need for nursing care made treatment costly and unavailable except to a fortunate few.

The search for simpler, less cumbersome methods of treatment led to the development of occlusive dressings, stiffened at first with starch and later with plaster of paris. The ambulatory treatment of fractures was the direct result of these innovations. Four military surgeons—Dominique Larrey of France, Louis Jean Seutin of Belgium, Antonius Mathijsen of the Netherlands, and Nikolai

Ivanovitch Pirogov of Russia—were responsible for the introduction of the new techniques.

Dominique Jean Larrey (1768–1842) was born in a small town in southern France (figure 3.1). He first studied medicine with his uncle, a surgeon in Toulouse. From there he went to Paris and became a student of Desault at l'Hôtel Dieu. After a short tour of duty as a naval surgeon, he returned to Paris, where he was soon caught up in the turmoil of the Revolution, being present at the storming of the Bastille. From this time forward, he made his career as a surgeon in France's revolutionary and Napoleonic armies, which he accompanied throughout Europe and the Middle East. Larrey as a result accumulated a vast experience in military medicine and surgery, much of which he describes in his *Mémoires de chirurgie militaire.*[1] In the fourth volume of this work, for example, he describes the use of an undisturbed occlusive dressing. Among his patients after the Battle of Borodino was an infantry officer whose arm was amputated at the shoulder. The patient was evacuated from the field immediately following the operation and passed from Russia through Poland and Germany. On his arrival at his home in France, some three and one-half months later, the original dressing was removed and the wound was found to be healed![2]

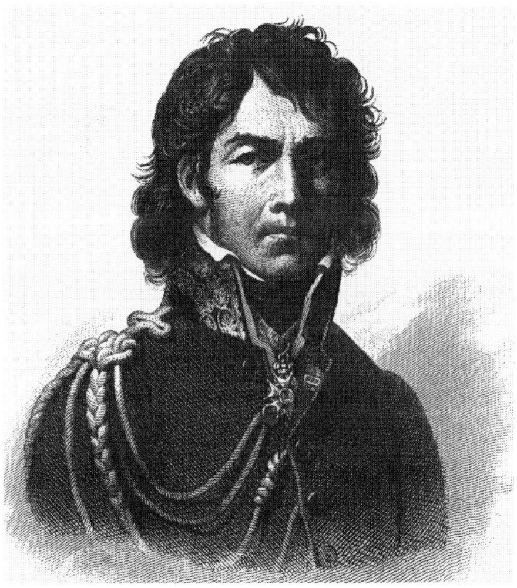

Figure 3.1 Dominique Jean Larrey (1768–1842), surgeon to Napoleon. From Paul Triarire, *Dominique Larrey et les campagnes de la révolution et de l'empire,* (Tours: Alfred Mame et Fils, 1902), frontispiece.

After the wars ended, Larrey continued to advocate the use of infrequent dressing changes and rigid immobilization in the treatment of open fractures.[3] Larrey stiffened and congealed his dressings by soaking the bandages as they were applied in a solution of camphorated alcohol, lead acetate, and egg whites beaten in water. His methods were fully described by his son, Félix Hippolyte Larrey (1808–1895) in his thesis *Traitement des fractures des membres par l'appareil inamovible*, which he presented to the faculty of medicine in Paris in 1832.[4] Although Dominique Larrey had demonstrated that occlusive dressings could be used safely, his method of making them rigid was far from ideal. The search for a more satisfactory *appareil inamovible* continued.

An improved method of applying rigid dressings that could be left undisturbed for long periods was introduced by Louis Jean Seutin (1793–1865) of Brussels in 1835.[5] Seutin had served in the allied armies in the wars against Napoleon and was on the field of Waterloo. At the time of the development of the starched bandage, he was the chief surgeon of the Belgian army. Seutin's *bandage amidonnée* consisted of cardboard splints and bandages soaked in a solution of laundry starch and applied wet. These dressings required two or three days to dry, depending upon their thickness and the ambient temperature and humidity. The substitution of dextrine for starch, advocated by Velpeau, reduced the drying time to six hours, but even this was too long.[6] These methods did not escape the attention of surgeons in the United States, and their use was advocated by A. F. Dulin of Baltimore.[7] J. H. James referred approvingly to the starch apparatus in his retrospective address on surgery, delivered in Liverpool in 1839: "Perhaps there are few additions to modern surgery of more importance than this."[8] A good description of the technique was provided by Sampson Gamgee.[9] Gamgee had learned it from Seutin himself in Florence during the winter of 1851–52, and promoted its use in Britain.

The requisite materials for making this apparatus are firstly, cotton, wool, or soft tow, and lint, or linen rag, to make pads for the bony prominences; secondly, common bandages; thirdly, pasteboard for making splints; fourthly, starch, made according to the fashion of laundresses.

The pasteboard should be thick and porous, so as readily to soften on immersion in water, and be easily moulded to the shape of the limb.

Let us suppose a case of recent simple fracture of both bones of the leg, a little above the ankle joint; the tibia being broken obliquely, so as to allow of projection of the upper fragment forwards. The requisite materials being at hand, three splints are required; a straight one to be placed at the back, and to reach from half an inch above the heel to four inches above the knee; and two lateral splints, reaching from the same point above the foot, to fit which, each splint requires to be cut with a foot piece. From the commencement, one assistant is charged with the duty of making extension from the foot while another counter extends from above. Reduction having been affected, the tendo Achilles, the instep, the ball of the great toe, and the proximal end of the fifth metatarsal bone being well padded with wool, a dry bandage is applied from the root of the toes, over the heel, and up the leg, with the precaution to reverse at the back and not over the crest of the tibia, where the ridges caused by the reverses would be very liable to occasion painful pressure. The crest of the tibia may be additionally protected by a strip of cotton wool placed immediately over it; . . . The bandage is continued over the knee to a little below the middle of the thigh, care having been previously taken to pad with cotton wool the head of the fibula, the tuberosity of the tibia, the patella, and the tendons of the hamstring muscles. The surface of this bandage is now smeared uniformly with starch, in doing which the open hands will be found more expeditious and effectual, though some less neat and agreeable, than a brush.

At this stage, the splints, previously softened by soaking in warm water and smeared with starch on both surfaces, are applied to the limb. The back one should not reach further down than half an inch from the heel; but the foot pieces of the lateral ones require to be moulded so as to embrace the outer and inner edges of the foot, respectively, and turn in to the sole. These three splints should extend on to the thigh as far as the first bandages; care must be taken that they do not overlap anywhere, and that neither of the lateral ones reach as far forward as the crest of the tibia. The assistant who holds them in position, manipulates them, so as to mould them accurately to the limb, while the surgeon fixes them

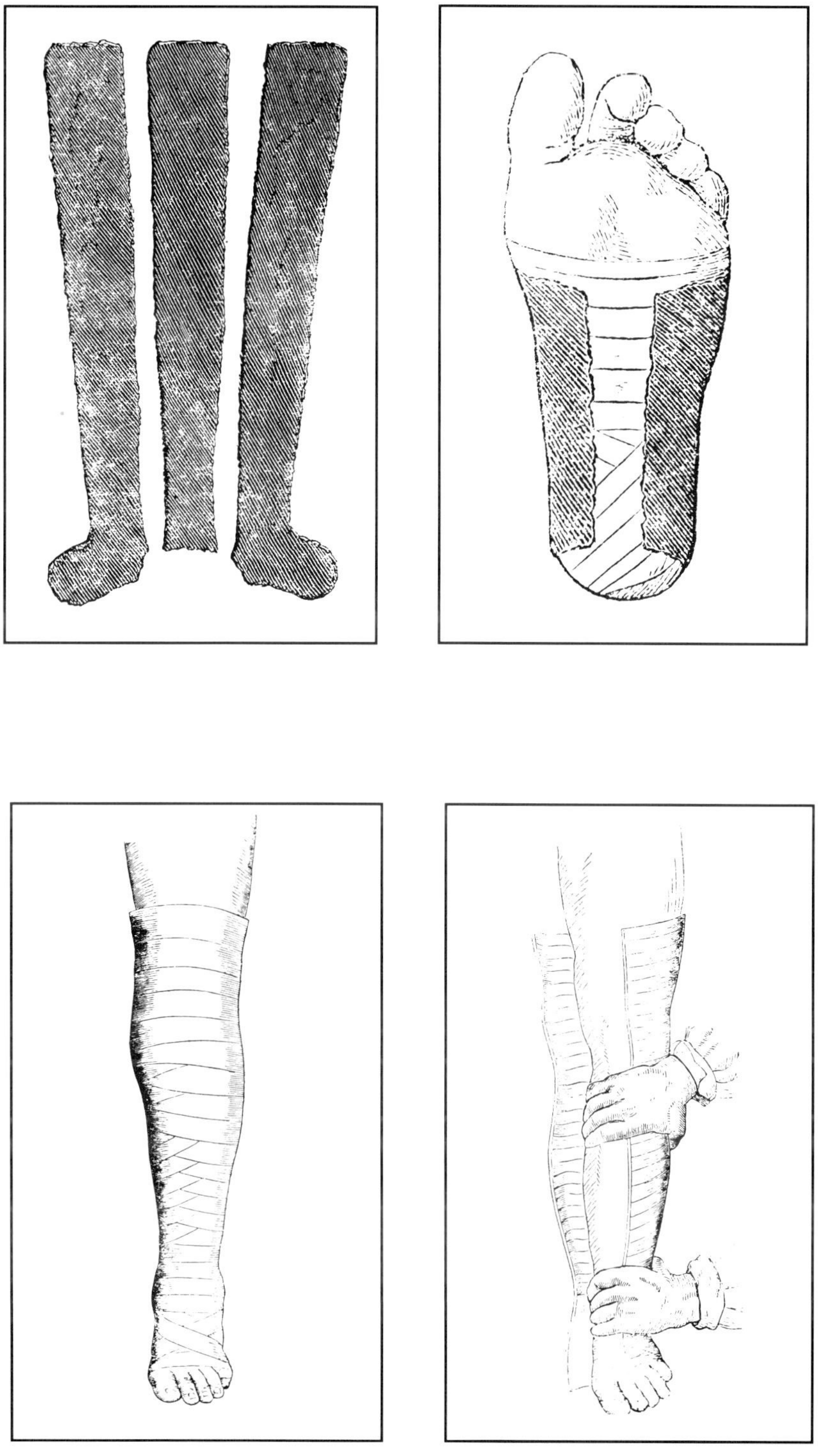

Figures 3.2a,b,c,d Details of the application of the starch apparatus. From Gamgee, *On the Advantages of the Starched Apparatus in the Treatment of Fractures and Diseases of the Joints* (London: H. K. Lewis, 1853), 4–6, 8, 10.

by a bandage applied with moderate and even pressure from below upwards. The apparatus is completed by starching the outside of the last bandage.

As a preventative against displacement, so long as the apparatus is moist, a couple of dry pasteboard splints may be placed laterally and fixed with a bandage. If the individual is very muscular, a sand bag varying from four to eight pounds in weight, may be placed over the front of the apparatus to a little above the seat of the fracture, as an additional precaution during the drying stage—the first thirty-six hours.

So soon as dry, the bandages are cut along the front and in the middle line of the sole of the foot to admit of the limb being examined[10] (figures 3.2a,b,c,d).

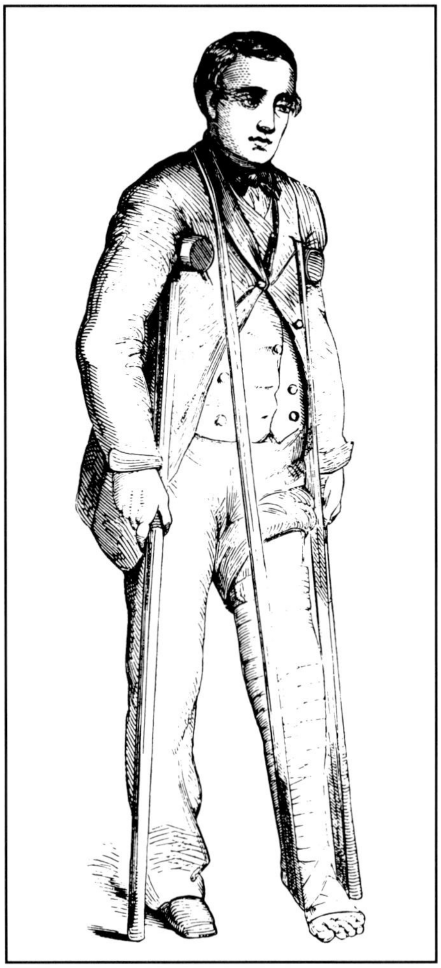

Figure 3.3 Ambulation in the starched apparatus. From Gamgee, *On the Advantages of the Starched Apparatus.*

Seutin's technique for the application of the starch apparatus formed the basis for the development of dressings made of plaster of paris, and many of his basic principles are still invoked by physicians today.

The use of Seutin's method led to the early mobilization of patients with fractures of the extremities and to a marked reduction in the period of hospitalization required for their treatment (figure 3.3). This progress is demonstrated nicely in the report of thirty such patients treated by the starch apparatus in Queen's Hospital, Birmingham.[11]

Although starched bandages were an improvement over Larrey's method, they were far from ideal. They required a long time to apply, and they dried too slowly. The differences in drying times between the thick and thin parts of the dressing resulted in distortion and shrinkage. It was also difficult to cut windows in the dressings, and they did not absorb drainage from wounds. After being in vogue for twenty to thirty years, they disappeared quickly following the introduction of bandages containing plaster of paris.

A great deal of interest had been aroused in Europe around 1800 by a British diplomat's description of a method of treating fractures that he had observed in Turkey:

I saw in the eastern part of the empire a method of setting bones practiced, which appears to me worthy of the attention of surgeons in Europe. It is by enclosing the broken limb, after the bones are put in their places, in a case of plaster of Paris (or gypsum) which takes exactly the form of the limb, without any pressure, and in a few minutes the mass is solid and strong. If it be a compound fracture, the place where the wound is, and out of which an exfoliated bone is to come, may be left uncovered, without any loss to the strength of the plaster encasement. The substance may be easily cut with a knife, and removed, and replaced with another. If, when the swelling subsides the cavity is too large for the limb, a hole or holes being left, liquid gypsum plaster may be poured in,

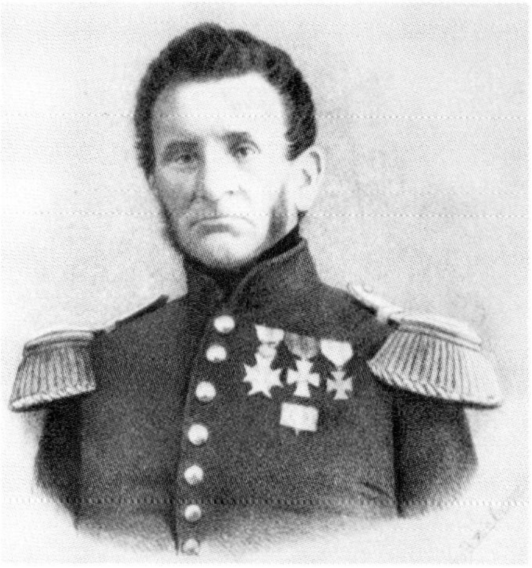

Figure 3.4 Antonius Mathijsen (1805–1878), pioneer of plaster of paris bandages. From G. J. Bremer, *The Plaster of Paris Bandage* (Nieuwkoop: B. DeGraaf, 1962), frontispiece.

which will perfectly fill up the void, exactly fitting the limb. A hole may be made at first by placing an oiled cork or a bit of wood against any point where it is required and when the plaster is set, it is to be removed. There is nothing in gypsum injurious, if it be free of lime; it will soon become very light and dry, and the limb may be bathed with spirits, which will penetrate through the covering. Spirits may be used instead of water, or mixed with it (or vinegar) at the first making of the plaster.

I saw a case of a most terrible compound fracture of the leg and thigh by the fall of a cannon, cured in this manner. The person was seated on the ground and the plaster case extended from below his heel to the upper part of his thigh, whence a bandage, fastened into the plaster, went round his body. He reclined back when he slept as he could not lie down. During the cure, where they saw matter or moisture appear through the plaster coating, they cut a hole with a knife to dress the wound or let out the matter more freely.[12]

Adapting the use of plaster of paris in this manner to hospital practice took some time.[13] In 1828 Otfried Foerster and Kluge at La Charité in Berlin were treating fractures of the leg by aligning them in a long, narrow box that was then filled with firmly packed, moist sand.[14] The substitution of plaster of paris for sand was an obvious next step. One of the chief proponents of this method was Johann Friedrich Dieffenbach, whose technique was described as follows:

When the box had been prepared, its inner surface was smeared with oil or with ointment to prevent adhesion to it of the plaster and a similar unction was applied for the same purpose, to the leg. The leg was then placed in the box in such a manner that it came nowhere in contact with its walls and extension, and such other manipulations as were necessary to reduction were now performed.

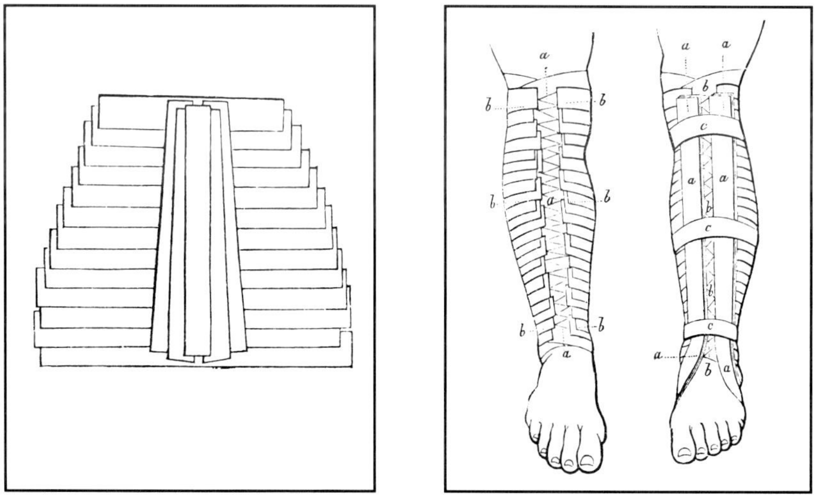

Figures 3.5a,b Details of Mathijsen's plaster of paris bandages. From Bremer, *Plaster of Paris Bandage*, 33.

Liquid plaster of Paris was then gradually and cautiously poured in until, filling the box evenly and exactly, it was brought nearly to the level of the anterior surface of the limb. The limb was to be nearly, but not fully covered in, so as to leave a certain portion of its anterior surface uncovered, in order without detracting from the solidity of the apparatus to have the advantage of having the site of the fracture always open to view. As soon as the mass of plaster had sufficiently set, the box was unhooked and removed.

The removal of the apparatus at the end of the period of retention was done by cutting away, with a mallet and chisel, the upper portion of the plaster until the leg could be readily lifted out.[15]

It is easy to see why such plaster casts, of which there were several variations, did not succeed. Not only were they heavy and cumbersome, but they confined the patient to bed.

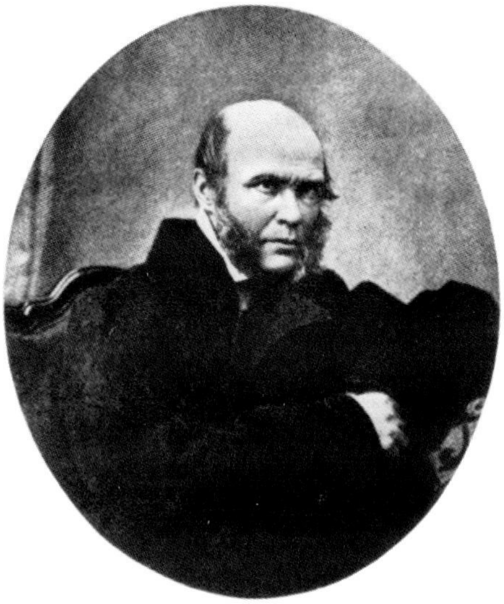

Figure 3.6 Nikolai Ivanovitch Pirogov (1810–1881), the leading Russian surgeon of his era, made many innovations in surgical technique, including his own method of making plaster of paris bandages. From S. S. Yudin, "The Treatment of War Fractures of the Femur," *SGO* 78(1944): 1.

Plaster of paris dressings were introduced into the treatment of fractures by two army surgeons, one at a peacetime home station and the other on active service at the front. Antonius Mathijsen (1805–1878) was born in Budel, the Netherlands, where his father was the village doctor[16] (figure 3.4). He was educated in Brussels, Maastricht, and Utrecht, obtaining the degree of Doctor of Medicine at Giessen in 1837. He spent his entire career as a medical officer in the Dutch army. It was while he was stationed in Haarlem in 1851 that he developed his method of applying plaster of paris bandages. A brief initial note describing his method was published on January 30, 1852; it was followed shortly by more complete accounts.[17] In these papers Mathijsen emphasized that plaster of paris bandages required only simple materials and could be quickly applied without assistants. The bandages hardened rapidly, provided an exact fit to maintain reduction, and could be windowed or bivalved easily. The plaster was porous and absorbent. Mathijsen used coarsely woven materials, usually linen, into which dry, powdered plaster of paris had been rubbed thoroughly. The bandages were moistened with a wet sponge or brush as they were applied and rubbed by hand until they hardened. Four different types of bandages were used: rollers, the Scultetus many-tailed bandage, a "clamshell" made of two splints, and a mould[18] (figures 3.5a,b). Mathijsen's work soon received strong support from Johannes van de Loo, who did much to popularize the technique.

Plaster of paris dressings were first employed in the treatment of mass casualties in the 1850s during the Crimean War by Nikolai Ivanovitch Pirogov (1810–1881) (figure 3.6). Pirogov was born in Moscow and he received his early education there. After obtaining his medical degree at Dorpat, he studied in Berlin and Göttingen before returning to Dorpat as a professor of surgery. In 1840 he became the professor of surgery at the Academy of Military Medicine in St. Petersburg. Pirogov introduced the use of ether anesthesia into

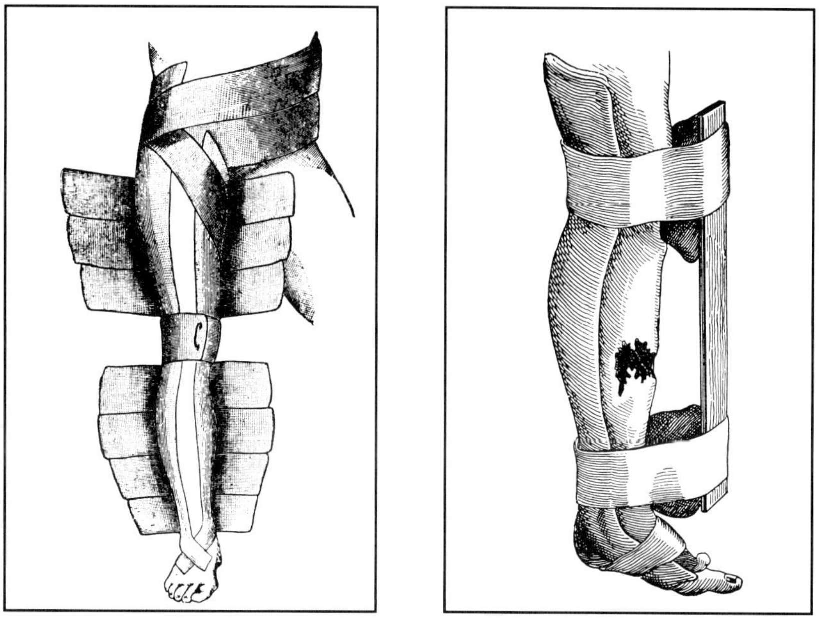

Figures 3.7a,b Details of Pirogov's plaster of paris dressings. From N. Senn, *Practical Surgery for the General Practitioner* (Philadelphia: W. B. Saunders, 1901), 548.

Russia and made important contributions to the study of cross-sectional human anatomy. He was in charge of the Russian medical service during the siege of Sebastopol in 1854. With the help of his patron, the Grand Duchess Helene Pavlovna, he introduced female nurses into the military hospitals at the same time that Florence Nightingale was beginning a similar program in the British military hospitals. As the leading Russian surgeon of his time, his extensive publications were translated into German and disseminated widely.

Plaster of paris casts had been used for the treatment of fractures in Russia as early as 1816.[19] Seutin himself had traveled in Russia demonstrating his starched bandage, and his technique had been adopted by both the Russian army and navy in 1837.[20] Pirogov had observed the use of plaster of paris bandages in the studio of a sculptor who used strips of linen soaked in liquid plaster of paris in making models. Pirogov went on to develop his own methods independently, although he was aware of Mathijsen's work. Pirogov's method consisted of using coarse cloth, either in large pieces or in strips that were immersed in a liquid mixture of plaster of paris immediately before applying them to limbs protected by stockings and cotton pads.[21] Large dressings might be reinforced by pieces of wood (figures 3.7a,b). On the basis of his wartime experience, Pirogov believed that all patients with fractures due to missile wounds should not be evacuated from the forward dressing stations until the limb had been immobilized in a proper dressing of plaster of paris. Mathijsen and Pirogov watched their methods slowly

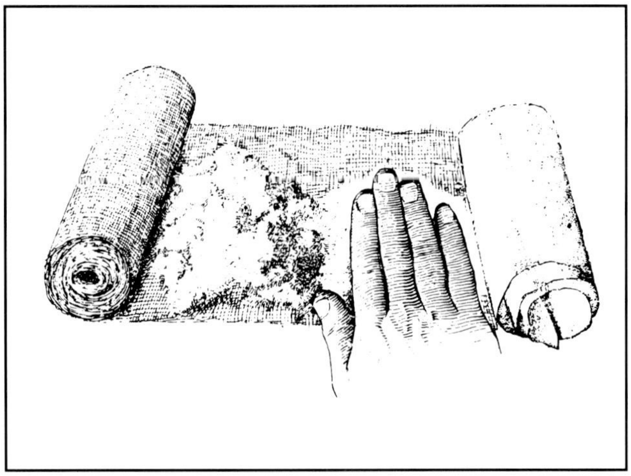

Figure 3.8 Preparing the plaster of paris bandage by hand. From M. W. Ware, *Plaster of Paris and How to Use It* (New York: Surgery Publishing Co., 1911), 2.

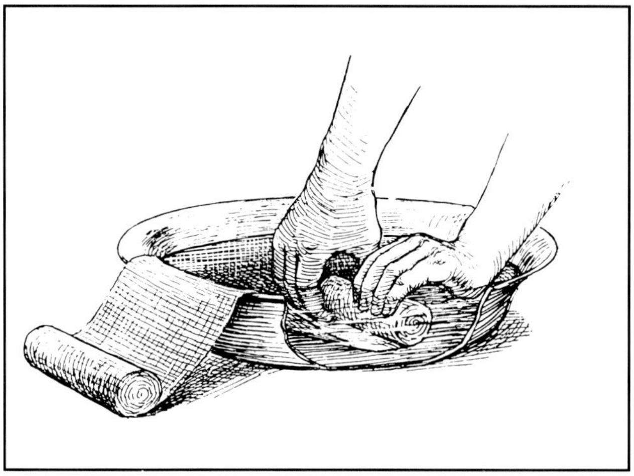

Figure 3.10 Calot's method of preparing a plaster of paris bandage, a modification of Pirogov's technique, required immersing and rerolling the bandage in a cream consisting of three parts water and four parts plaster of paris. From Ware, *Plaster of Paris*, 5.

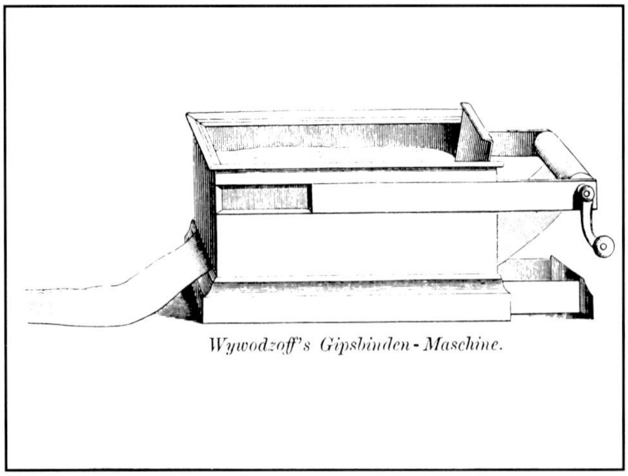

Figure 3.9 A machine for making plaster of paris bandages. From F. Esmarch, *Handbuch der Kriegschirurgischen Technik* (Hanover: Rumpler, 1977), 139.

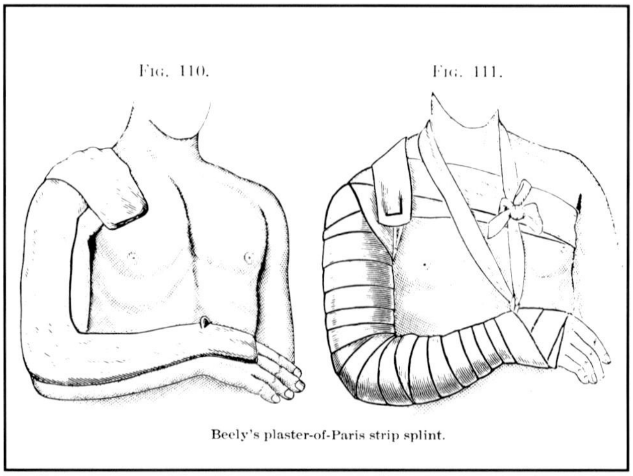

Figure 3.12 A technique utilizing splints made of plaster of paris bandages. From E. von Bergmann and P. Bruns, *A System of Practical Surgery* (New York: Lea Brothers, 1904), 173.

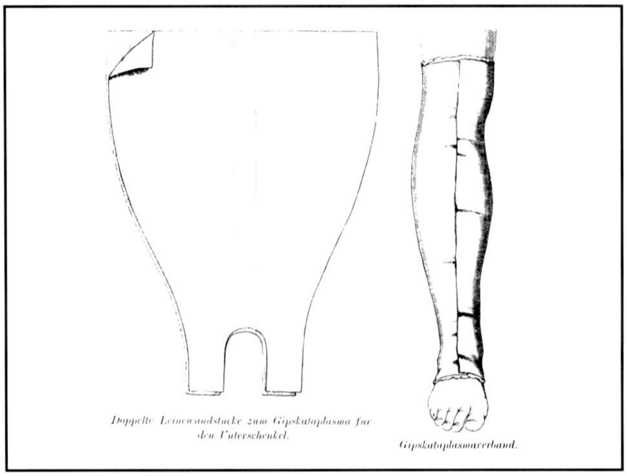

Figure 3.11 An example of a pattern plaster of paris bandage technique. From Esmarch, *Handbuch*, 138.

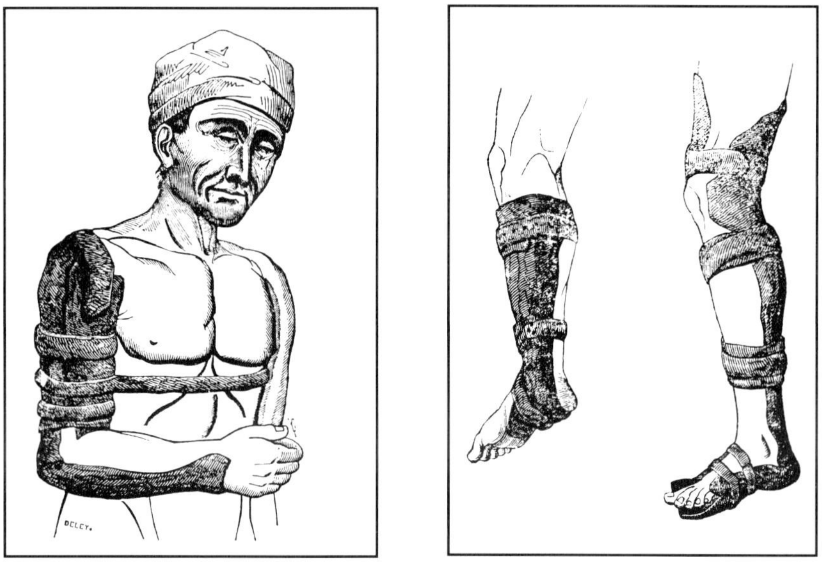

Figures 3.13a,b Splints made of gutta percha. From A. Utterhoeven, *De l'application de la gutta percha* (Brussels: J. B. Tircher, 1857), 17, 44.

win adoption by military and civilian surgeons throughout Europe until by 1870 they were in general use.

Plaster of paris bandages were not used to any great extent in the American Civil War (1861–65), although the United States Sanitary Commission circulated to army surgeons a pamphlet prepared by James Laurence Little of the New York Hospital describing the technique.[22] Frank Hastings Hamilton, the recognized expert on the treatment of fractures in the United States at that time, was not enthusiastic about the use of the starched bandage and in the early editions of his book on fractures did not mention the use of plaster of paris bandages at all.[23] By 1875, however, he had accepted the method and recommended its use, particularly for open fractures.[24]

At the Bellevue Hospital in New York, Lewis A. Sayre began to use plaster of paris bandages in the treatment of fractures, and by 1874 he could report favorably on a vast experience.[25] At this time he was also using body jackets made of plaster of paris bandages for the treatment of spinal tuberculosis.[26] Lewis A. Stimson of New York also promoted the use of plaster of paris bandages in the treatment of fractures, as did Charles Locke Scudder at Boston City Hospital.[27] In Europe, Richard Volkmann was a pioneer in the use of plaster of paris bandages for the treatment of fractures in civilian practice.[28]

The use of plaster of paris bandages was never popular in Liverpool, however. Hugh Owen Thomas believed it to be "a convenient method requiring much labor at first and little care after," but condemned its use: "Confining a lesion in plaster of Paris, or by compressing bandages, is not rest, but the opposite of it, and a method of starving and injuring a diseased part, which is already below the normal standard of viability."[29] Thomas's opposition

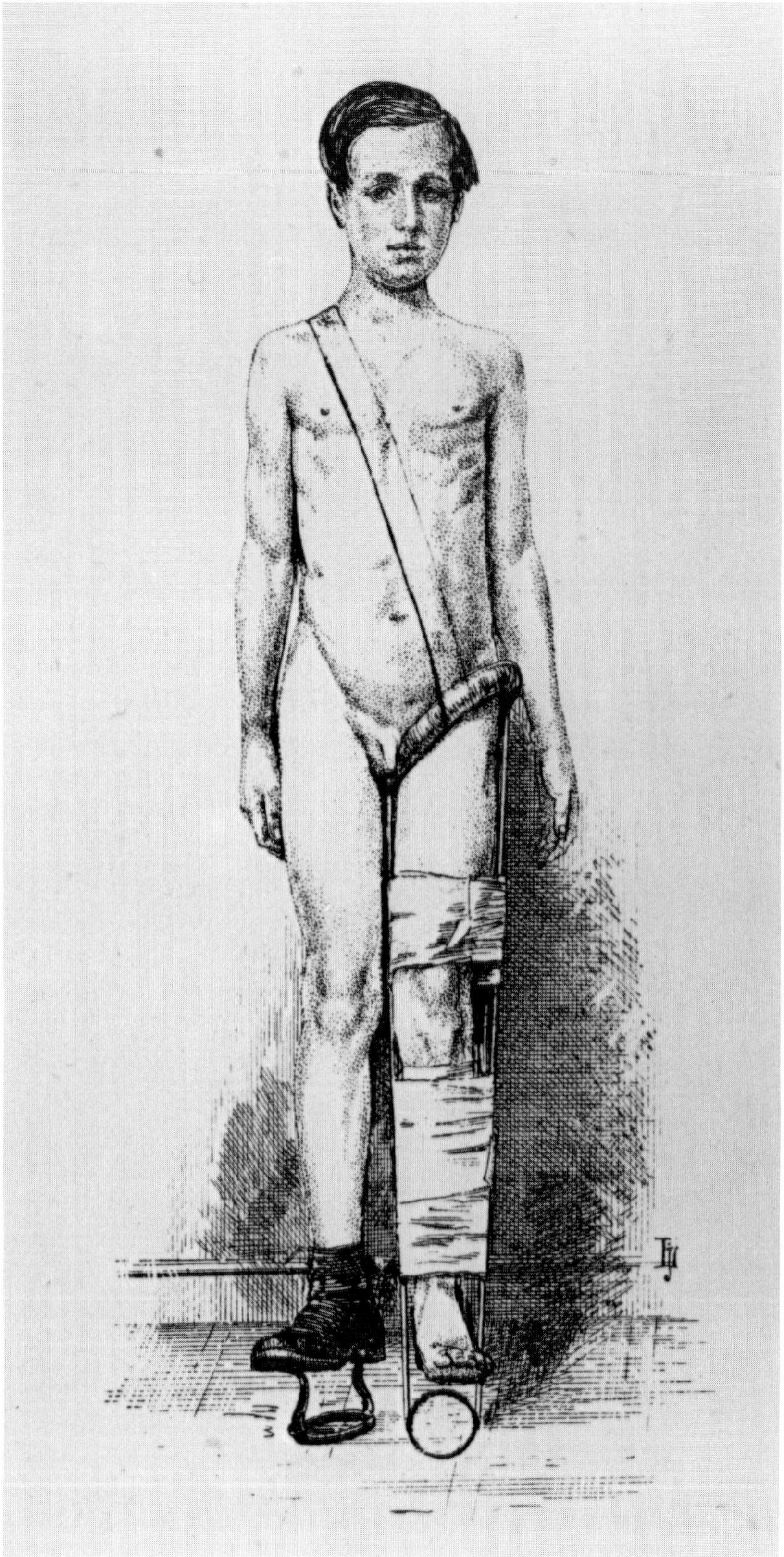

Figure 3.14 The original Thomas splint, designed for the treatment of tuberculosis of the knee. From Hugh Owen Thomas, *Diseases of the Hip, Knee, and Ankle Joints* (Liverpool: T. Dobb & Co., 1875), plate 16.

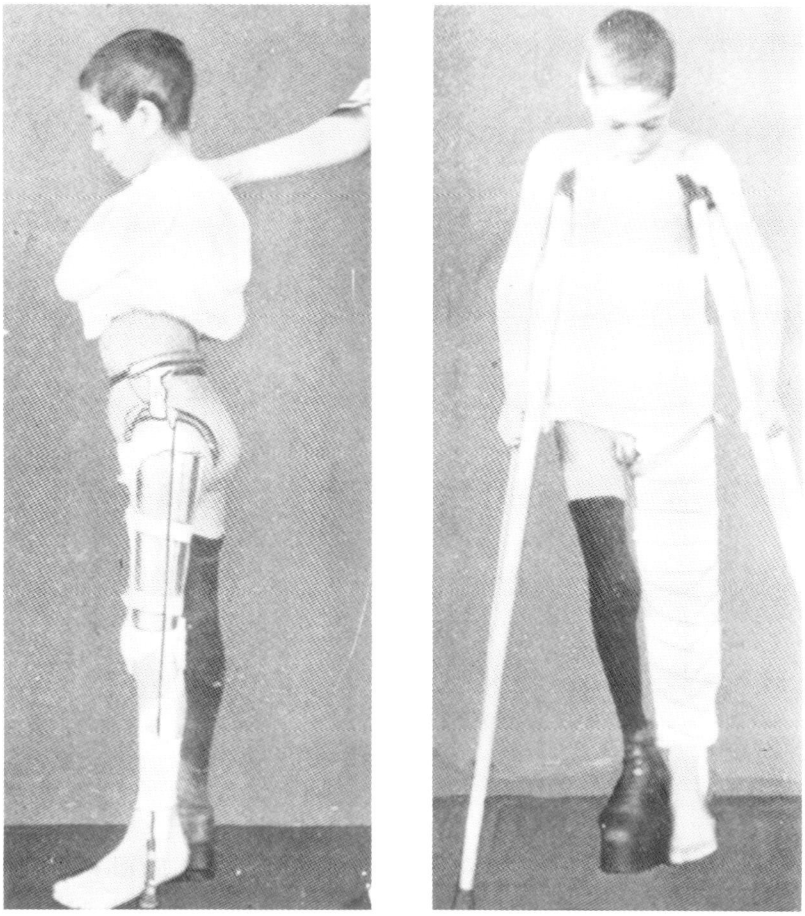

Figure 3.15 The Thomas splint used for the ambulatory treatment of a fracture of the femur, according to Thomas's directions. Note the addition of the pelvic band and the absence of the patten. From E. H. Bradford, "Ambulatory Treatment of Fractures in Children," *Ann Surg* 24(1896): 481.

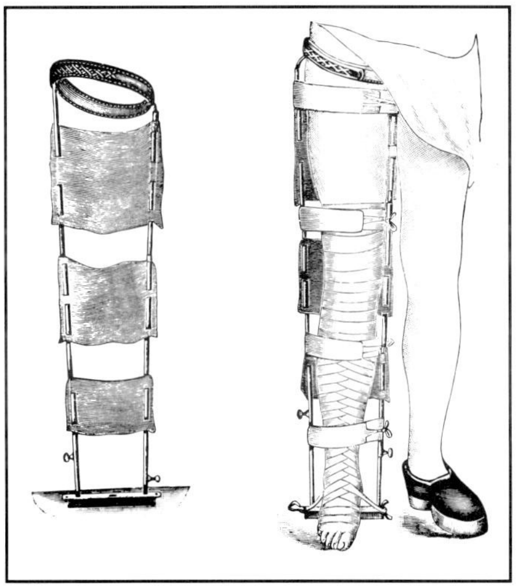

Figure 3.16 Bruns's modification of the Thomas splint. From von Bergmann and Bruns, *A System of Practical Surgery*, 543.

might have had negligible effect except for the influence of his nephew Robert Jones. Writing about the treatment of fractures in 1913, Jones did not mention the use of plaster of paris bandages at all, preferring instead to recommend the use of wooden and metal splints.[30] Thomas and Jones objected to the use of the plaster of paris bandage because they believed that it interdicted the use of concurrent physical therapy and that preventing exposure of the limb to the air caused atrophy and deterioration of the skin.[31]

Many improvements in technique were made as surgeons gained experience in the use of plaster of paris bandages. Pirogov's method gave way gradually to that of Mathijsen, and the use of bandages and splints impregnated with dry powdered plaster of paris became general (figures 3.8, 3.9, 3.10, 3.11, 3.12). Among the improvements suggested as early as 1860 was the not unexpected one of making the dressings resistant to water by painting the dried plaster of paris with a mixture of shellac dissolved in alcohol.[32]

Surgeons experimented with the use of other types of materials for use as splints. One of the earlier plastic-like materials was gutta

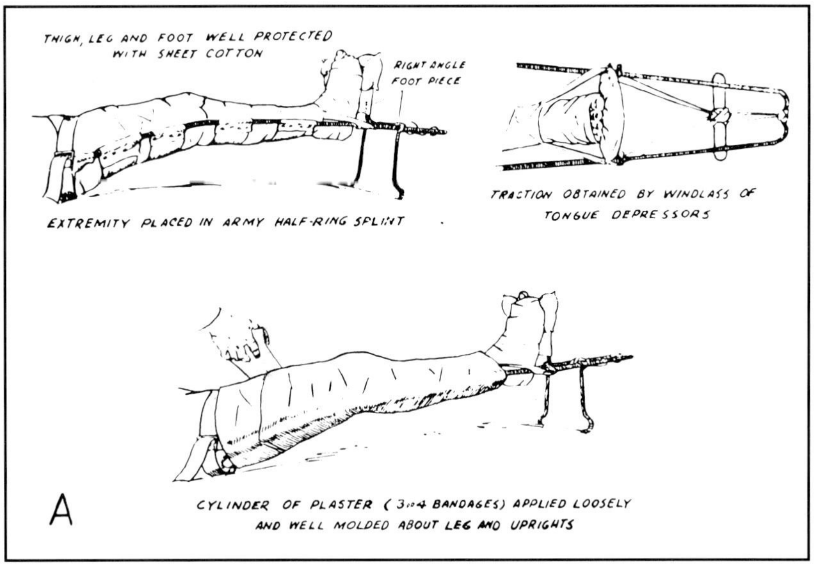

Figure 3.17 The Tobruk splint. From O. P. Hampton, *Wounds of the Extremities in Military Surgery* (St. Louis: C. V. Mosby Co., 1951), 101.

percha, obtained from the latex of several trees found in Malaya. It resembled rubber but contained more resins. When dry, it was hard and inelastic, but when warmed it became soft and malleable. In 1851 Utterhoeven described the use of splints made from this material for the treatment of fractures[33] (figures 3.13a,b). Gutta percha was the forerunner of the wide variety of plastic materials subsequently introduced for use in the treatment of fractures.

Surgeons recognized that the treatment of patients by prolonged recumbency in bed was associated with serious complications, and they were also concerned about the high cost of such methods. They therefore greeted with enthusiasm new techniques that allowed patients to leave their beds and get about with crutches. Whether to permit full, partial, or no weight bearing became an important question.

The use of braces for the ambulatory treatment of ununited fractures was described by H. H. Smith in 1851.[34] These braces of moulded metal and leather were too expensive for general use. On the other hand, the simple leg splint introduced by Hugh Owen Thomas in 1875 for the ambulatory treatment of tuberculosis of the knee was easy to make and cheap[35] (figure 3.14). It was the first satisfactory ischial weight-bearing splint. Although Thomas did not describe its use for the ambulatory treatment of fractures of the femur until 1890, he in fact used it for this purpose much earlier[36] (figure 3.15). The Thomas splint was used for the ambulatory treatment of fractures in Russia by Reyher and Kasimir Smirgrodski,[37] in Germany by Paul Bruns and Koenig,[38] and in the United States by Edward Hickling Bradford[39] (figure 3.16). Their techniques consisted of using the splint according to Thomas's instructions, attaching an

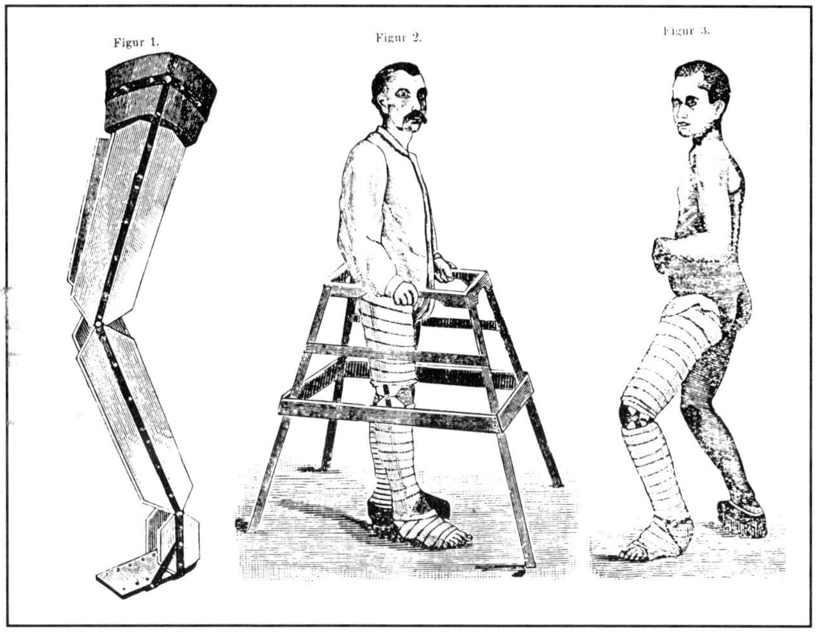

Figure 3.18 Heusner's splint for the ambulatory treatment of fractures of the femur. From Heusner, "Ueber Behandlung der Oberschenkelbruche im Umhergehen," *Dtsch med Wschr* (1890): 845.

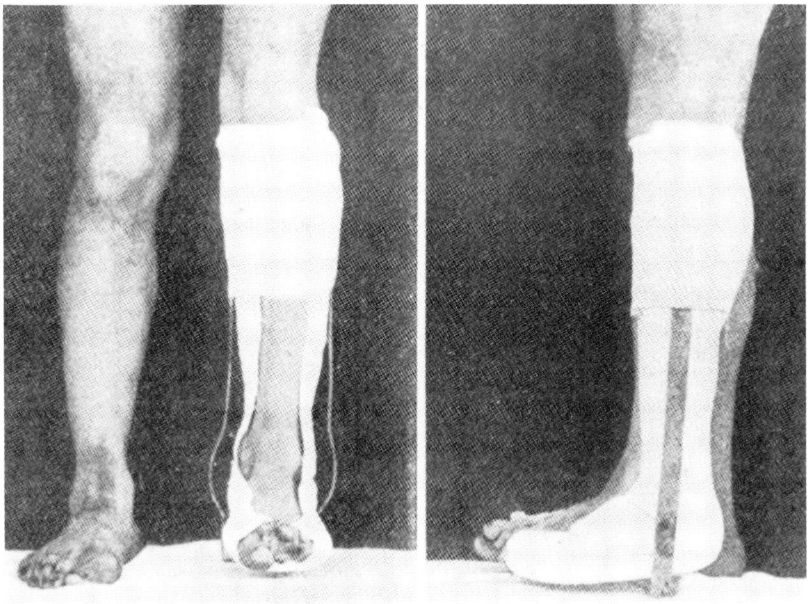

Figure 3.19 The walking plaster of paris dressing devised by Reclus. All weight is borne on the flare of the upper end of the tibia and fibula. From J. Tanton, "Fractures du membre inférieur," in Part IV of *Nouveau traité de chirurgie*, A. LeDentu and Pierre Delbet, eds. (Paris: J. B. Baillière et Fils, 1916), 2:283.

ischial ring to a completed long-leg plaster dressing, or incorporating the entire splint into a plaster of paris dressing. This latter method was revived briefly in World War II at the siege of Tobruk to stabilize fractures of the femur in wounded soldiers awaiting evacuation[40] (figure 3.17). Other types of braces for the ambulatory treatment of

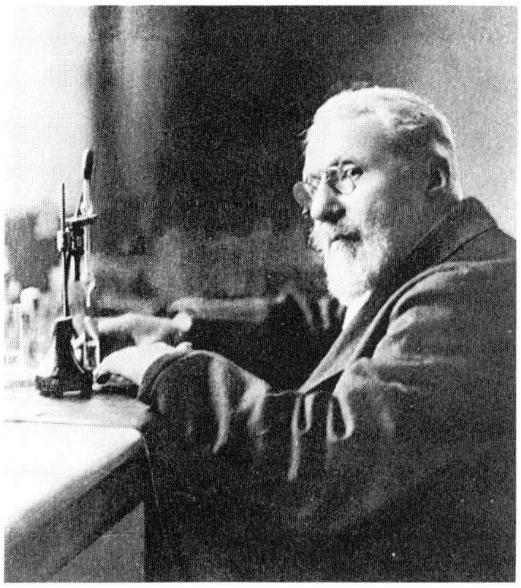

Figure 3.20 Pierre Delbet (1861–1925). From Delbet, *L'oeuvre scientifique de Prof. Pierre Delbet* (Paris: Masson, 1932), frontispiece.

femoral shaft fractures were described by Harbordt, Liebermann, and Heusner.[41] Heusner's splint was made with an ischial weight-bearing ring and knee and ankle joints. It was constructed of sheet metal and steel rods, padded with leather, and bound in place with paper bandages (figure 3.18).

The introduction of the "walking cast" in the treatment of fractures of the tibia and fibula was the work of Fedor Krause (1857–1937), one of Volkmann's assistants[42]. Later in his career he distinguished himself as one of the pioneers of neurosurgery. Krause's work was stimulated by Smirgrodski's report on the use of early ambulation in a "cast brace" in the treatment of fractures of the leg.[43] Krause's method was based on a very careful technique employing a minimal amount of padding and a carefully applied plaster of paris bandage. He also devised a "cast shoe" for the patient to wear over the dressing. Two years later, Korsch described a similar dressing applied without any padding—that is,

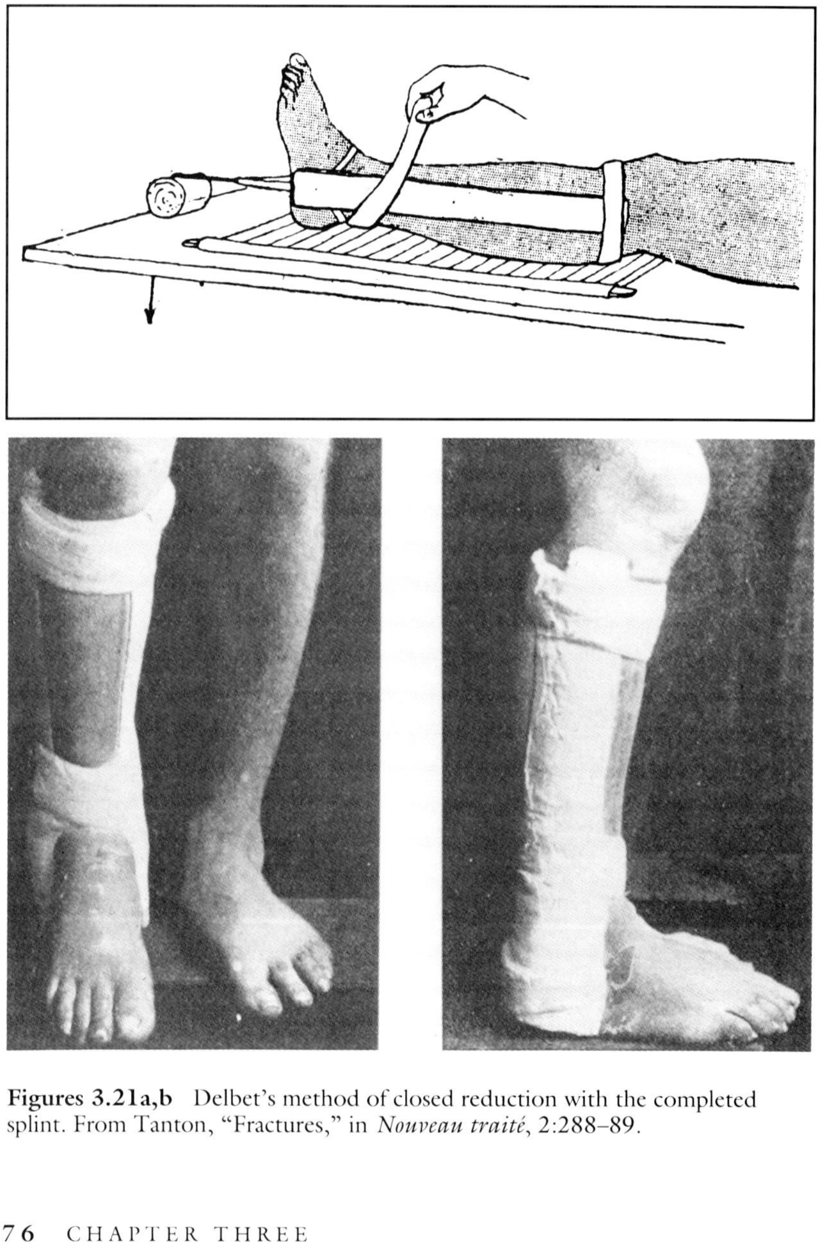

Figures 3.21a,b Delbet's method of closed reduction with the completed splint. From Tanton, "Fractures," in *Nouveau traité*, 2:288–89.

one that was "skintight."[44] Albers continued the work of Korsch in Bardeleben's clinic in Berlin and reported the results of the management of seventy-eight patients with fractures of the tibia by this method in 1894 before the Deustche Gesellschaft für Chirurgie.[45] Julius Dollinger modified the method further by insisting that all such plaster dressings be bivalved immediately following their application.[46]

These reports met with widespread interest in the United States and resulted in an editorial article in the *Annals of Surgery* in 1895 that discussed the work of the German surgeons and the experience of J. P. Warbasse of Brooklyn.[47] This editorial was followed in 1896 by a long article by one of the editors, Lewis S. Pilcher, that offered these conclusions:

> *In the hands of surgeons who may have considerable technical skill and experience in the use of the plaster bandage, it is evident that most fractures of the lower extremity may be safely treated by apparatus which will early permit the injured limb to be actively used in locomotion; as a result the tedium and disadvantage of prolonged detention from the activities of life may be avoided, the amount of muscular atrophy and joint stiffness incident to disuse of the limb may be much lessened, and the restoration of the full function of the limb after consolidation may be expedited, a more vigorous state of nutrition in the injured parts will be maintained, and the possibilities of delayed or non-union will be lessened; in the aged and in alcoholics the ability to early get patients up and about will tend to prevent the development of the hypostatic congestions and the nervous disturbances to be feared in such patients; and, finally, the beds of hospitals, which otherwise would be encumbered by such patients for many weeks, may be emptied after a few days, and the opportunity for the reception of new patients made.*[48]

However, Charles L. Scudder discussed the experience of Massachusetts General Hospital and Boston City Hospital with this method of treatment in an article in 1898, and pronounced it only a qualified success.[49] Stimson, in New York, shared Scudder's lack of enthusiasm.[50]

At a meeting of the Surgical Society of Paris on March 17, 1897, Paul Reclus presented a patient with a fracture of the tibia being treated by this method in which the major stress of weight bearing was borne on the flare of the upper end of the tibia[51] (figure 3.19). His colleague Just Lucas-Championnière did not approve. It was Pierre Delbet (1861–1925) (figure 3.20) who popularized the ambulatory treatment of fractures of the tibia in France. His technique involved, first, an accurate closed reduction obtained by skin traction (figures 3.21a,b), and second, the application of two plaster of paris splints, one on either side of the leg in such a manner that pressure was spread proximally over the flare of the tibia and distally over the malleoli[52] (figure 3.22).

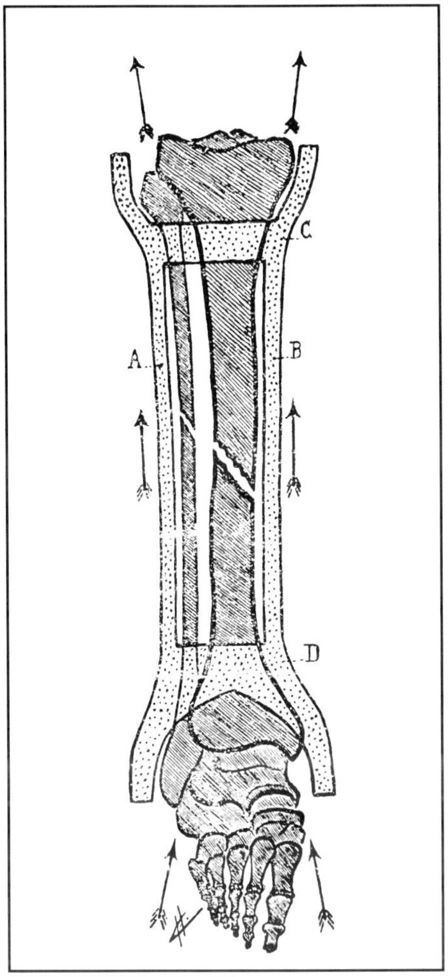

Figure 3.22 Details of the Delbet splint. From H. Colleu, "Fractures diaphysaires de jambe," *Presse méd*, December 22, 1920, 925.

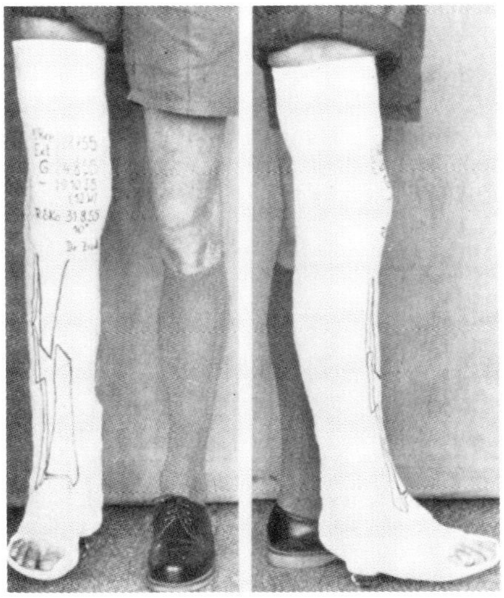

Figure 3.23 The skintight plaster of paris dressing used by Böhler. From Böhler, *The Treatment of Fractures* (New York: 1958), 1729.

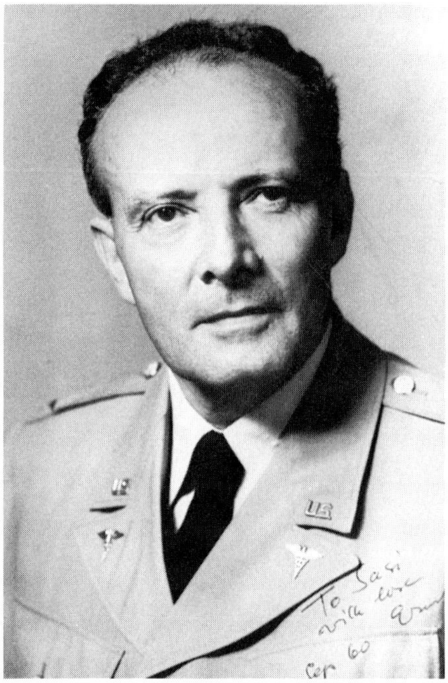

Figure 3.24 Ernst Dehne (1905–1983).

The champion of closed reduction, plaster of paris dressings and active ambulation between World Wars I and II was Lorenz Böhler of Vienna.[53] Building on the work of his predecessors, Böhler developed a system of fracture treatment that was adopted by many fracture clinics throughout the world. It was based on three principles: The displaced fragments must be reduced properly, using skeletal traction if necessary; the reduction must be maintained; and the fracture must be immobilized by means of a skintight plaster of paris dressing (figure 3.23).

During the period of fracture immobilization, the Böhler program of treatment called for active exercise of all the body except for the immobilized portion. Reduction, immobilization, and active exercises were thus the cornerstones of his system. In his lecture room hung a chart that epitomized his approach:

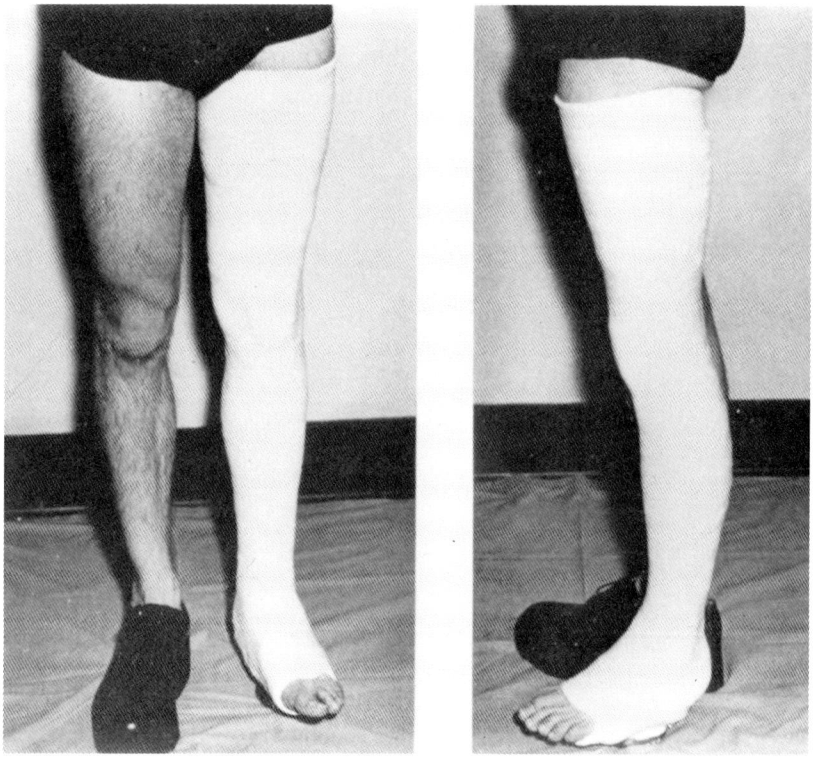

Figure 3.25 An example of the type of plaster of paris dressing used by Dehne. Note the similarity to Böhler's technique. From P. W. Brown, and J. G. Urban, "Early Weight-Bearing Treatment of Open Fractures of the Tibia," *J Bone Joint Surg* 51A(1969): 59.

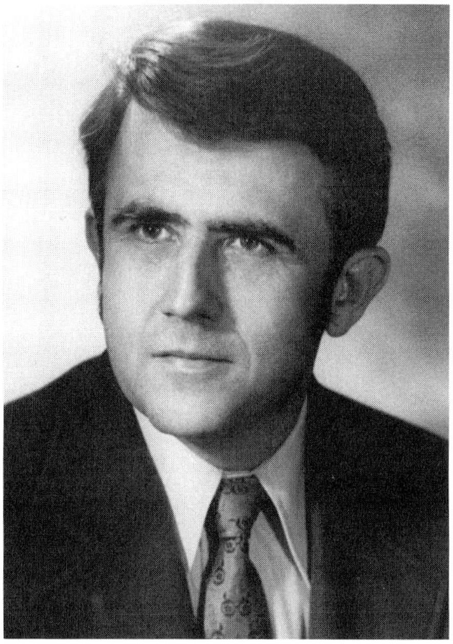

Figure 3.26 Augusto Sarmiento (b. 1924).

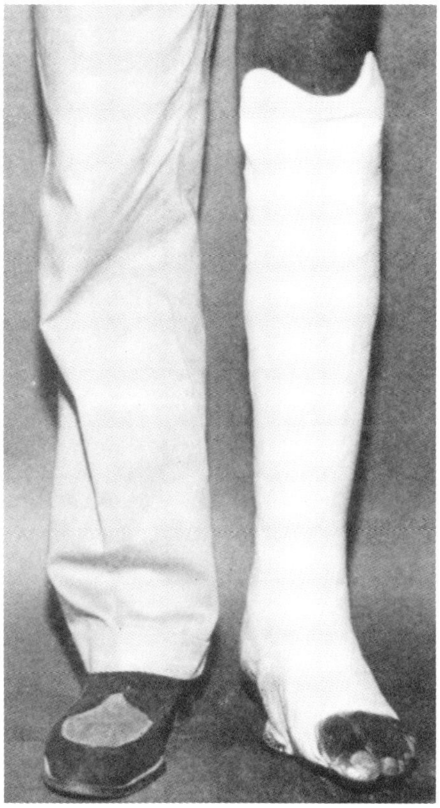

Figure 3.27 The below-the-knee plaster of paris dressing designed by Sarmiento for the ambulatory treatment of tibial fractures. From Sarmiento, "A Functional Below the Knee Cast for Tibial Fractures," *J Bone Joint Surg* 49A(1967): 855.

What heals the fractured bone?
The organism itself or NATURE

What does NATURE require for healing?
TIME

What should the physician do during this time?
After reduction of the fracture he should
provide for uninterrupted REST

And at the same time provide for good
CIRCULATION

By elevation of the extremity and active
use of the whole body including the injured
limb, under supervision and with
AVOIDANCE OF PAIN[54]

The success of Böhler's system depended on a high standard of technical excellence in the application of the plaster of paris dressings. Complications and failures with his method were frequent in the hands of others, but were almost always due to poor technique. In his Fracture Oration before the 1939 annual meeting of the American College of Surgeons, Fraser B. Gurd discussed the ambulatory treatment of fractures of the tibia in plaster of paris dressings and advocated the method strongly.[55] Only the British hung back, with both Watson-Jones and Charnley delaying weight-bearing for at least ten weeks after fracture.[56]

After World War II, reduction, plaster of paris dressings, and early ambulation with full weight-bearing, especially in open fractures, were re-emphasized by Ernst Dehne (figure 3.24). In June 1950 at the 98th General Hospital in Munich, Dehne began to treat fractures of the tibia by the aggressive implementation of such a program.[57] His method fulfilled these criteria: "The method should be applicable to all fractures of the tibia without exception, be simple and easy to learn, and lead to early union and optimal functional rehabilitation."[58] It consisted of reduction of the fracture and immobilization in a snug, long-leg plaster of paris dressing with the knee in full extension, followed by immediate full weight-bearing. Ten years later, he and his colleagues reported excellent results in the management of 207 patients.[59] P. W. Brown and J. G. Urban described the use of this method in the treatment of 63 patients with open fractures of the tibia in 1968, also with excellent results[60] (figure 3.25).

Surgeons from Böhler to Dehne had used a close-fitting long-leg plaster dressing with the knee fixed in full extension. The return to the short-leg dressing or brace was the result of the application to fracture treatment of principles developed in the design of prostheses for below-knee amputations by Augusto Sarmiento (b. 1924)[61] (figure 3.26). In 1967 Sarmiento used a modified short-leg plaster of paris dressing that controlled rotation at the fracture site and

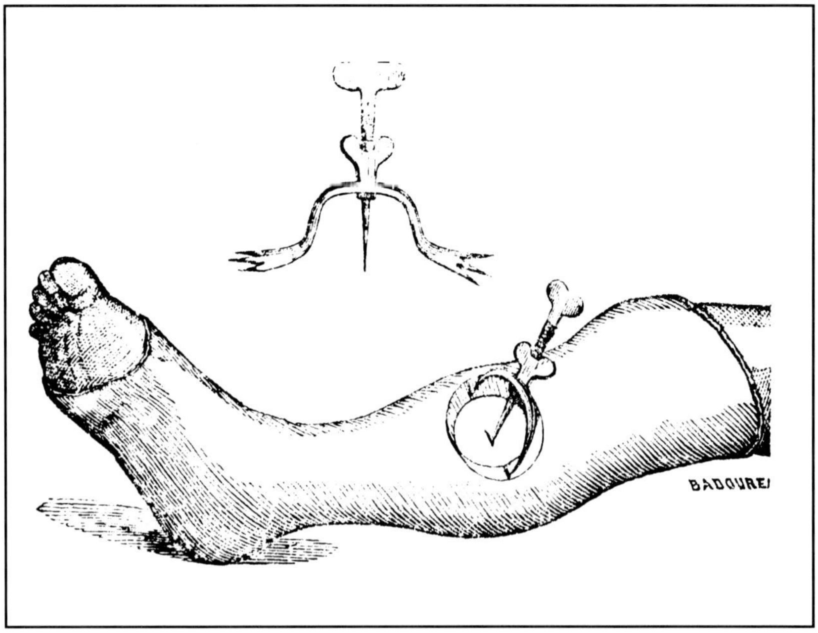

Figure 3.28 Malgaigne's point as modified by Ollier for use with a plaster of paris bandage. From Louis Ollier, *Du traitement des fractures diaphysaires des os longs par les points métalliques* (Paris: Adrien Delahaye, 1870), 8.

permitted full weight-bearing without restricting knee motion[62] (figure 3.27). By applying similar principles derived from orthotics, V. Mooney and his colleagues developed a "cast brace" for use in the treatment of femoral shaft fractures.[63] Further experience with orthotic and prosthetic devices, coupled with the emergence of a new generation of plastic materials, led to the development of an effective system of "cast braces."[64]

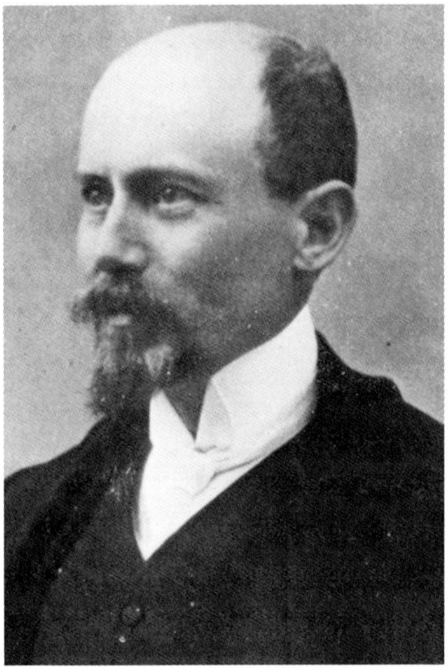

Figure 3.29 Alessandro Codivilla. From F. Delitalia, "The inventor of Direct Skeletal Traction: Alessandro Codivilla, 1861–1912," *Sci med ital* 4(1956): 537.

It did not take long for some of the old techniques to be adopted for use with plaster of paris dressings. In 1870 Louis Xavier Edouard Leopold Ollier described as a "nouveau appareil" a modification of Malgaigne's point that could be incorporated into a plaster dressing[65] (figure 3.28). A variation of this method was reported as recently as 1941 by H. K. Christie.[66] Alessandro Codivilla (1861–1912) initiated the use of the technique of "pins in plaster," and also made a significant contribution to the development of skeletal traction[67] (figure 3.29). Codivilla was a versatile and brilliant surgeon who limited his practice to orthopedics after becoming director of the Rizzoli Institute in Bologna. In 1903 he described his method for correcting malunited femoral shaft fractures by applying strong skeletal traction by means of a pin placed through the *os calcis.*[68] The procedure was carried out under a general anesthetic and sometimes included an osteotomy. When correction had been obtained, the patient was enveloped in a hip spica or plaster of paris dressing that incorporated the pin. This technique was quickly exploited by Codivilla's colleagues in Milan.[69] In Austria, Böhler introduced a method of using skeletal traction to obtain the reduction of tibial fractures that were then immobilized in unpadded plaster of paris dressings, sometimes incorporating one or more of the pins.[70]

The technique of "pins in plaster" was used particularly with open fractures. One of its proponents, H. Winnett Orr, emphasized the importance of primary reduction and immobilization in the treatment of open fractures and believed that this method achieved these goals without interfering with wound management.[71] His ideas were supported by Kellogg Speed.[72] However, when bicycle spokes or wires were used as pins, some sort of a bail had to be incorporated in the dressing.[73] To solve this problem, Roger Anderson developed a sophisticated "fracture robot," which used transfixation pins to control the reduction of the fracture, after which a plaster of paris dressing was applied incorporating the pins.[74] He also designed a smaller "table-ette" for use in the reduction of fractures of the forearm.[75] These methods were used with some success.[76] However, after World War II Anderson abandoned the use of pins in plaster in favor of external skeletal fixation.

Notes

1. Dominque Jean Larrey, *Mémoires de chirurgie militaire et campagnes* (Paris: J. Smith, 1812–17).

2. Robert G. Richardson, *Larrey: Surgeon to Napoleon's Imperial Guard* (London: John Murray, Ltd., 1974), 160–61.

3. Larrey, "Mémoire sur une nouvelle manière de réduite ou de traiter les fractures des membres compliquées de plaies," *J compl dict sci méd* 20(1824): 193.

4. Félix Hippolyte Larrey, *Traitement des fractures des membres par l'appareil inamovible* (Paris: Didot le Jeune, 1832).

5. L. J. G. Seutin, *Du traitement des fractures par l'appareil inamovible* (Bruxelles, 1835); id., *Du bandage amidonnée* (Brussels: Société Encyclographique des Sciences Médicales, 1840).

6. A. Velpeau, *Mode générale d'application du bandage dextrine; Leçons orales de clinique chirurgicale faites à l'Hôpital de la Charité* (Paris: Germer Baillière, 1841), 2:542–54.

7. A. F. Dulin, "The 'Immovable Apparatus' Used in the Treatment of Fractured Extremities," *Boston Med Surg J* 22(1840): 85.

8. J. H. James, *The Retrospective Address in Surgery from July 1836 to July 1839* (Worcester: Henry Deighton, 1839).

9. J. S. Gamgee, *On the Advantages of the Starched Apparatus in the Treatment of Fractures and Diseases of the Joints* (London: H. K. Lewis, 1853); id., *Researches in Pathological Anatomy and Clinical Surgery* (London: H. Bailliere, 1856).

10. Gamgee, *Advantages*, 4–5

11. B. Hunt, "The Modern Treatment of Fractures," *Assoc Med J* (1855): 341, 622, 699, 836.

12. W. Eton, *A Survey of the Turkish Empire*, 2d edition (London: Cadell and Davies, 1799), 225–27.

13. Lorenz Böhler, "Apparate zum Einrichten von Knochenbruchen unter Schraubenzug" *Münch med Wschr* 75(1928): 2047.

14. A. L. Richter, *Theoretisch-praktisches Handbuch der Lehre von de Bruchen und Verrenkung der Knochen* (Berlin: Enslin, 1828), 450–51; id., *Lehrbuch von den Bruchen und Verrenkungen der Knochen* (Berlin: Enslin, 1833), 274–78.

15. L. W. Bacon, "On the History of the Introduction of Plaster of Paris Bandages as a Fixation Dressing," *Bull Soc Med Hist* 3(1923): 122.

16. G. J. Bremer, *The Plaster of Paris Bandage: Its Invention by Antonius Mathijsen and its First Applications* (Nieuwkoop: B. DeGraaf, 1962), 12–15.

17. Antonius Mathijsen, *Nieuwe Wijze van Aanwending van het Gips-Verband bij beenbreukin. Eene bijdrage tot de militaire chirurgie* (Haarlem: van Loghem, 1852); id., *Du bandage plâtre et de son application dans le traitement des fractures* (Liege: L. Grandmont-Donders, 1854).

18. C. J. Cessner, *Handbuch der chirurgischen Instrumenten und Verbandlehre*, 2d edition (Wien: L. W. Seidel, 1855), 427–28.

19. C. I. P. W. Hubenthal, "Neue Behandlungs weise der Knochenbruche," *Russ Samm Naturw Heilk* 1(1816): 592–96.

20. Gamgee, *Advantages.*

21. N. I. Pirogov, *Der Gypsklebeverband bei einfachen und complicirten Knochenbruchen; Klinische Chirurgie: Eine Sammlung von Monographien über die wichtigsten gegenstande der praktischen Chirurgie*, Vol. 2 (Leipzig: Breitkopf & Hartel, 1854); id., *Kriegs Sanitats-Wesen und die Private-Hulfe auf dem Kriegsschauplataze in Bulgarien und im Rucken der Operitenden Armee 1877–78* (Leipzig: F. C. W. Vogel, 1882).

22. J. L. Little, *On the Use of Plaster of Paris Splints in Military*, published for the United States Sanitary Commission (Washington, D.C.: Surgery Sanitary Commission, 1864).

23. Frank Hastings Hamilton, *A Practical Treatise on Fractures and Dislocations* (Philadelphia: Blanchard and Lea, 1860); id., *A Treatise on Military Surgery and Hygiene* (New York: Bailliere Brothers, 1865).

24. Hamilton, *A Practical Treatise on Fractures and Dislocations*, 5th ed. (Philadelphia: Henry C. Lea, 1875), 58–59.

25. Lewis A. Sayre, "Report on Fractures," *Trans Am Med Assoc* 25(1874): 301.

26. Sayre, *Lectures in Orthopedic Surgery and Diseases of the Joints* (New York: D. Appleton, 1876), 372–77.

27. Lewis A. Stimson, *A Treatise on Fractures* (Philadelphia: Henry C. Lea, 1883), 170–79; C. L. Scudder, "The Ambulatory Treatment of Fractures," *Boston Med Surg J* 138(1898): 102.

28. Richard Volkmann, "Verletzungen der Knochen (Knochenbruchen und Knochenwunden)," in *Handbuch der allgemeinen und speziellen Chirurgie*, Vol. 2, ed. Pitha and Billroth (Erlangen: Ferdinand Enke, 1865).

29. Hugh Owen Thomas, *The Principles of the Treatment of Fractures and Dislocations* (London: H. K. Lewis, 1886), 24.

30. Robert Jones, "An Orthopedic View of the Treatment of Fractures," *Am J Orthop* 11(1913): 314.

31. E. M. Bick, *Source Book of Orthopaedics* (New York: Hafner, 1968), 287.

32. A. Mitscherlich, "Ueber wasserfeste Verbande," *Arch klin Chir* 1(1860): 457; id., "Weitere Erfahrungen über die Anwendung wasserfeste Verbande," *Arch klin Chir* 2(1861): 585.

33. A. Utterhoeven, *De l'application de la gutta-percha au traitement des fractures* (Brussels: J. B. Tircher, 1851).

34. H. H. Smith, "On the Treatment of Permanent Pseudarthrosis by an Apparatus Which Permits Use of the Limb and Obviates Amputation," *Am J Med Sci* 21(1851): 106; id., "On the Treatment of Ununited Fractures by Means of Artificial Limbs," *Am J Med Sci* 29(1855): 102.

35. Hugh Owen Thomas, *Diseases of the Hip, Knee, and Ankle Joints* (Liverpool: T. Dobb & Co., 1875), 51–52.

36. Thomas, *Fractures, Dislocations, Deformities, and Diseases of the Lower Extremities* (London: H. K. Lewis, 1890), 45.

37. J. Treuberg, "Zur Behandlung der Frakturen der unteren Extremitaten (Aus der chirurgischen Klinik des Prof. C. Reyher)," *Zentralbl Chir* (1883): 254; K. Smirgrodski, "Die Grenzen der Anwendung der Ruhe und der Nutzen der Bewegung bei der Heilung von Knochenbruchen," *Zentralbl Chir* (21 February 1891): 161.

38. P. Bruns, "Über den Gehverband bei Frakturen und Operationen an den unteren Extremitaten," *Bruns Beitr klin Chir* 10(1893): 499; Koenig, "Moderne

Behandlung der Fracturen der unteren Extremitaten," *Zeit ärztl Landprax* 3(1894): 363.

39. E. H. Bradford, "Ambulatory Treatment of Fractures in Children," *Ann Surg* 24(1896): 481.

40. W. R. Bristow, "Some Surgical Lessons of the War," *J Bone Joint Surg* 259(1943): 524.

41. Harbordt, "Eine neue Schiene zur Behandlung von Oberschenkelbruchen ohne dauernde Bettlage," *Dtsch med Wschr* (1889): 764; Liebermann, "Demonstration einer Extensionsschiene zur ambulanten; Behandlung der Coxitis, von Knochenbruchen und anderen schweren Erkrankungen der unteren Extremitaten," *Verh Dtsch Ges Chir* (1894): 103; Heusner, "Ueber Behandlung der Oberschenkelbruche im Umbergehen," *Dtsch med Wschr* (1890): 845–47.

42. Fedor Krause, "Beiträge zur Behandlung der Knochenbrucke der unteren Gliedmaassen im Umhergehen," *Dtsch med Wschr* 17(1891): 457–60.

43. Smirgrodski, "Die Grenzen der Anwendung," 161; Krause, "Beiträge zur Behandlung," 457–60.

44. Korsch, "Ueber den ambulatorischen Verband bei Knochenbruchen der Unter and Oberschenkels, sowie bei complicirten Bruchen," *Berl klin Wschr* 30(1893): 29.

45. Albers, "Ueber Gehverbande bei Bruchen der unteren Gliedmassen," *Verh Dtsch Ges Chir*, 23d Congress (1894): 75–91.

46. J. Dollinger, "Ein einfacher abnehmbarer Gipsverband zur ambulanten Behandlung der Unterscheknelfracturen," *Zentralbl Chir* 20(1893): 995.

47. "The Ambulant Treatment of Fractures of the Lower Extremity," editorial, *Ann Surg* 21(1895): 187; J. P. Warbasse, "The Ambulant Treatment of Fractures of the Tibia and Fibula," *Brooklyn Med J* 9(1895): 285.

48. Lewis S. Pilcher, "The Ambulatory Treatment of Fractures of the Lower Extremity," *Ann Surg* 24(1896): 69.

49. Scudder, "Ambulatory Treatment of Fractures."

50. Stimson, *A Practical Treatise on Fractures and Dislocations* (New York: Lea Brothers, 1905), 92–94.

51. Paul Reclus, *Bulletins et mémoires de la société de chirurgie de Paris* 23(1897): 267.

52. J. Tanton, "Fractures du membre inférieur," in Vol. 4 of *Nouveau traité de chirurgie*, eds. A. LeDentu and Pierre Delbet (Paris: Baillière et Fils, 1916).

53. Lorenz Böhler, *Technik der Knochenbruchbehandlung* (Vienna: W. Maudrich, 1929), 137–41; id., *The Treatment of Fractures* (New York: Grune and Stratton, 1956).

54. Böhler, *The Treatment of Fractures* (New York and London: Grune & Stratton, 1956), 1:43.

55. Fraser B. Gurd, "The Ambulatory Treatment of Fractures of the Lower Extremity," *SGO* 70(1940): 385.

56. John Charnley, *The Closed Treatment of Common Fractures* (Edinburgh: E. & S. Livingstone, 1950), 150; R. Watson-Jones, *Fractures and Joint Injuries* (Baltimore: Williams and Wilkins, 1944), 2:754.

57. Ernst Dehne, personal communication, 1982.

58. Dehne et al., "Nonoperative Treatment of the Fractured Tibia by Immediate Weight Bearing," *J Trauma* 1(1961): 514–33.

59. Dehne et al., "Nonoperative Treatment," 514.

60. P. W. Brown and J. G. Urban, "Early Weight-Bearing Treatment of Open Fractures of the Tibia: An End Result Study of 63 Cases," *J Bone Joint Surg* 51A(1968): 59.

61. Augusto Sarmiento, personal communication, 1983.

62. Sarmiento, "A Functional Below-the-Knee Cast for Tibial Fractures," *J Bone Joint Surg* 49A(1967): 855.

63. V. Mooney et al., "Cast Brace Treatment for Fractures of the Distal Part of the Femur," *J Bone Joint Surg* 52A(1970): 1563.

64. Sarmiento and L. L. Latta, *Closed Functional Treatment of Fractures* (Berlin: Springer-Verlag, 1981), 297–309.

65. Louis Ollier, *Du traitement des fractures diaphysaires des os longs par les pointes métalliques* (Paris: Adrien Delahaye, 1870).

66. H. K. Christie, "A Simple Appliance for the Correction of Gross Displacement in Tibial Fractures," *J Bone Joint Surg* 23(1941): 955.

67. Alessandro Codivilla, "Ueber Nagelextension," *Zeit orthop Chir* 27(1910): 404; F. Delitala, "The Inventor of Direct Skeletal Traction: Alessandro Codivilla (1861–1912)," *Sci med ital* 4(1956): 537.

68. Codivilla, "Sulla correzione della deformità da frattura del femore," *Bull sci med Bologna*, 8th ser., 3(1903): 246; id., "On the Means of Lengthening in the Lower Limbs, the Muscles and Tissues which are Shortened Through Deformity," *Am J Orthop Surg* 2(1905): 352.

69. A. Anzoletti, "Zur Codivilla'schen Methode der Nagel-extension am Knochen," *Zentralbl Chir* 63(1909): 985; Baldo Rossi, discussion, Atti del Congresso della Società Italiana di Orthopaedia e Traumatologia 3(1906): 111.

70. Böhler, "Apparate," 137–41.

71. H. Winnett Orr, "The Treatment of Fractures by Means of Skeletal Devices: with Fixation in Plaster-of-Paris Casts," *JAMA* 98(1932): 947; id., *Wounds and Fractures: A Clinical Guide to Civil and Military Practice* (Springfield, Ill.: Charles C Thomas, 1941), 11–36.

72. Kellogg Speed, "Plaster Embedded Skeletal Traction," *SGO* 51(1930): 854.

73. J. W. White, "Plaster Cast, Bone Pin Method in Fractures of the Lower Leg," *South Med J* 25(1932): 218; R. M. Carter, "Fixed Skeletal Traction in Fractures of the Leg," *J Bone Joint Surg* 15(1933): 737.

74. Roger Anderson, "An Automatic Method of Treatment for Fractures of the Tibia and Fibula," *SGO* 58(1934): 639; id., "An Ambulatory Method of Treating Fractures of the Shaft of the Femur," *SGO* 62(1936): 685; id., "Subtrochanteric and High Shaft Fractures of the Femur," *South Surg* 8(1939): 159.

75. Anderson, "Fractures of the Radius and Ulna: A New Anatomical Method of Treatment," *J Bone Joint Surg* 16(1934): 379.

76. Howard A. Swart, "An Analysis of the Treatment of Sixty-Eight Cases of Fractures of the Shafts of the Tibia and Fibula with the Roger Anderson Splint," *South Med J* 33(1940): 1081; A. F. Voshell and D. Verda, "Fractures of the Femur Treated by the Automatic Ambulatory Method of Roger Anderson," *Am J Surg* 49(1940): 175–76.

CHAPTER FOUR

The Treatment of Open Fractures

OPEN FRACTURES ARE fractures associated with a wound of the soft tissues that permits communication between the fracture site and the outside environment. The important element in this association is the wound, with its predisposition to infection and the complications of local and systemic sepsis. The treatment of the wound is of paramount importance, since the prognosis for healing of the fracture is poor without controlling infection and healing the soft tissue envelope. Treatment of the wound is complicated by the mechanical instability introduced by the fracture as well as by the proclivity of bone for sequestration and chronic suppuration. Delayed union and nonunion frequently occur. The difference in the prognosis betweeen a closed and an open fracture was recognized in the earliest times, as shown in Case 37 from the *Edwin Smith Papyrus.*

A FRACTURE OF THE HUMERUS WITH RUPTURE OF OVERLYING SOFT TISSUE

Title

Instructions concerning a break in his upper arm, with a wound over it.

First Examination

If thou examinest a man having a break in his upper arm, over which a wound has been inflicted, [and] thou findest that that break crepitates under thy fingers, [conclusion follows in diagnosis].

First Diagnosis

Thou shouldst say concerning him: "One having a break in his upper arm, over which a wound has been inflicted. An ailment with which I will contend."

First Treatment

Thou shouldst make for him two splints of linen; thou shouldst bind it with ymrw; [and] thou shouldst treat it afterward [with] grease, honey, [and] lint every day until thou knowest that he has reached a decisive point.

Second Examination

If, however, thou findest that wound which is over the break, with blood issuing from it, and piercing through to the interior of his injury, [conclusion in second diagnosis].

Second Diagnosis

Thou shouldst say concerning him: "One having a break in his upper arm, over which a wound has been inflicted, piercing through. An ailment not to be treated."[1]

Almost 2,500 years later, Hippocrates had accumulated a good deal more information and experience.[2] He gave patients with open fractures a bad prognosis—and a worse prognosis if the fractures were in the larger bones close to the trunk. In such cases death typically resulted from tetanus, gangrene or septicemia. Hippocrates treated fractures that opened from the inside out through minor soft tissue wounds by cleansing and sealing the wounds with pitch or balsam and then wrapping the limb in compresses soaked in wine. As an example of such a balsam, we can cite Jeremiah 46:11 (writing in the sixth or seventh century B.C.) for his mention of the balm of Gilead, an oleoresin obtained from fir trees growing in eastern Palestine; a similar preparation, balsam of Peru, is still used today. Hippocrates concentrated his initial treatment on the wound, applying warm compresses of a "black, austere wine," or a warm cerate or wax to which balsam or pitch had been added. After the condition of the wound had stabilized, generally after seven to ten days, he reduced the fracture. Sometimes this was accomplished by means of short iron levers introduced into the wound as prys, a technique recommended for the reduction of closed fractures of both bones of the forearm as recently as 1936.[3] If the ends of the bones protruded from the wound and could not be reduced, they were cut off. In some cases the bone was allowed to protrude and to sequestrate.

Succeeding authors adhered closely to the methods of treatment expounded by Hippocrates, except for the observation by Celsus that amputation was usually required in open fractures of the femur.[4]

Ambroise Paré's account of his experience with his own open fracture of the tibia is an interesting description of the method of treating open fractures in the middle of the fifteenth century.

To better instruct the young Surgeon I will give a history that was very dear to me.

The misfortune overtook me in the presence of the late M. Nestor, Regent Physician of the Faculty of Medicine and of Richard Hubert, King's Surgeon-in-Ordinary (whose name is well known).

We were going to visit some patients at the town of Bons-Hommes, near Paris. On wishing to cross the water, in putting my horse on the boat, I switched him across the rump. The excited beast kicked me, entirely breaking the two bones of the left leg, four fingers above the ankle. Having received the blow and fearing the horse would kick me again, I stepped back a pace, but suddenly fell down. The broken bones came out through the flesh, stocking and boot, from which I felt as much pain as a man can endure.

My bones thus broken and the foot distorted, I feared greatly that it would be necessary to amputate the leg. Turning my eyes and my mind to Heaven, I called my God and prayed Him in His benign grace to help me in my extreme necessity. Immediately I was carried into the boat to cross the river to make my dressing, but the movement almost killed me, as the ends of the bone sawed against the flesh and those who carried me could not help it.

Finally I was carried to a village house with more pain than I had endured in the boat, for one held my body, another the foot and in walking one pulled to the left, the other bore to the right. Finally they laid me on a bed to catch my breath and I found my clothing soaked with perspiration from a generalized sweat, and if I had been thrown into the water I would have been no more wet. Then they treated me with such a medication as we could get in such places, composed of egg white, flour and chimney soot with fresh melted butter.

Then I begged M. Richard Hubert not to spare me more than any stranger in his care; that in reducing the fracture, he forget the friendship he bore me. Moreover I admonished him (even though he knew his Art well) to strongly pull the foot straight and that if the wound was not large enough, to open it with his razor and let him easily put the bones in their normal positions, and that he search the wound carefully with his fingers, which are better than any instrument (for the sense of touch is more certain than any instrument) for removing the fragments and pieces of bone that can be widely separated. Also that he express and force out the blood which was abundant around the wound. He should bandage and place the leg as he knew how to do, in doing this to use three bands as we have described above, and that he start to bandage the wound itself; then splints are added, some three fingers wide, the others two and half a foot long and bent to better lie around the leg; they also should be less large at the ends and about a finger width apart. These are tied with little bands of thread like those women tie in their hair. All this is done to the end that the fractured area be supported and held better than otherwise.

After the leg was thus bound, I had them fill the cavity of the knee-joint and that between the saddle of the leg and the ankle with compresses made of flax wrapped in cloth. Then were applied two splints or torches made of straw in which were placed little rods to hold the straw firm and round and enclosed in a half-shroud, then applied to the sides of the leg extending from the heel to the groin, tied in four places to prevent the leg from turning from side to side. And afterward it was put into a straight and not curved position, and raised a little, gently and slowly, to prevent pain, dislocation, inflammation and other accidents.

But it should be noted that if one sets the leg badly he makes the patient lame, because if the foot is left too high the fracture remains concave in front. Contrarily, if it is left too low, it will be convex or gibbous in front.

Moreover you should observe that if one fails to fill well the concave place between the saddle of the leg and the ankle, the heel will suffer greatly from long pressure which causes great pain (which I know from having felt it myself), because the spirits cannot move well and often they make a strange heat. When hunting the cause of such pain, often I lift the heel a little to give it air so the spirits can flow and some vapor transpire.

And to tell it in a word, my leg was rested on a pillow, banded and tied with struts of straw as you see in the accompanying figure [figure 4.1].

To return to my misfortune, my leg was treated point by point as described. I was taken to my house where I was disabled of three palettes by the left basilic. At the second dressing and others following, I was cared for by my companions and friends, Sworn Surgeons of Paris.

Rose ointment was applied around the wound and its neighboring parts. This is strongly praised by the ancients for fractures, since it quiets pain and prevents inflammation. It repels humors from the injured part, since it is quite cold, astringent and repressive. It is made of oil of omphacin, rose water, a little vinegar and white wax. Its use is continued to the sixth day.

The compresses and bands were treated with oxycrat in some coarse astringent wine to strengthen the part. This was especially recommended by Hippocrates for fractures with wounds to dry and drive out the humors. When they are dry, I irrigate them with oxycrat, alternating with oxyrhodinum. For when they are too dry, pain and inflammation return to the part, since they squeeze more when moist. Some surgeons

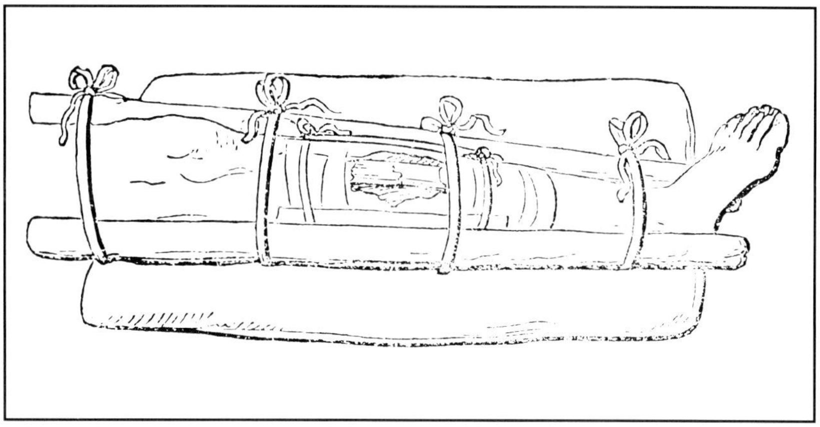

Figure 4.1 Splint and dressing for the treatment of an open fracture of the tibia, similar to that used by Paré. From Paré, *Oeuvres complètes d'Ambroise Paré*, ed. J.-F. Malgaigne (Paris: J. B. Baillière, 1840), 2:332.

use only astringent medications and ointments from beginning to end in such a case, unlike the method of Hippocrates and Galen. They consider that with astringents and ointments, they stop the skin pores of the part. This increases the strange heat, with severe pruritis and itching. This engenders under the skin a certain serous, acrid and morbid moisture which makes ulcers. This makes it well to remember not to continue such medications more than five or six days. In place of these one should use ointments described later.

And to return to my story, I was treated from the start of my illness with such an extreme diet that for nine days I ate no more each day than a dozen Damas plums with six morsels of bread and drank a pint of hippocras water. At other times I had boiled water with syrup Capil, Vener, or Divine Drink. These are all mixed in glass bottles or other drinking vessels. Sometimes I used a bolus of cassia with a little rhubarb. At other times soap suppositories were used to stimulate the bowel; I dreaded this greatly because when I went some time without a bowel movement, I developed a great heat in the kidneys.

Even such an exquisite regimen could not protect me against the fever that seized me on the eleventh day, with drainage which caused me an abscess which suppurated a long time. I believe all of this happened because of some humor retained in the part, as well as not having been able to stand having the wound tightly enough bandaged at first, as well as for some comminuted fragments separated from the ends of the bones, made both by the fracture and its reduction. For the ends were not quite equal and when some little fragments separated, they could not unite and agglutinate. So they changed and decayed, which often is why an abscess and other complications develop.

But the signs that let me know that some bone had separated was that the wound gave out a clear discharge and swelled, while its edges were greatly enlarged and the flesh lax and moist like a sponge. Beyond such causes, it seems to me that the principal occasion of the fever and the abscess came when one night while asleep, the muscles contracted with such great violence that I raised my leg in the air, in such a way that the bones got out of position and pressed the edges of the wound. So it was necessary to pull them out again to reduce them. This hurt even more than when it was first dressed.

This fever continued seven days, at the end of which it terminated partly by drainage, partly by profuse sweating. It was another month before I could get the foot to the ground without support. This was painful at first, because the callus held the muscles. For, before the movement can be free, it is necessary that the tendons and the membranes became loosened little by little where attached to the scar. Finally, thanks to God, I was entirely healed without limping in any way.[5]

The treatment of open fractures had not changed for 2,000 years! Paré's generation witnessed a gradual change in management as amputation of severely injured extremities as a life-saving procedure became more common.

The development and widespread use of firearms during the fifteenth, sixteenth, and seventeenth centuries led to a great increase in the number of missile wounds complicated by disruption of bone—the worst type of open fracture. These wounds were characterized by severe soft tissue damage, injuries to vessels and nerves, and comminution with splintering of the bone. Missile fragments, bullets, wads and bits of clothing were introduced into these wounds at the time of injury. Under these conditions, infection followed by loss of limb and life was a foregone conclusion. It was in response to this challenge that operations for amputation were perfected. The evolution of these procedures has been recounted by Billroth and more recently by the Wangensteens.[6] The introduction by Paré in 1564 of the use of the ligatures to control hemorrhage in amputations and the invention of the screw tourniquet by Jean-Louis Petit in 1718 made the operation more feasible technically but did nothing to control infection.

It was recognized that the treatment of open fractures must be individualized. In 1676 Richard Wiseman advised reduction of the fracture and stitching of the wound, followed by immobilization in a dressing for some open fractures.[7] In other cases he recommended immediate amputation. In lectures delivered in 1786, John Hunter advocated similar treatment of open fractures, ranging from dressing the wound with a poultice soaked with a solution of subacetate of lead after reducing and splinting the fracture, to amputation.[8] The case of Percivall Pott, as related by his biographer James Earle, illustrates the ambivalence of surgeons called upon to apply their judgment in a particular situation.

In the year 1756, an accident befell Mr. Pott; which, though of little consequence in itself, yet as it displays the vigour and firmness of his mind, and seems to have had considerable influence on his future life, deserves to be recorded in this place: . . . As he was riding in Kent-street, Southwark, he was thrown from his horse, and suffered a compound fracture of the leg, the bone being forced through the integuments. Conscious of the dangers attendant on fractures of this nature, and thoroughly aware how much they may be increased by rough treatment, or improper position, he would not suffer himself to be moved until he had made the necessary dispositions. He sent to Westminster, then the nearest place, for two chairmen, to bring their poles; and patiently lay on the cold pavement, it being the middle of January, till they arrived. In this situation he purchased a door, to which he made them nail their poles. When all was ready, he caused himself to be laid on it, and was carried through Southwark, over London bridge, to Watlingstreet, near St. Paul's where he had lived for sometime—a tremendous distance in such a state! I cannot forbear remarking that on such occasions a coach is too frequently employed, the jolting motion of which, with the unavoidable awkwardness of position, and the difficulty of getting in and out, cause a great and often a fatal aggrevation of the mischief.

At a consultation of surgeons, the case was thought so desperate as to require immediate amputation. Mr. Pott, convinced that no one could be a proper judge in his own case, submitted to their opinion; and instruments were actually got ready, when Mr. Nourse, who had been prevented from coming sooner, fortunately entered the room. After examining the limb, he conceived there was a possibility of preserving it; an attempt to save it was acquiesced in, and succeeded. This case, which Mr. Pott sometimes referred to, was a strong instance of the great advantage of preventing the insinuation of air into the wound of a compound fracture; and it probably would not have ended so happily, if the bone had not made its exit, or external opening, at a distance from the fractures; so that when it was returned into the proper place, a sort of valve was formed, which excluded air. Thus no bad symptom ensued, but the wound healed, in some measure, by the first intention.[9]

The attitudes of these English surgeons regarding the indications for various methods of treatment and the means by which care should be effected were shared generally with their colleagues in other countries.

After the development of amputation, the next significant improvement in the treatment of open fractures was the development of mechanical cleansing of the wound and the release of tension. The idea was first enunciated by Pierre-Joseph Desault, chief surgeon of l'Hôtel Dieu in Paris, and tested in practice by his student, Dominique Jean Larrey on battlefields all over Europe. It is the procedure we call *debridement.*

Pierre-Joseph Desault (1744–1795) was born in a small town in Haute-Saône, one of fourteen children[10](figure 4.2). He obtained his primary education locally and then studied in the military hospital at Belfort. From there he moved to Paris and by 1766, at the age of 22, was teaching private classes in anatomy. His success as a teacher brought him pupils, fame, and the envy of many of his colleagues. After serving as the chief surgeon at the Charité for several years, he was appointed chief surgeon at l'Hôtel Dieu in 1786. In the 1780s, l'Hôtel Dieu had four hundred surgical patients, and more operations were carried out in this hospital than in any other hospital in Europe. Almost without exception, the operations were performed by Desault. It was Desault who introduced bedside teaching rounds into medical education. In addition to these daily rounds, he lectured to hundreds of students and performed operations in an amphitheater seating three hundred spectators. Desault continued to carry on his work during the most turbulent years of the French Revolution. On one occasion, he was arrested by soldiers and marched off to prison. Accused by a committee of "citizen students of surgery" of failing to provide instruction for all of the students who desired it, he answered in a letter that gives an insight into the problems that beset him and his hospital.[11] One of his students, Xavier Bichat, published a collection of Desault's lectures and an appreciation of his chief in 1801, six years after his death.[12]

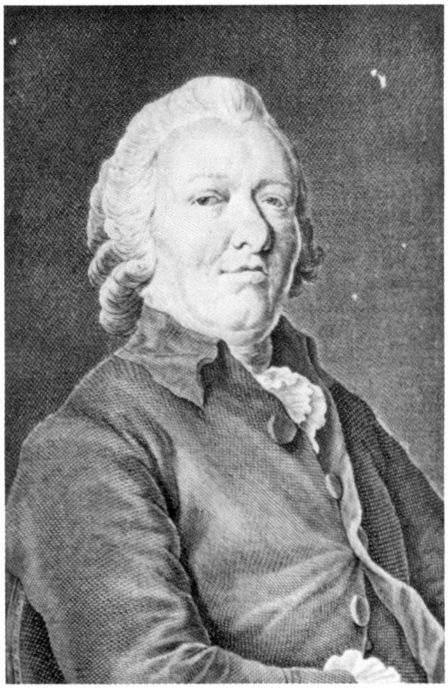

Figure 4.2 Pierre-Joseph Desault (1738–1795) who first enunciated the concept of *debridement.* From Desault, *Oeuvres chirurgicales; ou, Exposé de la doctrine et de la pratique de P.-J. Desault par Xav. Bichat* (Paris: Méquignon, An. IX (1801), frontispiece.

It was while attending a course of Desault's lectures in 1789 that Larrey heard him expound on the treatment of wounds. Larrey gives this account:

From the period of my return to Paris, at the commencement of the memorable winter of 1789, to that of my first campaign in the countries bordering on Germany, many remarkable events transpired in this capital, to which I was a witness. I shall confine myself to a succinct account of those connected with the healing art.

The first storms of the revolution were followed by violent commotions in the suburb Saint-Anthony; an insurrection took place among the workmen of the manufacturer Reveillon, and a sanguinary contest ensued, between them, a party of the inhabitants of the suburb, and two regiments of cavalry which had been sent there to restore order. In this conflict a great number were wounded on both sides, but principally on that of the inhabitants, of whom a part were transported to the Hôtel Dieu, where I attended a course of clinical surgery under M. Desault, who practised with so much zeal and success. The illustrious practitioner embraced this occasion to give us the result of his experience on several points of military surgery.

1st. It was the custom to use spirits in the dressing of all gunshot wounds. Desault taught us that their use was pernicious, and that it was necessary to return to the emollients, recommended and used by Ambroise Paré: vegetomineral water had also been used.

2nd. Desault likewise taught us, by examples, that extensive incision of these wounds produced muscular hernia.

3rd. It was a prevalent opinion that incisions changed the nature of gunshot wounds. Desault taught us, that in order to change the nature of wounds, from a complicated to a simple state, it was not sufficient to make the part bleed: that in order to attain this end, it was necessary to remove the bruised edges with a sharp knife, and then to unite the wound with a suture; and that this method is practicable only in wounds of the face, and in solutions of continuity of the soft parieties of the mouth. In my campaigns in Germany and Egypt, I have profited by the practical lessons of this man of genius, who appears to have here made one of the most important discoveries in surgery.[13]

The second precept of Desault as given by Larrey is as follows: "Il nous démontra également, par des exemples, que le trop grand débridement des ces plaies a l'inconvénient de produire des hernies musculaires."[14] The etymology of the term *debridement* would be much easier to understand if it were derived from the verb *desbriser*, "to break apart," "to fragment," and we could explain the process of debridement simply as removing all of the debris from the wound. Unfortunately, it is more complex than that. Debridement is derived from the verb *débrider*, "to unbridle," and in a surgical sense, "to release constriction and tension in a wound by incision." As the term is understood by surgeons today, *debridement* is the surgical procedure of mechanically cleansing the wound by excising dead and devitalized tissue and removing foreign materials from a wound. What it meant to Larrey can be appreciated by these two case reports taken from his account of the campaign in Egypt:

M. Duroc, first aide de camp to the commander-in-chief, had nearly died from an enormous wound in the right thigh, caused by the bursting of a bomb, which carried away a great portion of the integuments of the thigh, near its external side, the aponeurosis and fascia lata. Many nervous branches were wounded and the crural vessels laid bare. Excision of the ragged portions, dilating the wound and division of the parts strangulated or distended, gentle dressings and most assiduous care, prevented the fatal effects which appeared likely to ensue, and perfected his cure.

I washed the wound, removed all foreign bodies, cut off all disorganized and ragged parts, and applied the ligature on the vessels I had opened.[15]

Hippocrates had advised the removal of loose bone splinters from the wounds of open fractures, and Leonardo Botallo, in his book *De curandis vulneribus scleptorum*, published in Lyons in 1560, had emphasized the removal of all foreign matter from the wounds along with bone fragments, bits of contused and lacerated tissue, and blood clots.[16] Unfortunately, Botallo had few followers and it remained for

Desault and Larrey to develop and popularise the procedure of debridement.

As used by Pierre François Percy, surgeon in chief to Napoleon's Grand Army, "the primary purpose of the operation is to change the nature of the wound, as nearly as possible, into an incised wound."[17] His emphasis was on dilation of the missile tract and removal of the foreign bodies, and he designed an instrument for this purpose. George James Guthrie, Wellington's surgeon in Spain and at Waterloo, discussed exploring, incising and removing foreign bodies from wounds and cited historical precedents and current opinion at considerable length.[18] He had definite indications for his surgical exploration of the wound and preferred to wait a few days rather than operate immediately. Guthrie was concerned primarily with the removal of foreign material from the wounds. An American military surgeon, John B. Porter, on the basis of a similar review of contemporary literature and his personal experience in the war with Mexico (1845–1848), concluded: "The knife may be required to remove foreign bodies, to secure bleeding vessels, to incise tense fascia, and to evacuate deep-seated matter, and to relieve engorgement of vessels. I would recommend, in all cases, that a ball or other foreign body be at once removed, if it can be felt, no matter how deeply it may be situated."[19]

The experience of the British army in the Crimean Wars was described by George H. B. Macleod, who practiced the immediate removal of all foreign bodies and loose bone splinters and the enlargement of the wounds in cases of gunshot fractures.[20] He believed that many lives were lost by trying to save the limbs. In a group of 174 gunshot fractures of the femur, 96 came to amputation. The overall survival rate of the entire group was 63 percent. In a similar group of 144 tibial fractures, 91 amputations were performed. The survival rate for this group was only 19 percent. It is doubtful if the results of civilian surgeons in comparable cases were better than those of their military colleagues. Malgaigne, in a statistical study of amputations carried out in Parisian hospitals, noted that the mortality rate for major amputations for trauma was 63 percent.[21] Although these results do not appear to be good, the results during the U.S. Civil War were no better. In a group of 6,576 cases of gunshot fractures of the femur about which data was collected by the Surgeon General, the survival rate of those undergoing amputation and those treated by debridement and subsequent dressing and splinting were the same, approximately 50 percent.[22] In addition, the function of the limbs that were preserved was frequently grossly impaired. Frank Hastings Hamilton set forth the indications for treatment of gunshot fractures of the femur as follows:

> *We are prepared to say, however, that the surgeon ought not to attempt to save the thigh after a gunshot fracture, when any of the following conditions obtain:*

When the patient has to be carried far over rough roads and without adequate support to the limb.

When the bones are greatly comminuted.

When the patient suffers great pain, or violent spasms continue in spite of opiates and rest.

When the soft parts have suffered great contusion, as in case of a fracture from a solid shot or shell.

When there is very extensive laceration of the soft parts.

When the principal arteries or nerves are involved in the injury.

When the fracture implicates the knee-joint, or even when it is near the knee-joint; experience having shown that amputations near the knee-joint give a better percentage of recoveries than any other thigh amputations; while, on the other hand, attempts to save the limb in these cases give a worse percentage of success than in any other fractures of the thigh.

Under the following circumstances we would not, as a rule, resort to amputation:

When the ball has entered the head, neck, or trochanteric portion of the femur. Owing to the more spongy nature of the femur in these parts, and the presence of a less amount of solid lamellated structure, there is usually here less comminution than in gunshot injuries of the shaft. The great vascularity of the trochanteric portion, and the firmness with which the bone is attached to the adjacent tissues, diminish the danger of necrosis and exfoliation. The cases to which we have already referred seem to justify this conclusion. If any surgical operation is demanded in these cases, it is usually excision.

When the fracture is just below the trochanters; experience having shown that very few recover after these amputations. We think we have seen during the last three years more femurs united after gunshot fractures in the upper third of the shaft, than we have seen successful amputations after the same injuries.

When the fracture is caused by a pistol ball, by a round musket ball; or by any missile, whose force is nearly spent.

It will be understood that the last observation has reference solely to the less degree of comminution which these missiles usually occasion.

The following conditions must be added as essential to success:

All pieces of bone which are only slightly attached to the soft parts must be removed.

All foreign bodies, such as fragments of balls or other missiles, pieces of cloth, wadding, etc., must be carefully taken away.

Whatever binds or obstructs the external opening and prevents the free escape of blood or of pus, must be divided or removed.

The limb must be placed in a position of absolute rest. It must not be confined by tight bandages, or forcibly extended by apparatus.

If the knee-joint is implicated it must be laid freely open and placed at perfect rest, without adhesive straps, bandages, or other means of compression.

During the whole treatment the limb must be handled with great care, and not lifted roughly or carelessly.

When sinuses form, the matter must be let out by direct or counter-openings, and not by violent pushing and thumbing.

When spicules of bone present themselves, they must be removed.

The patient must be supplied with a good, nourishing diet.[23]

MacLeod noted that the difference between theory and practice in military and in civilian life is especially sharp as it concerns the treatment of open fractures:

That military surgery does not differ from the surgery of civil life is an assertion which is true in letter, but not in spirit. As a science, surgery, wherever practiced, is one and indivisible; but as an art, it varies according to the peculiar nature of the injuries with which it has to deal, and the circumstances in which it falls to be exercised. To the surgeon practicing in the camp, many accidents are presented which seldom or never come within the observation of the civil practitioner; while not a few of the cases which are daily treated in domestic life rarely come under the charge of a military surgeon. The two classes of practitioners may be said to be engaged in separate departments of the same professions, which, though uniting occasionally, are yet tolerably distinct from one another.[24]

Contrasting with these accounts by military surgeons is that of Astley Cooper, writing in 1822 and describing the treatment of open fractures in a civilian practice:

The first question which arises upon this subject is the following: Is amputation generally necessary in compound dislocations of the ankle? My answer is, certainly not. Thirty years ago it was the usual practice to amputate limbs for this accident, and it was then thought absolutely necessary for the preservation of life, by some of our best surgeons; but so many limbs have been of late years saved, indeed, I may say, so great a majority of cases, that such advice would now be considered not only injudicious, but cruel. It is far from being my intention to state that amputation is never required; but only to observe that in by far the greater number of these accidents this operation is unnecessary.

But before I give the proofs of what I have advanced, I shall state the mode of treatment which is to be pursued in these cases.

When the surgeon examines the limb, he finds a wound of greater or less extent, according to the degree of the injury. The extremity of the tibia projects, if the dislocation of the tibia be inwards; and the tibia and fibula are protruded, if the dislocation be at the outer ankle. The ends of the bones are often covered with dirt, from their having reached the ground. The foot is loosely hanging on the inner or outer side of the leg, according to the direction of the dislocation. Sometimes, though very rarely, a large artery will be divided; and it is surprising that the posterior tibial artery so generally escapes laceration; the anterior tibial being the only vessel I have known to be torn. The arrest of hemorrhage is the first object; and for this purpose, if the anterior tibial artery be wounded, it must be secured by ligature. The extremity of the bone is to be washed with warm water, as the least extraneous matter admitted into the joint will produce and support a suppurative process, and the utmost care should be taken to remove every portion of it adhering to the end of the bone.

If the bone be shattered, the finger is to be passed into the joint, and the detached pieces are to be removed; but this is to be done in the most gentle manner possible, so as not to occasion unnecessary irritation: and if the wound be so small as to admit the finger with difficulty, and small loose pieces of bone can be felt, the integuments should be divided with a scalpel, to allow of such portions being removed without violence; the incision should be so made as to leave the joint with as much covering of integument as possible. The integuments are sometimes nipped into the joint by the projecting bone; and then it cannot be reduced, without making an incision, to allow of the skin being brought from under the bone; and when the edges of the incised wound are afterwards brought together, no additional evil arises from the extension of the wound.

The mode of reducing the bone is (in other respects) similar to that which I have already described, when speaking of simple dislocation, by bending the leg upon the thigh, so as to relax the muscles before the extension is made. When the bone has been reduced, a piece of lint is to be dipped in the patient's blood, and applied wet over the wound, upon which the blood coagulates, and forms the most natural, and as far as I have seen, the best covering for the wound.[25]

Robert Liston, a prominent London surgeon, writing twenty years later, has this to say:

In compound fractures, when the wound is so small and clean that adhesion readily takes place, the cure is as rapid as in the simplest form of accident; but when the soft parts are much lacerated, the breach in them must be repaired by granulation; there will be profuse discharge from the wound, with the risk of deep suppuration, and union of the bone will be slow. To accomplish reduction, long and sharp pieces of bone may require to be removed by means either of the saw or of the forceps, or else the wound must be dilated; both proceedings may be necessary in some cases. Detached portions of bone and foreign bodies, if any must be taken away; and the edge of the wound may be approximated when a reasonable chance of adhesion exists. The limb must then be properly placed and secured.[26]

Every surgeon knew that the introduction of air into the fracture site led to the disasters of local and systemic sepsis. John Hunter had discussed the problem extensively in 1769.[27] When possible, he dressed the "puncture compound" fracture with lint soaked in the patient's blood to seal the wound. This was an effort to promote "scabbing" or healing and epithelization of the wound under a scab, a natural occlusive dressing.

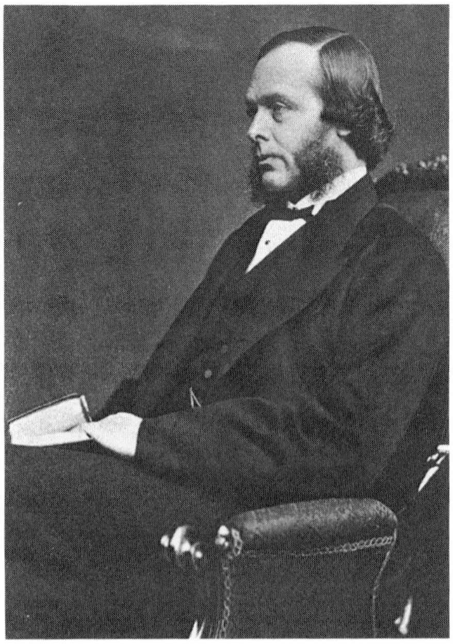

Figure 4.3 Joseph Lister (1827–1912). From R. J. Godlee, *Lord Lister* (London: Macmillan, 1927), facing p. 209.

Why did occlusive dressings, and the exclusion of air from the wound, in particular, prevent infection when it could be accomplished? The answer to this question was provided by Louis Pasteur (1822–1895). In his study of diseases of beer and wine, Pasteur established that yeasts and bacteria suspended in the air were the causative agents.[28] The exclusion of the organisms prevented fermentation. The germ theory of disease evolved from these experiments. While Spencer Wells (1818–1897) had in 1864 called attention to Pasteur's work and its possible applications in surgery, it remained for Joseph Lister (1827–1912) to perfect a practical system for the prevention of airborne infection in wounds.[29]

Joseph Lister was the son of a Quaker merchant and well-known amateur microscopist[30] (figure 4.3). He studied medicine at the University of London, where he was particularly influenced by Thomas Graham, professor of chemistry, and William Sharpey, professor of physiology. His first scientific contributions consisted of observations on the contractile tissue of the iris, the first description of the *erectus pilae* muscles, and a description of the structure of involuntary muscle fibers.[31] He also studied blood coagulation and the process of inflammation in the web space of the frog. For his surgical training, he studied with James Syme (1799–1870), professor of surgery at the University of Edinburgh, and the foremost teacher of surgery of his day. Lister worked with Syme for eight years and during this time married Syme's daughter. In 1860, at the age of thirty–three, Lister was made professor of surgery at the University of Glasgow. It was while he was at Glasgow that he began his work on the prevention of surgical infections. In 1864 Pasteur's work came to his attention. After assimilating Pasteur's observations and ideas, Lister formulated these basic principles. Germs must be prevented from getting into the wound during or after operations. Secondly, germs should be killed outside the wound if possible. Finally, if germs are present in the wound they must be killed before they can spread and secure a foothold.

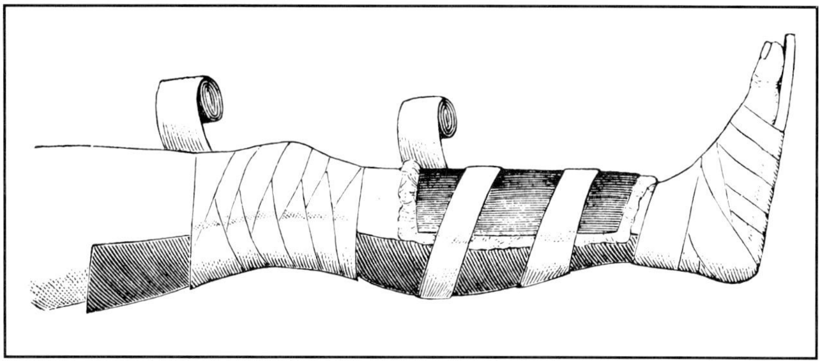

Figure 4.4 A Lister dressing and plaster of paris splint. The wound was covered with a putty containing phenol and backed with a sheet of tin to hold it in place. From Stimson, *A Treatise on Fractures* (Philadelphia: Henry C. Lea's Son, 1883), 190.

It is characteristic of Lister that his first step was to carefully repeat and confirm the work of Pasteur. Not until he had familiarized himself with the nature and growth of bacteria did he attempt to apply his principles to a patient. During this preliminary work, he devised the first technique for obtaining pure cultures of bacteria by a dilution method. All laboratory procedures in bacteriology at this time relied on sterilization by heat. Lister turned to the study of chemical compounds to find another method of killing bacteria, and eventually was led to choosing carbolic acid (phenol) as an antiseptic agent.

Lister applied his antiseptic principles for the first time in March 1865, in a patient with an open fracture. He sterilized the air about the wound with a fine spray of a solution of carbolic acid. The hands of the surgeon and his instruments were washed and soaked in the same solution. There followed a long period of experimentation and improvisation of dressings and techniques for carrying out his antiseptic principles. The revolution did not come overnight. His first paper, "On a New Method of Treating Compound Fractures, Abscess, etc., with Observations on the Condition of Suppuration," appeared in 1867 and reported eleven cases of compound fractures.[32] In five patients the wound healed by primary intention; there was one death from secondary hemorrhage, a mortality rate of 9 percent!

Lister's technique accomplished two things. First, bacteria were kept out of the wound by purifying the air and everything coming into contact with the wound. The wound was closed, if possible, and sealed with an antiseptic barrier (figure 4.4). Second, bacteria already in the wound were destroyed by the direct application of an antiseptic solution by swabbing or irrigation of the injured and exposed tissues.

Lister's ideas spread slowly through the surgical community, but spread they did.[33] In 1884 Frederic S. Dennis of New York published a paper entitled "The Treatment of Compound Fractures, Including a Report of One Hundred and Forty-Four Cases Without a Death from Septic Infection, and One Hundred Cases Without a Death from Any Cause." Dennis described his technique as follows:

It will be the aim of this paper to demonstrate by the results of a large number of cases that the treatment of compound fractures is best accomplished by adherence to three well-recognized and established principles.

1st. Absolute cleanliness.

2nd. Immediate fixation.

3rd. Provision for free drainage when necessary.

The treatment which has been employed for the most part in the cases to be reported is in brief as follows:

The patient having been taken to the operating theatre, is placed upon the table, and if the exigencies of the case demand, an anesthetic is at once administered. Anesthesia relaxes the muscles, and affords the surgeon an opportunity to explore thoroughly the extent of the injury without inflicting pain. The injured limb is washed with soap and warm water and scrubbed well with a brush. The dirt, debris, and blood are thus removed, and the hair on the extremity is cleanly shaved, and then the limb is irrigated for a few minutes with a solution of carbolic acid (1–40) or with a solution of corrosive sublimate (1–2,000) or with any other well-known disinfectant. Gentle traction is made upon the extremity, while at the same time counterextension is employed with a view to bringing the broken fragments into coaptation. If the bones protrude through the wound and cannot be reduced without the exercise of too much violence, the projecting end is removed by a chainsaw. It has been my custom when the protruding bones cannot be reduced without the exercise of undue violence, to divide subcutaneously all tendons and thus overcome all resisting forces. This operation secures physiological rest during the repair of the fracture.

Attention now must be directed to the wound itself. Any loose fragments or spiculae of bone are removed, except where they are adherent to periosteum, in which case these detached pieces are preserved, and they seldom exfoliate owing to the blood-supply through the periosteum. The interior of the wound is thoroughly irrigated by a syringe, or by a tube from an Esmarch's wound-douche. Having cleansed the limb, including even the fingers and toes, and having adjusted the fragments and having washed and disinfected the interior of the wound, the application of a splint is now made. The limb is elevated, and under it are placed towels saturated in some disinfectant solution, which keeps the limb from coming in contact with the covering upon the operating-table, or from the opposite limb, or from any part of the body. If the wound is small a piece of surgically clean adhesive plaster is placed over the seat of fracture, and then collodion is painted over the plaster. If the wound communicating with the seat of the fracture is too large to hermetically seal in the manner already described, a part of the wound can be closed by catgut suture, and a drainage-tube is introduced into the bottom of the wound. Decalcified bone drainage-tubes are used, as they seem to answer the purpose in the most satisfactory manner. Into the wound, and over, and around the wound is sprinkled a layer of idoform and then over this any of the many differently prepared dressings, such as corrosive sublimate gauze, or Idoform gauze, or absorbent cotton. The limb is now ready for the splint. A roller of Gamgee's absorbent cotton is heated which causes it to swell, and this is now made to envelope the entire limb. Heating the cotton seems to permit it to expand, and any dressing, such as plaster of Paris bandage, can be snugly applied over it, and the cotton will not lose its wonderful elasticity. During the application of the bandage, extension and counter-extension should be employed, the patient being at the same time well under the influence of ether. The bandage is now permitted to dry, and great care must be exercised while the bandage is drying, lest the patient while returning to consciousness, disturb the setting of the plaster and consequently the wound. The patient is placed in a suitable bed after the plaster of Paris bandage is firm. If there is no irritation or unpleasant sensation at the seat of the fracture, if the toes or fingers are free from any numbness or cyanosis, if the respiration, pulse and temperature are normal, the first dressing is left undisturbed. In many cases the plaster of Paris bandage is worn until the fracture is repaired and healing by primary intention has been obtained.[34]

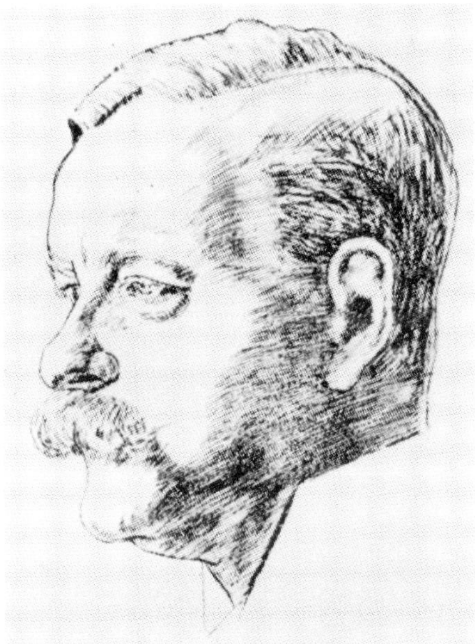

Figure 4.5 Paul Leopold Friedrich (1864–1916) using experimental wounds in guinea pigs that he contaminated with dirt and manure, observed the length of time it took for local infection to become established in a contaminated wound and the effects of a surgical excision of the wound on this process. From V. Worm, "Paul Leopold Friedrich," *Zentralbl Chir* 101(1976): 568.

Dennis's report set a high standard for the management of open fractures in a civilian urban environment.

As experience accumulated and the science of microbiology matured, it became possible to address experimentally questions of great clinical significance such as, "How long does a wound remain not infected, but only contaminated?" The answer to this question was important because it set the indications and contra-indications for primary wound closure within a time frame. Critical animal experiments to answer this question were carried out by Paul Leopold Friedrich (1864–1916) in Carl Thiersch's clinic in Leipzig[35] (figure 4.5). Friedrich had studied microbiology with Robert Koch in Berlin and was well qualifed to undertake this work. Later in his career, as a collaborator of Ferdinand Sauerbruch in Griefswald, he was to make important contributions to the development of thoracoplasty in the treatment of pulmonary tuberculosis. Using experimental wounds in guinea pigs that he contaminated with dirt and manure, sometimes sterile and sometimes contaminated with pure cultures of staphylococci and streptococci and clostridia, Friedrich observed the length of time it took for local infection to become established in a contaminated wound and the effects of a surgical excision of the wound on this process. From these observations he concluded:

In an untreated wound, infection is initially a local process and remains so for at least six hours, often longer, and many times indefinitely. This is due to the incubation time of the bacteria. During this time, careful and exact debridement with excision of damaged tissue is the best treatment. When this cannot be accomplished, the wound should be treated open. Antiseptic solutions are useful only when the cavity of the wound is accessible, when they are applied during the period of germination of the bacteria or after the demarcation of the infectious process. They are useless and even detrimental in the presence of invasive or systemic infection. Their use is often little more than a preliminary to open wound treatment.[36]

There was no question that the ideal treatment of an open fracture should consist of immediate cleansing and debridement of the wound, reduction of the fracture, primary closure of the wound and immobilization of the limb in a splint or rigid dressing. When the wound healed primarily, the complications of acute or chronic suppuration and delayed or nonunion of the fracture were avoided. Dennis's experience and Friedrich's experiments demonstrated that this ideal could be achieved in many patients, given prompt and proper treatment. Some patients with open fractures could not be treated safely by this method, however. These were patients coming to treatment late, patients with grossly contaminated wounds and extensive soft tissue and bony injuries and patients in whom healing by primary intention did not occur. These patients required other methods of wound treatment. In these methods, the wounds remained open, slowly healing in by the formation of granulation tissue, scar contraction and epithelization from the wound edges. Open methods of wound management generally took one of two forms, although these forms were not always distinct and were sometimes used in combination. One method attempted to exclude bacteria from the wound by using occlusive dressings, changed infrequently; it relied on the properties of the granulation tissue to suppress invasive infection. The other method attacked bacteria in the wound directly by the continuous or intermittent application of antiseptic, bactericidal solutions.

During the Napoleonic Wars, Larrey had extensive experience with the treatment of soft tissue wounds by means of occlusive dressings. During peacetime he applied this principle to the treatment of open fractures. The wounds were first cleaned and debrided. Bleeding was controlled by ligatures and particular care was taken to remove all blood from the wound. The fracture was then reduced. The edges of the wound were brought together with strips of tape and the wound covered with an occlusive dressing soaked with wine or camphorated vinegar. The limb was then immobilized in a rigid dressing which was not changed for several weeks or longer. In 1824 Larrey reported good results with this method in ten patients.[37] In 1832 William Beaumont, an English surgeon, reported the results of some experiments in rabbits in which he produced open fractures of the tibia and radius.[38] The fractures were treated solely by immobilization in plaster casts and healed without complication. On the basis of his experiments he proposed that patients be treated by a similar method.

In 1872 Louis Ollier (1830–1900) of Lyons gave this description of his method in a paper entitled "Occlusion and Immobility as a General Method of Wound Treatment in a Surgical Hospital":

> *The immovable occlusion to which I refer depends upon two essential principles of equal importance: the protection of the wound by a material which forms a barrier to infectious germs, and, immobility, complete and absolute, permanently fixing the region of the wound by means of a rigid splint to prevent the effects of any motion on the divided tissue.*[39]

Ollier used cotton wadding for the dressing and a silicate dressing for the fixation. In cases of joint resection, Ollier lightly packed the wound open with an oiled or waxed gauze.[40]

German surgeons also had good results with occlusion and immobilization in the treatment of open fractures:

> *It was with this principle of the aseptic occlusive dressing that von Bergmann and his assistant, Reyher, obtained such brilliant results in the Russo-Turkish War. We must admit that in the case of a compound fracture, pathogenic organisms may obtain entrance to the wound along the protruding spicula of bone even through the medium of the bullet. But it is a fact that under the occlusive dressing an unfavorable result has seldom been seen. Almost invariably these injuries run a course unattended by reaction, in case of a gunshot wound the missile becoming quietly encapsulated. In the hospital of a city with the population of a million, gunshot injuries and compound fractures are by no means rare, and still in the von Bergmann clinic we cannot recall an instance in which a simple gunshot wound or fracture with small external opening had not healed properly under the aseptic occlusive dressing. In the battle of Groni Dubnik of the Russo-Turkish war, von Bergmann selected, from a number of cases of gunshot injury to the knee, fifteen of the most serious, in which aside from the opening of the knee joint, there was extensive comminution of the bone. These patients were treated with the aseptic occlusive dressing after a disinfection of the skin in the region of the wound, salicylic gauze being applied and the limb immobilized in plaster-of-Paris, and with but a single exception perfect recovery took place, notwithstanding the fact that the patients were exposed for days to pouring rain, and had to be transported across plains over muddy roads.*[41]

This approach to the treatment of open fractures was used successfully in civilian hospitals in the United States.[42]

The treatment of an open fracture presents two problems: the treatment of the wound and the treatment of the fracture. Ollier's method of *l'occlusion inamovible* addressed these problems by preventing the innoculation of the wound by bacteria from the environment and by providing optimum conditions for soft tissue and bone healing. In spite of the value of the method, it was not used extensively during World War I.

H. Winnett Orr (1877–1956), a graduate of the University of Nebraska, obtained his M.D. degree from the University of Michigan in 1899 (figure 4.6). He returned to Lincoln, Nebraska and entered general practice. However, he obtained some special training and became an orthopedic surgeon through the help of John Ridlon, professor of orthopedic surgery at Northwestern University Medical School. In 1905 he was instrumental in the establishment of the first state-supported hospital for the care of crippled children in the United States. In 1917 he was selected by Joel Goldthwait as one of the initial group of orthopedists sent to Europe after the entry of the United States into World War I. Orr's experience in France, where he was responsible for evacuating thousands of American soldiers with open fractures back to the United States by boat, convinced him of the value of rest in the treatment of such cases: "Rest for the wound means infrequent dressings; rest for the injured or inflamed part of the body means protection against movement, relief from muscle spasm, relaxation in correct position—that is to say efficient immobilization."[43]

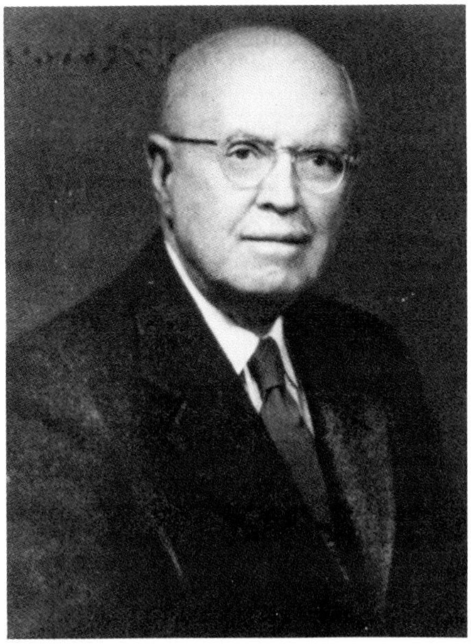

Figure 4.6 H. Winnett Orr (1877–1956) developed a treatment for open fractures consisting of thorough debridement, reduction of the fracture, and usually, maintenance of the reduction by the technique of pins transfixing the fragments and incorporated into the plaster. From "H. Winnett Orr," obituary, *J Bone Joint Surg* 39A(1957): 466.

Resuming civilian practice with its accent on children's orthopedics, Orr had many opportunities to develop his technique in the treatment of acute hematogenous osteomyelitis. It consisted of evacuation of pus, removal of sequestra, provision for drainage by lightly packing the wound open with vasoline gauze, and immobilization of the limb in a plaster of paris dressing. Subsequent dressing changes were made only at long intervals. In open fractures, this technique, in addition to thorough debridement, included reduction of the fracture and, usually, maintenance of the reduction by the technique of pins transfixing the fragments and incorporated into the plaster. Orr never had the opportunity to apply his methods in wartime. However, in 1941 he published a book outlining them for the use of military surgeons.[44]

By 1929, José Trueta (1897–1977), a Spanish surgeon, had treated over forty cases of osteomyelitis by using Orr's technique and had been much impressed by its success, particularly in two respects: first, the rarity of secondary infections, and second, the extraordinary ease and comfort experienced by the patient.[45] He argued that if the protection of the wound by a plaster cast can arrest an infection already in progress, it must have an even better chance of success if applied before the infective process had begun. He therefore began to treat some patients with open fractures by debridement and wound excision, followed by packing the wound open and immobilizing the limb in a plaster dressing. As his experience grew, he eliminated the vasoline and used only small quantities of fine meshed gauze. His first lecture describing his technique was delivered to the Italian Society of Surgery in 1934.

José Trueta was born and educated in Barcelona[46] (figure 4.7). In 1935, at the age of thirty-eight, he was appointed professor of surgery at the Autonomous University of Barcelona and chief surgeon of the Hopital de Sant Paua. The Spanish Civil War began the following year, and during these years Trueta had ample opportunity to develop his method and teach it to other surgeons as civilian and military casualties passed through his hospital. In 1938 he published his famous monograph *Tratamiento de las fracturas de guerra* describing his technique and its results.[47] Supporting the loyalist cause to the end, Trueta left Barcelona as it was being occupied by the troops of Francisco Franco. Invited to Oxford as a lecturer, Trueta remained there for twenty-seven years, succeeding Herbert John Seddon in the chair of orthopedic surgery at Oxford. After World War II he continued to make significant contributions in both the clinical and basic sciences.[48] After his retirement in 1966 he returned to Barcelona, where he participated in the intellectual life of his community until his death in 1977.

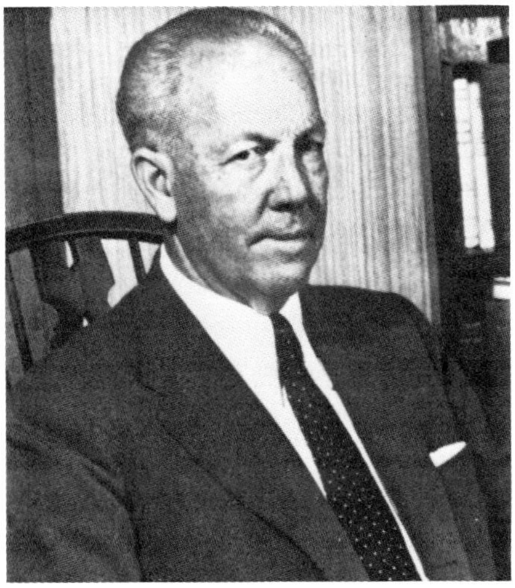

Figure 4.7 José Trueta (1897–1977) refined and improved Orr's technique for the treatment of open fractures and acute hematogenous osteomyelitis. From "José Trueta," obituary, *J Bone Joint Surg* 59A(1977): 243.

The work of Orr and Trueta established beyond a doubt that open fractures could be safely and successfully managed by simple methods. Adequate debridement and excision to cleanse the wound, occlusion to prevent reinnoculation of the wound with nosocomial organisms, reduction of the fracture, provision for drainage and rigid, uninterrupted immobilization are the key elements of their method. The methods of Orr and Trueta were simple, required very little special equipment, and could be taught easily to medical and paramedical personnel. As a result, they were widely used during World War II.

Sergei Sergeievich Yudin's work offered an example of what could be accomplished under difficult conditions; he described his experience with the treatment of five hundred gunshot fractures of the femur with a mortality rate of 5.9 percent. His operative technique consisted of 1) debridement and wound excision; 2) no drains; 3) continuous free drainage provided by large incisions; 4) skin edges sutured to deep fascia; 5) abundant washing of the wound with a soap solution; 6) dusting of the wound surfaces with a sulfanilamide-sulfathiazole powder; 7) reduction of the fractures; and 8) the application of a closed, nonpadded plaster of paris dressing. This treatment was accomplished by using a simple, portable orthopedic table moving through a conveyor-belt system run by a "thigh brigade," the term used by Yudin to refer to the team of surgeons and technicians who provided care for, on an assembly-line basis, the hundreds of wounded with open fractures of the femur. Using this system, one experienced surgeon with a large number of less-skilled assistants was able to treat a large volume of patients. The first stop

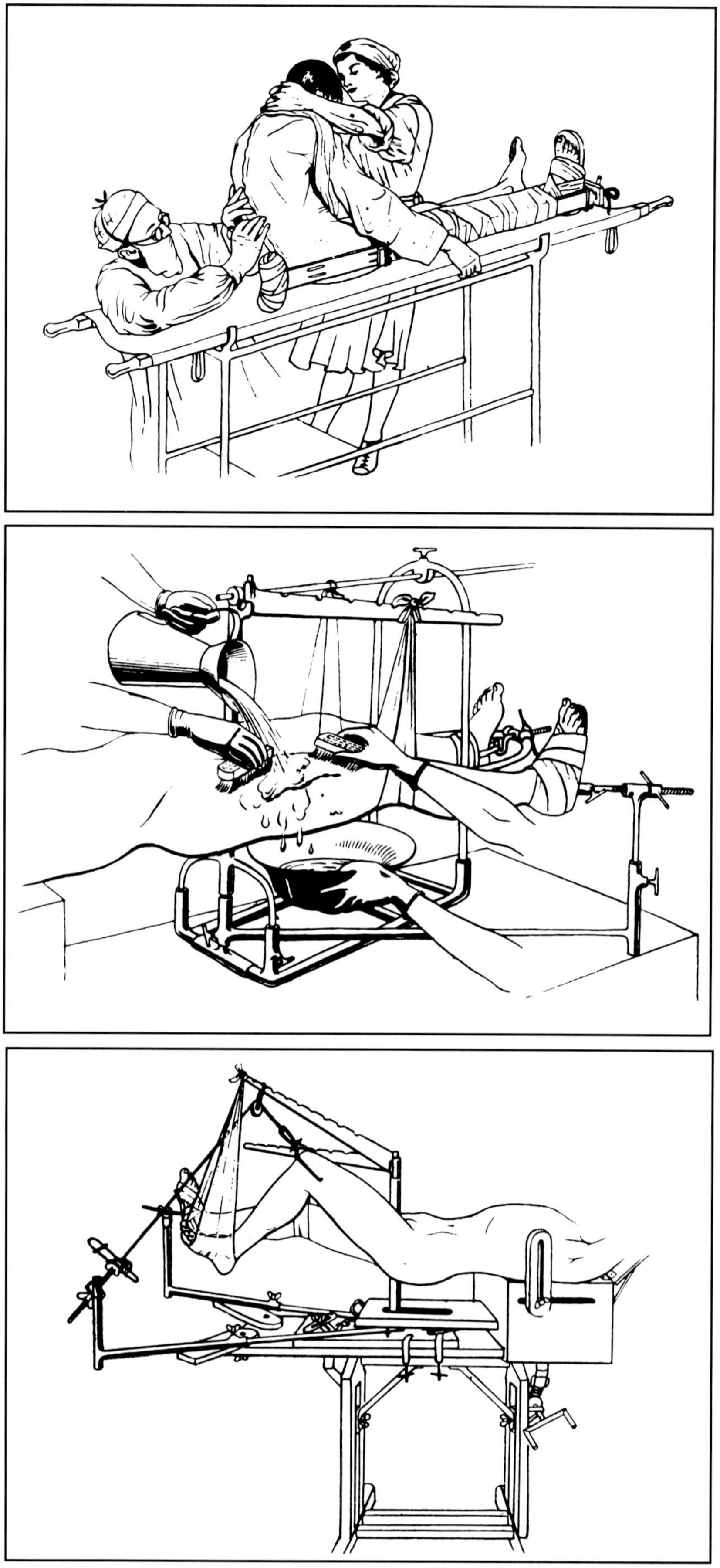

Figures 4.8a,b,c Details of Yudin's "thigh brigade": a) The administration of the anesthetic; b) The application of traction and cleansing; c) Ready for the application of the plaster dressing. From Yudin, "The Treatment of War Fractures," *SGO* 78(1944): 1.

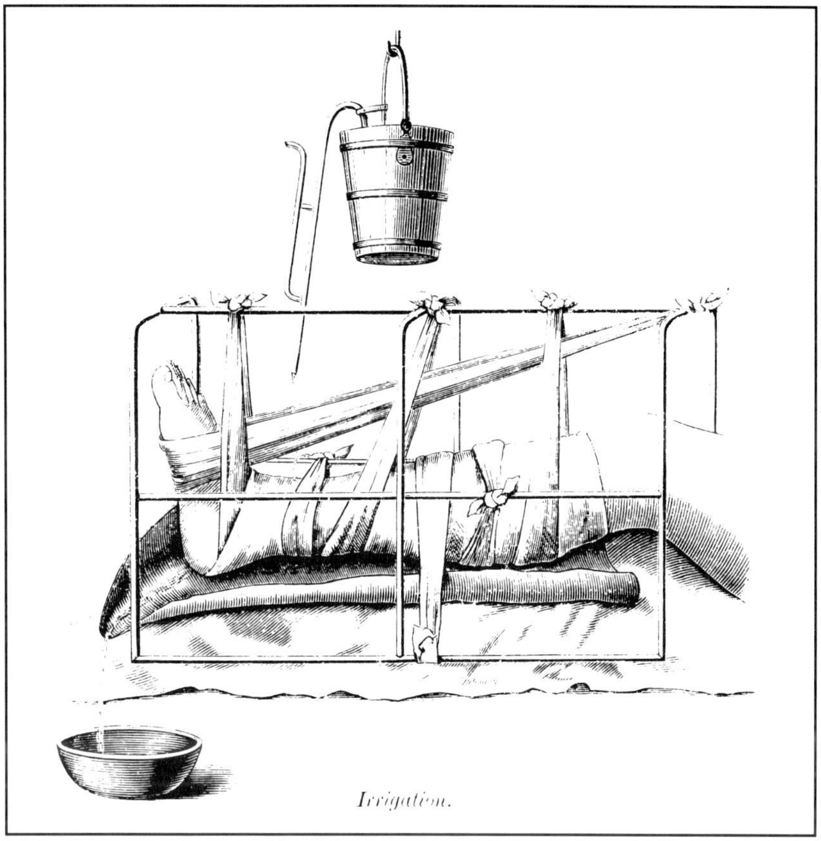

Figure 4.9 Equipment for intermittent irrigation of the wound or for moistening the dressings. From F. Esmarch, *Handbuch der Kriegschirurgischen Technik* (Hanover: Rumpler, 1877), 77.

was for the administration of a spinal anesthetic; the second, for the application of traction and cleansing; and the third, for the operation itself and the application of the plaster of paris dressing (figures 4.8a, b,c). Yudin closed his article with a tribute to Nikolai Pirogov, the Russian surgeon who had first used plaster of paris dressings in war casualties during the Crimean War ninety years before.[49]

The antiseptic method was based on the concept of destroying bacteria in the wound by the application of antiseptic or bactericidal solutions. Widely practiced before the elucidation of the germ theory, it received new impetus from the work of Pasteur and Lister.[50] The introduction of rubber drainage tubes for wound treatment by Edouard Pierre Marie Chassaignac in 1859 simplified the technique.[51] Sometimes the wounds were simply covered with wet dressings that were moistened at intervals (figure 4.9). Thomas Masters Markoe of New York devised a method that consisted of debridement, reduction of the fracture, and placement of perforated rubber tubes in the wound, which was closed loosely with silk suture.[52] The wound was covered by "carbolized gauze," and the leg was immobilized in a plaster of paris splint (figure 4.10). A solution of phenol (1:40) was instilled through the tubes several times each day.

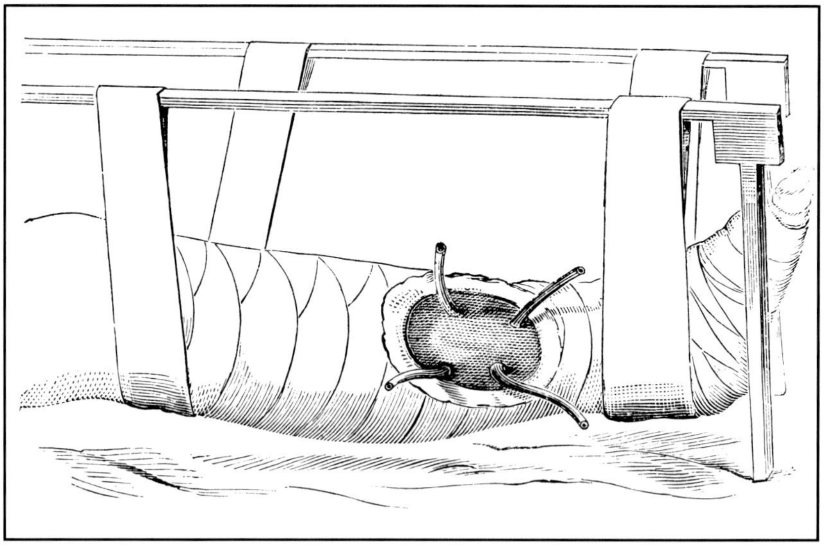

Figure 4.10 The method of wound irrigation used by Markoe. From Markoe, "Thorough Drainage in the Treatment of Open Wounds," *Am J Med Sci* 79(1880): 305–35.

The high-water mark of the antiseptic wound irrigation treatment of open fractures was reached during World War I with the use of the Carrel-Dakin technique. Henry D. Dakin (1880–1952), an American microbiologist, screened more than two hundred substances for use as a wound antiseptic before choosing a special solution of sodium hypochlorite (Dakin's solution) for the purpose.[53]

Alexis Carrel (1873–1944), so famous after World War I, so infamous after World War II, and his associates further developed this system of wound treatment.[54] It is fully described and illustrated in a manual by Carrel and Georges Dehelly.[55] The wounds were debrided and excised, perforated irrigation tubes were placed in the wounds, the fractures were reduced and immobilized, and the wounds were irrigated every two hours and inspected daily (figures 4.11a, b). An elaborate system of wound cultures was developed, and an estimate of the bacterial population on the surface of the wound made at regular intervals. Only when the wounds no longer contained bacteria was delayed primary closure or secondary closure of the wounds considered.

In contrast to the occlusive method of treating open fractures, in which the treatment of the wound and the fracture were given equal emphasis, the antiseptic treatment of the wound, requiring as it did daily dressing changes, took priority over the treatment of the fracture. The method was complicated in its application, requiring additional supplies and personnel and a bacteriological laboratory. The patients were subjected to a daily disturbance of their dressings and could not be moved or evacuated to distant hospitals easily.

While primary closure of the wounds in open fractures was carried out successfully in World War I in France and in Gallipoli, it was obvious that it could be done only in special circumstances and not

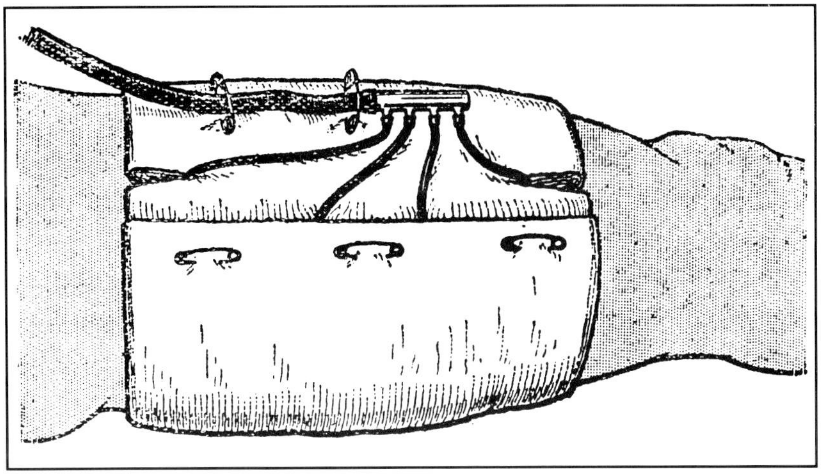

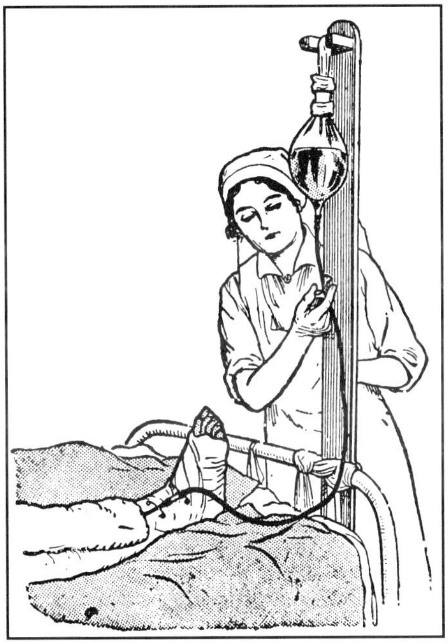

Figures 4.11a,b Details of the Carrel-Dakin technique: a) The arrangement of the tubes; b) The intermittent irrigation. From Carrel and Dehelly, *Infected Wounds* (New York: Paul B. Hoeber, 1917), 118, 136.

as a general practice.[56] The value of early wound closure was recognized, and the endpoint of the Carrell-Dakin technique was a wound sufficiently clean to permit closure. Eugene Hillhouse Pool thoroughly discussed the indications for primary closure, delayed primary closure, and secondary closure in a 1919 article.[57] Antoine Depage reported a series of forty-three open fractures of the femur, four of which were closed primarily with healing; thirty-nine were treated by delayed primary closure with successs in thirty cases.[58] In 1940 William Darrach described primary and secondary closure of wounds in the treatment of open fractures, and in addition advocated early skin grafting to cover granulating wounds.[59]

During World War II, British policies for the treatment of open fractures passed through three stages: 1) treatment by the closed plaster method; 2) initial treatment by the closed plaster method, followed by secondary closure; and 3) initial treatment by the closed plaster method, followed by excision and delayed primary closure.[60] In the European theatre of operations, the U.S. Army used the same approach, with an emphasis on early use of skin grafts where necessary.[61] Mather Cleveland and John Grove were able to report on 2,393 patients with open fractures treated by delayed primary closure, with successful healing in 93 percent.[62]

Gerhard Domagk introduced prontosil, the first drug to contain sulfanilamide, into clinical medicine in 1935.[63] Experience with the "sulfa drugs" grew rapidly, and in 1939 N. K. Jensen and his colleagues reported their use in the treatment of open fractures.[64] After debriding the wound and reducing the fractures, the wound surfaces were sprinkled lightly with sulfanilamide powder and the wound was closed primarily. They reported a series of thirty-nine patients with open fractures treated in this manner, all of whose wounds healed without infection. This was in contrast to a similar group of ninety-four patients in whom sulfanilamides were not used: 27 percent of the wounds in this group became infected. In a group of patients with open fractures treated at the Campbell Clinic in Memphis, the infection rate in patients treated by local implantation and oral administration of sulfanilamides was 19 percent. In contrast, a control group in which the drug was not used had an infection rate of 34 percent.[65] Frank Meleney, however, concluded that the sulfanilamides were of no value in preventing infection.[66] Böhler was of a similar opinion:

> *From 1941–1943 my assistants, during my absence strewed sulfanilamides into all wounds. Thereupon, the number of infections after excision and suture of fresh wounds increased from about 2 percent to 6 percent because the wound excision was carried out less thoroughly, reliance being placed on the new agents. Upon my return I stopped the use of sulfanimides and the number of wound infections dropped to 2%. Currently, [1966] we do not use topical agents on fresh wounds."*[67]

Valentine Herbert Ellis (1901–1953) was the first orthopedic surgeon to use penicillin in the treatment of patients with open fractures.[68] More than 1,500 wounded patients treated with penicillin were observed in his hospital. He carefully discussed the difference between wound contamination and wound infection and emphasized that an early and complete debridement was the most important element of treatment. He preferred administering the antibiotic systemically rather than applying it directly to the wound. His views on the use of penicillin in the treatment of open fractures were very similar to those expressed by M. J. Patazkis and his colleagues thirty years later.[69]

The current state of our knowledge and practice in the management of patients with open fractures has been ably summarized by Ramon B. Gustilo and John T. Anderson.[70]

Notes

1. James H. Breasted, *The Edwin Smith Papyrus* (Chicago: University of Chicago Press, 1930), 357-61.

2. Hippocrates, *The Genuine Works of Hippocrates*, trans. Francis Adams (Baltimore: Williams and Wilkins, 1939).

3. J. E. M. Thomson, "Fractures of the Forearm Reduced by Direct Leverage," *J Bone Joint Surg* 18(1936): 397.

4. Celsus, *De medicina*, trans. W. G. Spencer (Cambridge, Mass.: Harvard University Press, 1953), 3:549.

5. Ambroise Paré, *The Case Reports and Autopsy Records of Ambroise Paré*, comp. and ed. Wallace B. Hamby, trans. from J.-F. Malgaigne's *Oeuvres complètes d'Ambroise Paré* (Springfield, Ill.: Charles C Thomas, 1960), 82-85.

6. Theodor Billroth, *Historical Studies on the Nature and Treatment of Gunshot Wounds from the Fifteenth Century to the Present Time*, trans. C. P. Rhoads (New Haven, Conn.: Yale University Press, 1933); O. H. Wangensteen and S. D. Wangensteen, *The Rise of Surgery from Empiric Craft to Scientific Discipline* (Minneapolis: University of Minnesota Press, 1978).

7. Richard Wiseman, "Of Wounds," "Of Gunshot Wounds," "Of Fractures and Luxations," facsimile of Books 5, 6, and 7 from *Severall Chirurgical Treatises* (1676), ed. John Kirkup (Bath, England: Kingsmead, 1977), 420-21.

8. John Hunter, *Lectures on the Principles of Surgery, The Works of John Hunter F.R.S. with Notes edited by James F. Palmer*, Vol. 1 (London, 1835), 505-10.

9. Percivall Pott, *The Chirurgical Works of Percivall Pott, F.R.S., Surgeon to St. Bartholomew's Hospital . . . [with a] Short Account of the Life of the Author by Sir James Earle* (London: Wood and Innes, 1808), 1:xiii-xv.

10. F. L. Reichert, "The Historical Development of the Procedure Termed Debridement," *Bull Johns Hopkins Hosp* 42(1928): 93-104; L. M. Zimmerman and Ilza Veith, *Great Ideas in the History of Surgery* (Baltimore: Williams and Wilkins, 1961), 362-66.

11. Toby Gelfand, "A Confrontation over Clinical Instruction at the Hôtel Dieu of Paris during the French Revolution," *J Hist Med Allied Sci* 28(1973): 268-82.

12. Pierre Joseph Desault, *Oeuvres chirurgicales; ou, Exposé de la doctrine et de la pratique de P.-J. Desault par Xav. Bichat* (Paris: Méquignon, 1801).

13. Dominique Jean Larrey, *Memoirs of Military Surgery and Campaigns of the French Armies*, trans. Richard Willmott Hall (Baltimore: Joseph Cushing, 1814), 18-19.

14. Larrey, *Mémoires de chirurgie militaire et campagnes* (Paris: J. Smith, 1813), 1:50.

15. Larrey, *Memoirs of Military Surgery*, 176.

16. Ernest J. Gurlt, *Geschichte der Chirurgie und Ihre Ausubung* (Berlin: A. Hirchwald, 1898), 2:403-414.

17. Pierre François Percy, *Manuel du chirurgien à l'Armée; ou Instruction de chirurgie militaire* (Paris: Méquignon, 1790), 181.

18. George James Guthrie, *A Treatise on Gunshot Wounds, Etc.*, 3d edition, (London: Burgess and Hill, 1827).

19. John B. Porter, "Medical and Surgical Notes of Campaigns in the War with Mexico During the Years 1845, 1846, 1847, and 1848," *Am J Med Sci* 49(1853): 25-42.

20. George H. B. Macleod, *Notes on the Surgery of the War in the Crimea with Notes on the Treatment of Gunshot Wounds* (London: John Churchill, 1858).

21. Joseph-François Malgaigne, *Etudes statistiques sur les résultats des opérations dans les hôpiteaux de Paris* (Paris: Felix Locquin, 1858), 31.

22. *Medical and Surgical History of the War of the Rebellion*, Vol. II, Part III (Washington, D. C.: Government Printing Office, 1883), 175.

23. Frank Hastings Hamilton, *A Treatise on Military Surgery and Hygiene* (New York: Bailliere Brothers, 1865), 399-401.

24. Macleod, *Notes*, 87.

25. Astley Cooper, *A Treatise on Dislocations and on Fractures of the Joints* (London: Longman, Hurst, Rees, Orme and Brown, 1822), 253-55.

26. Robert Liston, *Elements of Surgery*, 4th American edition, with notes and additions by Samuel D. Gross (Philadelphia: Barrington and Haswell, 1846), 579-80.

27. Hunter, *A Treatise on Blood, Inflammation, and Gunshot Wounds* (London: G. Nichol, 1794).

28. Louis Pasteur, "Mémoire sur les corpuscles organisées qui existent dans l'atmosphère," *Ann sci nat* 16(1861): 5.

29. Spencer Wells, "Some Causes of Excessive Mortality after Surgical Operations," *Brit Med J* 2(1864): 384.

30. Rickman J. Godlee, *Lord Lister* (London: Macmillan, 1917).

31. Joseph Lister, *The Collected Papers of Joseph, Baron Lister* (Oxford: Clarendon Press, 1909), 9-14.

32. Lister, "On a New Method of Treating Compound Fractures, Abscess, etc., with Observation on the Condition of Suppuration," *Lancet* 1(1867): 326, 357, 387, 507; 2(1867): 95.

33. L. H. Toledo-Pereyra and M. M. Toledo, "A Critical Study of Lister's Work on Antiseptic Surgery," *Am J Surg* 131(1976): 736.

34. Frederic S. Dennis, "The Treatment of Compound Fractures, Including a Report of One Hundred and Forty-Four Cases without a Death from Septic Infection, and One Hundred Cases without a Death from Any Cause," *JAMA* 2(1884): 673-87.

35. V. Worm, "Paul Leopold Friedrich," *Zentralbl Chir* 101(1976): 568-69.

36. Paul Leopold Friedrich, "Die aseptische Versorgung frischer Wunden unter Mitteilung von Thier-Versuchen uber Auskeimungszeit von Infectionsrregern in frischen Wunden," *Arch klin Chir* 57(1898): 288-310.

37. Larrey, "Mémoire sur une nouvelle maniére de réduire ou de traiter les fractures des membres compliquées de plaies," *J compl dict sci méd* 20(1824): 193-200.

38. William Beaumont, "Observations and Experiments on a New Mode of Treating Fractures of the Leg and Forearm; Especially Compound Fractures," *Med-Chir Rev London* 16(1732): 247-51.

39. Louis Ollier, "De l'occlusion inamovible comme méthode générale de pansement des plaies dans la chirurgie hospitalière," *Congrès méd France* 11(1872): 192-219.

40. Ollier, "Des résections dans les plaies par armées de guerre et en particulier des résections du conde et de la diaphyse humérale," *Congrès méd France* 11(1872): 220-30.

41. C. Schimmelbusch, *A Guide to the Aseptic Treatment of Wounds*, trans. Frank J. Thornbury (New York: Putnams, 1900), quoted from H. Winnett Orr, *A New Era in the Treatment of Osteomyelitis and Other Infections* (St. Paul: Brune Pub. Co., 1930), 26-27.

42. W. G. LeBoutillier, "Results and Methods of Treatment of Compound Fractures at the J. Hood Wright Memorial Hospital," *Ann Surg* 30(1899): 297-316.

43. Orr, *Osteomyelitis and Compound Fractures and Other Infected Wounds: Treatment by the Method of Drainage and Rest* (St. Louis: C. V. Mosby, 1929), 36.

44. Orr, *Wounds and Fractures: A Clinical Guide to Civil and Military Practice* (Springfield, Ill.: Charles C Thomas, 1941).

45. José Trueta, *The Principles and Practice of War Surgery* (St. Louis: C. V. Mosby, 1943), 39.

46. "José Trueta," obituary, *J Bone Joint Surg* 59A(1977): 243-45.

47. Trueta, *El tratamiento de las fracturas de guerra* (Barcelona: Biblioteca Medica de Cataluña, 1938).

48. Trueta, *Studies of the Development and Decay of the Human Frame* (Philadelphia: W.B.Saunders, 1968).

49. S. S. Yudin, "The Treatment of War Fractures of the Femur,"*SGO* 78(1944): 1-8.

50. Malgaigne, *Traité des fractures et des luxations* (Paris: J. B. Baillière, 1847).

51. Edouard Pierre Marie Chassaignac, *Traité pratique de la suppuration et du drainage chirurgical* (Paris: Masson, 1859).

52. T. M. Markoe, "Thorough Drainage in the Treatment of Open Wounds," *Am J Med Sci* 79(1885): 305-35.

53. Henry D. Dakin, "On the Use of Certain Antiseptic Substances in the Treatment of Infected Wounds," *Brit Med J* 2(1915): 318-20.

54. Alexis Carrel, "Traitement abortif de l'infection des plaies," *Bull Acad Méd* (Paris) 74(1915): 361-68.

55. Carrel and G. Dehelly, *The Treatment of Wounds*, trans. Herbert Childs (New York: Paul B. Hoeber, 1917).

56. H. M. W. Gray, "Treatment of Gunshot Wounds by Excision and Primary Closure," *Brit Med J* 2(1915): 317. John Morley, "Surgery on the Gallipoli Peninsula," *Brit Med J* 2(1915): 461-63.

57. E. H. Pool, "War Wounds: Primary and Secondary Suture," *JAMA* 73(1919): 383-87.

58. Antoine Depage, "General Considerations as to the Treatment of War Wounds," *Ann Surg* 69(1919): 575-88.

59. William Darrach, "Compound Fractures," *AMA Arch Surg* 40(1940): 821-24.

60. Zachary Cope, ed., *Surgery*, in *History of the Second World War*, United Kingdom Medical Series (London: Her Majesty's Stationary Office, 1953).

61. J. B. Coates, Jr., ed., *Surgery in World War II*, in *Orthopedic Surgery in the European Theater of Operations* (Washington, D.C.: Office of the Surgeon General, Dept. of the Army, 1956).

62. Mather Cleveland and John A. Grove, "Delayed Primary Closure of Wounds with Compound Fractures," *J Bone Joint Surg* 27(1945): 452-56.

63. G. Domagk, "Ein Beitrag zur Chemotherapie den bacteriellen Infectionen," *Dtsch med Wschr* 61(1935): 250-53.

64. N. K. Jensen et al., "The Local Implantation of Sulfanilamide in Compound Fractures," *Surgery* 6(1939): 1-11.

65. Willis C. Campbell and Hugh Smith, "Fresh Compound Fractures: Treatment by Sulfonamides and by Internal Fixation in Selected Cases," *JAMA* 117(1941): 672-74.

66. Frank L. Meleney, *Treatise on Surgical Infections* (New York: Oxford University Press, 1948), 766.

67. L. Böhler and J. Böhler, *The Treatment of Fractures*, supplementary volume to the 5th English edition, trans. Alfred Wallner (New York: Grune and Stratton, 1966), 2311.

68. V. H. Ellis, "Orthopaedic Surgery and Fractures," in *Penicillin: Its Practical Application*, ed. Alexander Fleming (London: Butterworth and Co., Ltd., 1946); A. Innes and Ellis, "Battle Casualaties Treated with Penicillin," *Lancet* 1(1945): 524.

69. M. J. Patzakis et al., "The Role of Antibiotics in the Management of Open Fractures," *J Bone Joint Surg* 56A(1974): 532.

70. R. B. Gustilo and J. T. Anderson, "Prevention of Infection in the Treatment of 1,025 Open Fractures of Long Bones," *J Bone Joint Surg* 58A(1976): 453.

CHAPTER FIVE

The Internal Fixation of Fractures

INTERNAL FIXATION of fractures could not become a practical method of treatment until the introduction of antiseptic and aseptic techniques dispelled the spectre of infection. Although there had been anecdotal reports of the use of wire suture, cerclage, or ivory pegs in patients with open or ununited fractures before Lister, no real progress was possible until the safety of such surgical interventions could be assured.[1] As so frequently happens, the beginning of the new era was marked by a seminal work that recapitulated past experience and forecast future development. Such a work was the *Traité de l'immobilisation directe des fragments osseux dans les fractures* by Laurent Jean Baptiste Bérenger-Féraud (1832–1900), published in Paris in 1870[2] (figure 5.1). Bérenger-Féraud's book was the first work devoted to the treatment of fractures by internal fixation.

Bérenger-Féraud (figure 5.2) was born in the south of France, the son of a naval surgeon.[3] He received his early education in Algeria, where his father was stationed, returning to Toulon in 1850 to begin his medical education. During his studies, he observed two patients with open fractures of the tibia treated by Dr. Long, the chief surgeon of L'Hôtel Dieu Saint Esprit, who used wire sutures to stabilize the fragments. His thesis for the degree of medicine in Paris dealt with the treatment of comminuted fractures of the tibia.[4] He then became a medical officer in the French navy and served on tropical stations in equatorial Africa, where he became interested in tropical diseases. In 1870 he was recalled to serve with the French army during the Franco-Prussion War. He was present at the surrender at Sedan and later served with distinction as a surgeon at the military hospital, Val-de-Grace, during the siege of Paris. His book on fractures was published at this time, although he had published a

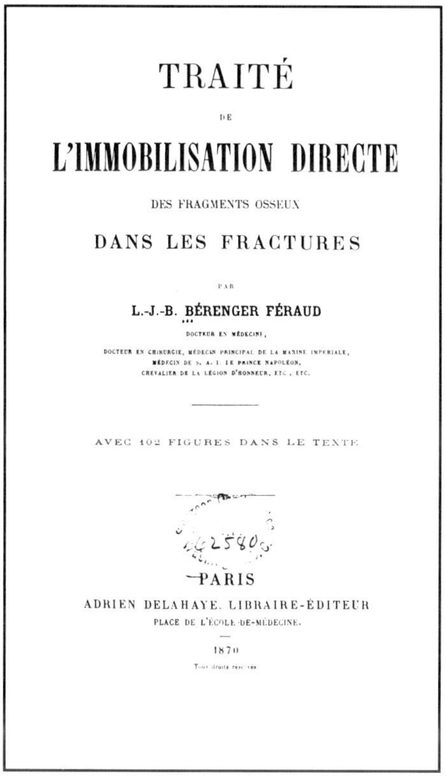
TRAITÉ

DE

L'IMMOBILISATION DIRECTE

DES FRAGMENTS OSSEUX

DANS LES FRACTURES

PAR

L.-J.-B. BÉRENGER FÉRAUD

DOCTEUR EN MÉDECINE,

DOCTEUR EN CHIRURGIE, MÉDECIN PRINCIPAL DE LA MARINE IMPÉRIALE,
MÉDECIN DE S. A. I. LE PRINCE NAPOLÉON,
CHEVALIER DE LA LÉGION D'HONNEUR, ETC., ETC.

AVEC 102 FIGURES DANS LE TEXTE

PARIS

ADRIEN DELAHAYE, LIBRAIRE-ÉDITEUR

PLACE DE L'ÉCOLE-DE-MÉDECINE.

1870

Tous droits réservés

Figure 5.1 The first book devoted to the internal fixation of fractures, *Traité de l'immobilisation directe des fragments osseux dans les fractures* by Laurent Jean Baptiste Bérenger-Féraud (Paris: Adrien Delahaye, 1870).

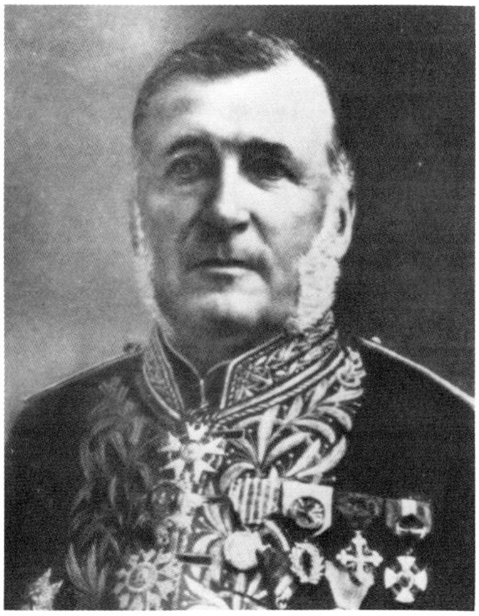

Figure 5.2 L. J. B. Bérenger-Féraud (1832-1900), pioneer in internal fixation and surgeon-in-chief of the French navy. From J. W. W. Stephens, *Blackwater Fever* (London: University Press of Liverpool, 1937), frontispiece.

short synopsis of his ideas six years previously.[5] After 1870, he concentrated on pursuing his naval career and the study of tropical medicine. His description of malaria complicated by dark urine, *fièvre bilieuse mélanurique*, was translated into English as "black water fever."[6] At the time of his retirement, Bérenger-Féraud had reached the rank of surgeon general of the Navy.

Bérenger-Féraud described six different methods for the direct fixation of fracture fragments: 1) the stabilization of fractures of the mandible by wiring or tying adjacent teeth together, as described by Hippocrates; 2) Malgaigne's point; 3) Malgaigne's clamp; 4) enclavement or impaction of a spike of one fragment into the marrow cavity of the other; 5) suture of the fragments; and 6) ligature or cerclage of the fragments[7] (figures 5.3, 5.4, 5.5, 5.6, 5.7, 5.8). Of these methods, he believed cerclage to be the most efficient. Bérenger-Féraud claimed no credit for devising any of these methods, and he provided extensive documentation of their use by others. Many of the methods had been used in the treatment of ununited fractures or pseudarthrosis. Bérenger-Féraud advised their application only in such cases, and in fresh open fractures where the risk of infection was already present. Following the operation, he gave the surgeon the choice of dressing the wound, which was left open, with dressings soaked with cold water, a mixture of alcohol and water, alcohol, wine, solutions of potassium permanganate, phenol, or creosote. He summarized the advantages of the direct fixation of fracture fragments as follows:

> *The direct immobilization of the fragments simplifies the pathology of the wound about the open fracture because the healing of the soft tissue is not impaired by motion of the bone fragments. The bones are less exposed to change caused by pyogenic or very dangerous putrid elements during the period when they are not protected by granulation tissue. And, finally, when the bones begin their inflammatory evolution, i.e. sequestration, callus, and involucrum formation, and the soft parts are already healing and well on their way to recovery, the patient who previously was very weakened by inflammation or suppuration of the soft parts can now easily support the phenomena accompanying bone repair.*[8]

If we examine carefully the six methods for the direct immobilization of fracture fragments described by Bérenger-Féraud, we can see in embryo concepts that contributed to the development and use of pins and nails, external skeletal fixation, intramedullary nailing, and cerclage.

It was the antiseptic system of wound treatment developed by Lister that ensured the safety of open reduction and internal fixation in the treatment of fractures and permitted these methods to develop. Lister began in 1865 by demonstrating in patients with open fractures that the wounds could heal without infection if they

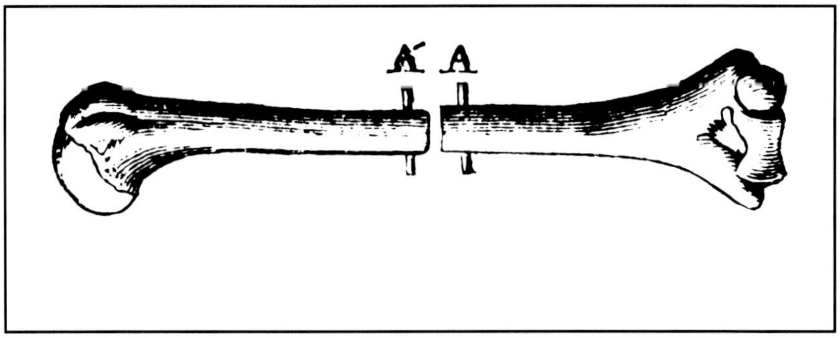

Figure 5.3 The direct fixation of a fracture using the Hippocratic principle of fixing fractures of the mandible by wiring adjacent teeth together. From Bérenger-Féraud, *Traité*, 264.

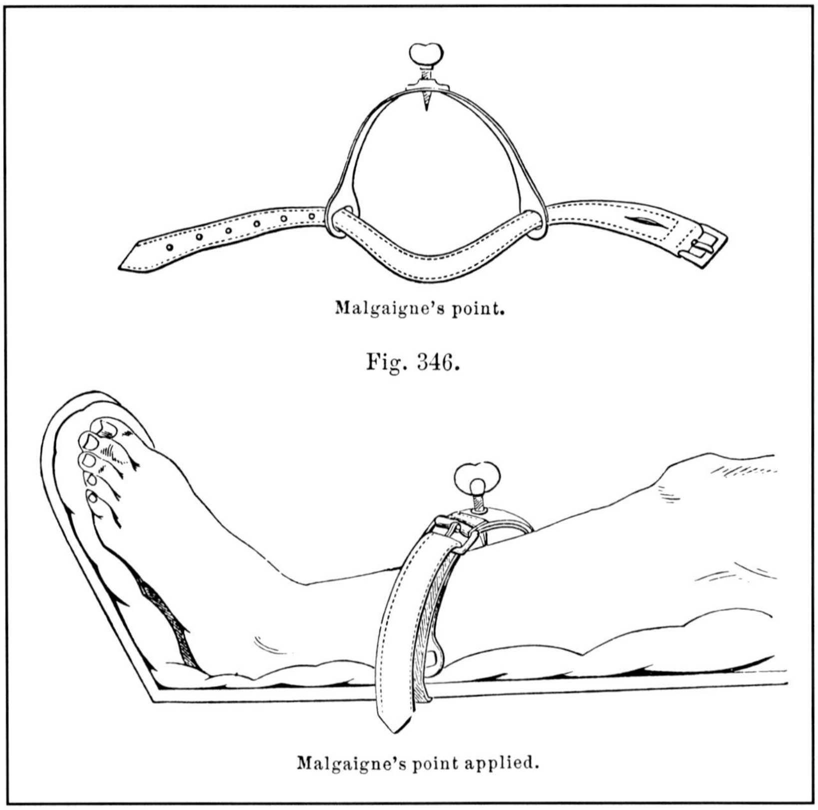

Figure 5.4 Malgaigne's point. From L. A. Stimson, *A Treatise on Fractures* (Philadelphia: Henry C. Lea's Son, 1883), 575.

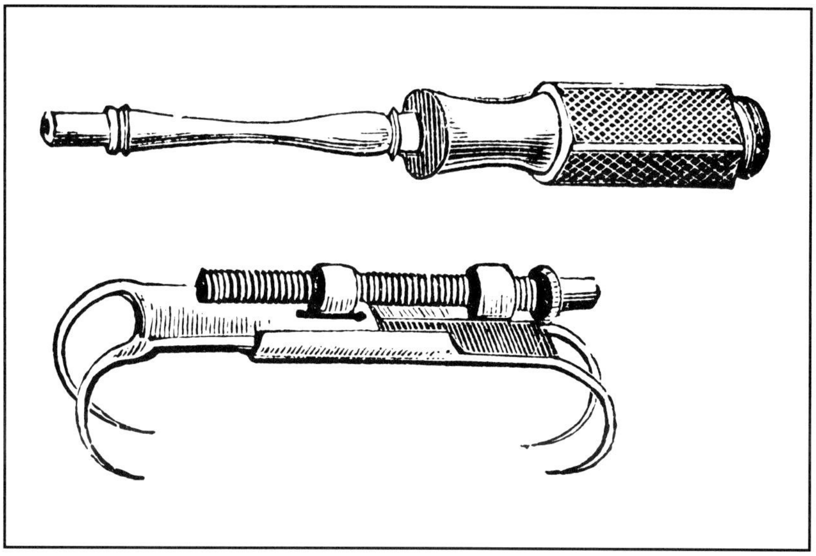

Figure 5.5 Malgaigne's hooks. From Stimson, *Treatise,* 460.

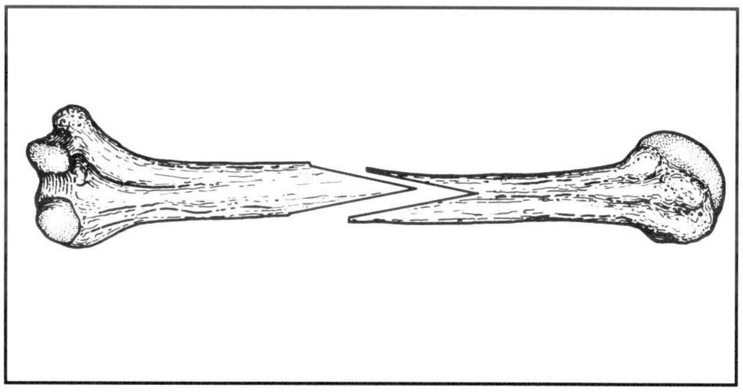

Figure 5.6 Enclavement, the stabilization of the fracture by inserting the pointed end of one fragment into the medullary canal of the other.

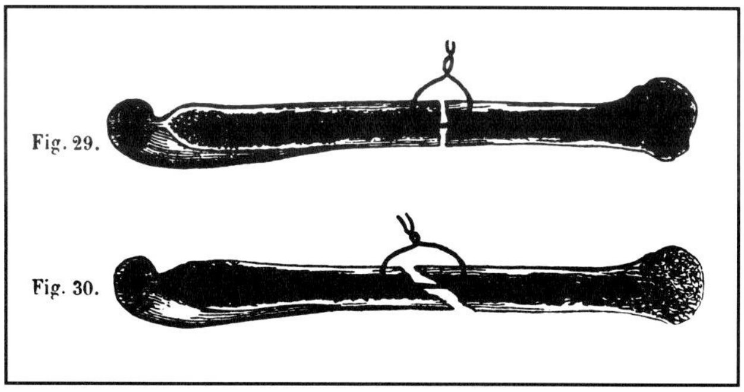

Figure 5.7 Bone suture. From Bérenger-Féraud, *Traité,* 264.

were covered carefully with an occlusive dressing containing phenol (carbolic acid). The next step, electively converting a closed fracture into an open one, was long delayed. Before it could be taken, Lister had to accumulate experience with the treatment of open fractures and with pseudarthrosis by operative methods. He also had to learn how to sterilize the instruments and materials that he used so that they did not infect the wounds. The simple decision to cut off sutures at the knot, leaving them buried in the wound was a crucial one. Finally, in October 1877, when he was confident of his technique, a patient with a closed fracture of the patella was admitted to his ward in King's College, London. Lister's resolve was strengthened by his knowledge of the success of his former colleague in Glasgow, Hector Cameron, who in March 1877 had repaired a displaced transverse fracture of the patella eight weeks old using a wire suture and antiseptic techniques.

After an initial attempt at closed treatment that did not completely reduce the fracture, Lister carried out an open reduction and internally fixed the fracture by means of a heavy silver wire (figure 5.9). The wound healed without infection and the wire was removed after eight weeks. Lister believed that this was the first case of a fresh fracture of the patella treated by "wire suture antiseptically applied."[9]

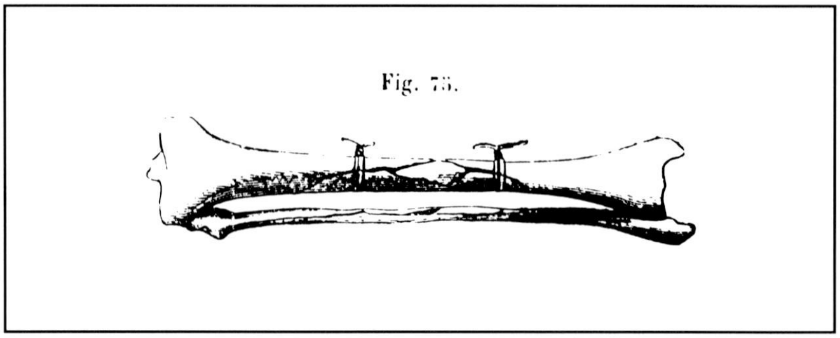

Figure 5.8 Bone ligature or cerclage. From Bérenger-Féraud, *Traité*, 407.

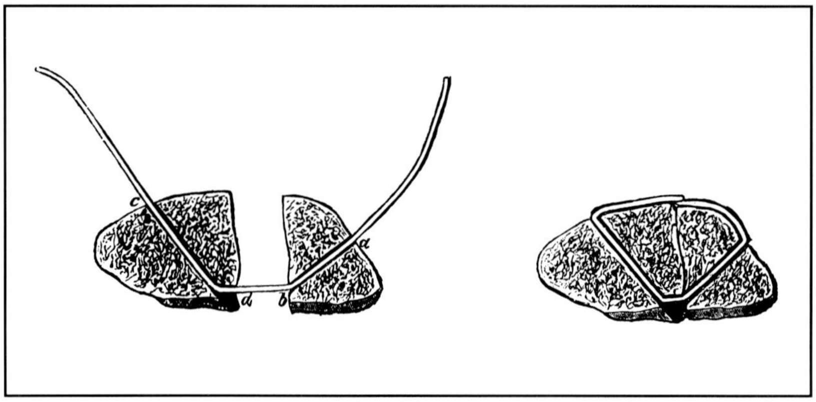

Figure 5.9 Joseph Lister's method of patellar suture using silver wire. From Lister, *The Collected Papers of Joseph, Baron Lister* (Oxford: Clarendon Press, 1919), 466.

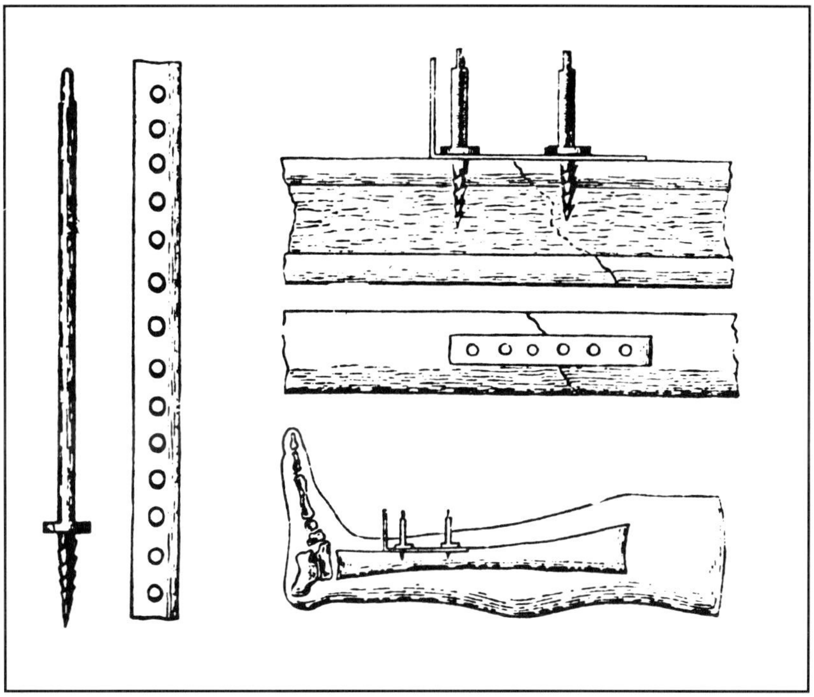

Figure 5.10 Hansmann's method. Note that the screws and the plate could be removed after the fracture had healed without reopening the wound. From Hansmann, "Eine neue Methode der Fixierung der Fragmente bei complicirten Fracturen," *Dtsch Ges Chir* 15(1886): 134–37.

He was unaware that Samuel Cooper in San Francisco had used a silver wire to successfully suture a fresh fracture of the patella in 1861.[10] Cooper's success was due to his use of antiseptic techniques that employed 50 percent and 75 percent alcohol.[11] In 1883 Lister was able to report good results in seven patients in whom he had wired fractures of the patella. Fifteen years later, the treatment of displaced closed fractures of the patella by open reduction and wiring was an established procedure.

> *That the operation has a well-fixed place in surgery seems plain. I believe it should done only by adepts in the surgical art, that it be confined to healthy individuals of suitable age, that its dangers and advantages should always be fully explained to the patient, that it should be reserved for fractures presenting a diastasis of over one-half of an inch or with extensive lateral tears of the capsule, and that it should always be supplemented by early massage and mobilization of the joint. The preferable form of operation is open arthrotomy. The suture of the soft parts should always be carefully made, such suture may be applied to the bone as the operator's judgement may dictate.*[12]

Displaced fractures of the olecranon were treated in the same manner as patellar fractures.

Protected to an increasing extent by antiseptic and, later, aseptic techniques, surgeons became bolder and treated an increasing number of closed fractures by open reduction and

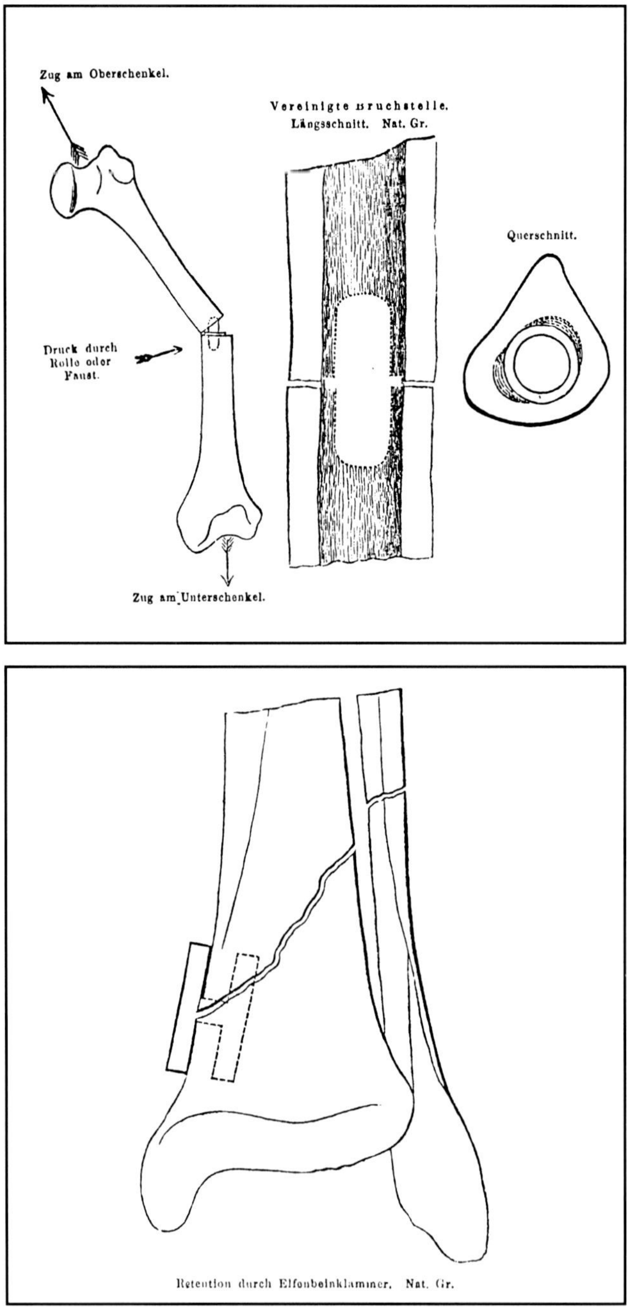

Figures 5.11a,b Bircher's methods of a) intramedullary ivory pegs for diaphyseal fractures and b) ivory "clamps" for metaphyseal fractures. From H. Bircher, "Eine neue Methode unmittelbarer Retention bei Fracturen der Rohrenkrochen," *Arch klin Chir* 34(1893): 410–22.

internal fixation. Fixation by means of a plate and screws designed in such a way that they could be removed after the fracture consolidated without reopening the wound, was introduced by Hansmann in 1886[13] (figure 5.10). Wiring techniques continued to improve.[14] Bircher developed some interesting

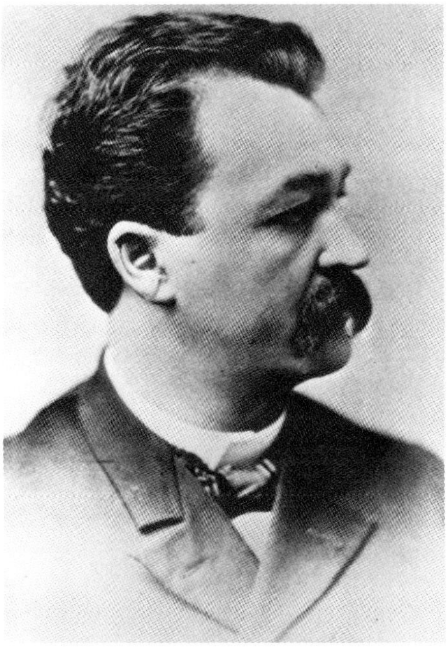

Figure 5.12 Nicholas Senn (1844–1908). From Mark Ravitch, *A Century of Surgery* (Philadelphia: J. B. Lippincott, 1981), 1:138.

ivory pegs and "clamps" for the intramedullary fixation of metaphyseal fractures[15] (figures 5.11a,b).

In 1893, Nicholas Senn (1844–1908) (figure 5.12) entitled his presidential address to the American Surgical Association "A New Method of Direct Fixation of Fragments in Compound and Ununited Fractures."[16] In a presentation reminiscent of Bérenger-Féraud's, he reviewed the status of the internal fixation of fractures and advanced his own ideas for the use of absorbable materials—cylinders made from the long bones of turkeys, chickens, and rabbits, and ferrules made from sections of ox bone (figures 5.13a,b). While his techniques were not widely used, Senn's espousal of internal fixation helped to promote its use in the United States. In 1897, at the very beginning of the new era heralded by Roentgen's discovery of X rays, Joseph Ransohoff suggested these postulates:

The conversion of a simple fracture is justifiable when other means to secure the best result fail. In fractures of the diaphysis of the tibia, femur, humerus, and clavicle, in which insurmountable longitudinal displacement or axial reduction cannot be otherwise effected, an early operation is justified. Fractures complicated with dislocations irreducible by other methods warrant operative interference. The involvement of a joint, except probably in the case of the knee and hip, do not, per se, militate against operation if this is otherwise indicated. Special precaution against infections must be taken, in connection with which

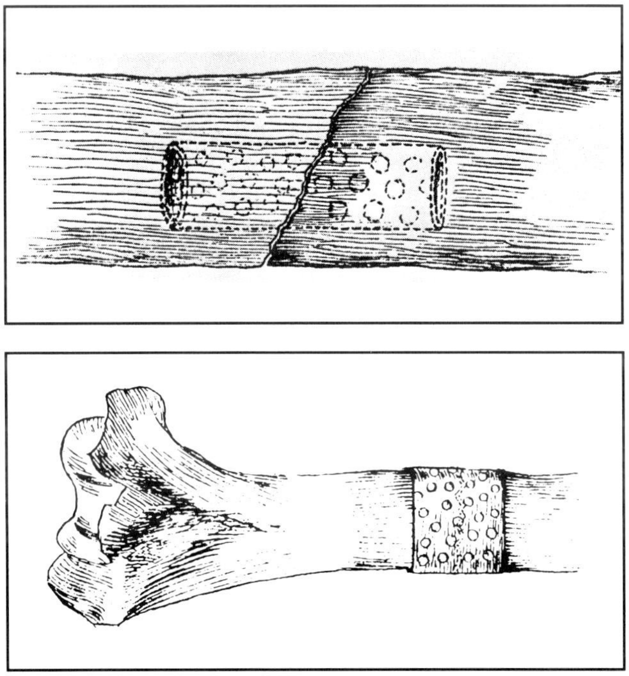

Figures 5.13a,b An intramedullary cylinder and an external ferrule used by Senn. These were made from biological absorbable materials—i.e., deossified animal bones. From N. Senn, "A New Method of Direct Fixation of the Fragments in Compound and Ununited Fractures," *Trans Am Surg Assoc* 11(1893): 125–51.

should be bourne in mind the dangers of too firmly closing a wound and the advantage of temporary tamponade and secondary suture. Reckless and indiscriminate resort to the operative relief of deformity in recent simple fractures is to be condemned, since there would be few fields of surgery, in the event of an unsuccessful intervention, in which the contrast could be greater between the good intended and the harm done.[17]

The first decade of the twentieth century saw the emergence of two strong and effective advocates for the internal fixation of fractures, one in London and the other in Belgium. William Arbuthnot Lane (1856–1943) was born on a British army post in Scotland[18]. His father, a regimental surgeon, moved his family with the regiment, and by the time "Willie" was sixteen he had lived in Africa, India, Corfu, Malta, Nova Scotia, and England. His early education was obtained along the way. His father's posting to Woolwich, south of London, gave him the opportunity to go to medical school. In 1872 he was enrolled at Guy's Hospital, where during his rotations he served as a surgical clerk on the service of Thomas Bryant, developer of "Bryant's traction." He progressed through the system, qualifying for the F.R.C.S. in 1882. Beginning as a demonstrator of anatomy at Guy's Hospital, he became an assistant surgeon and finally a surgeon on the staff of the hospital in 1903. A glance at his extensive bibliography reveals him to have been a general surgeon in the broadest sense. His interest in the treatment of fractures was but a small part of his work, which came more and more to focus on the problem of autointoxication due to chronic intestinal stasis. This led him to promote ileocolostomy as a treatment for a large number of degenerative diseases of the heart, kidneys, arteries, and brain. To combat chronic constipation, he popularized the use of mineral oil. Late in his life he founded a lay group, the New Health Society, to educate the public to improve their diet and to correct unhealthy habits. Lane was an innovative surgeon and a brilliant technician. His knowledge of anatomy allowed him to operate boldly. His strict adherence to a sterile, "no touch" technique in the operating room ensured his procedures a low rate of infection. This technique was made possible by the use of many instruments of his own design. Lane was a prolific writer and an effective promoter of his ideas. He was, for example, a frequent visitor to the United States, where his work on fractures became well known.

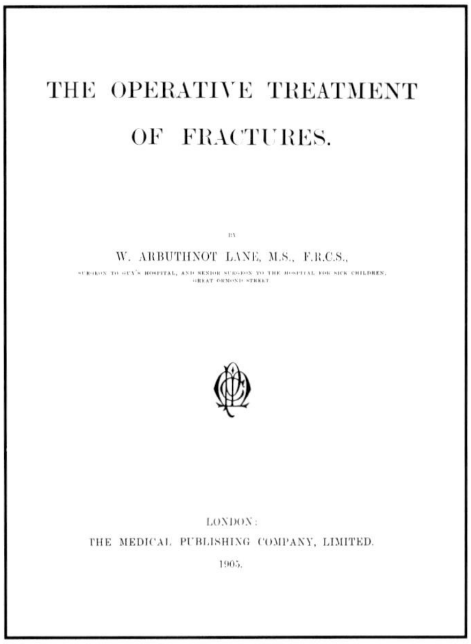
THE OPERATIVE TREATMENT
OF FRACTURES.

BY

W. ARBUTHNOT LANE, M.S., F.R.C.S.,

LONDON:
THE MEDICAL PUBLISHING COMPANY, LIMITED.
1905.

Figure 5.14 Lane's book on the operative treatment of fractures described and illustrated his techniques of using wires, screws, and staples.

Lane's attitude toward the treatment of fractures stemmed from his anatomical dissections, where he had observed the effects of mechanical stress on the skeleton and the traumatic arthritis associated with malunited fractures.[19] He became disenchanted with the result of the treatment of fractures by closed manipulation:

It was evident that the displaced fragments of a broken bone were never, or hardly ever, restored to their normal position, and that the so-called "setting of fractures" was a myth. In most cases the recognized explanation of the mode of production of the fracture was equally absurd, and the treatment by manipulation and splints was not based on any scientific or mechanical principle.[20]

Beginning in 1892, Lane began to operate on closed fractures and to internally fix them with screws and wires.[21] Even after a very short experience with this technique, he had the confidence to predict in 1894:

I think that you will find that in proportion, as the surgeon acquires confidence in the safety of his operative procedures, begotten of a thorough knowledge and careful application of the principles of aseptic surgery, so you will see him interfering actively with increasing frequency in the treatment of simple fractures of all kinds. . . .[22]

His book *The Operative Treatment of Fractures,* (figure 5.14) published in 1905, was illustrated with drawings, photographs, and X rays demonstrating the use of wires, screws, and staples.[23] The "Lane plate" made its appearance in 1907,[24] and in the second edition of his book, published in 1914, was the preferred method of fixation. However, Lane's methods were opposed by many of his colleagues as too risky and prone to failure.

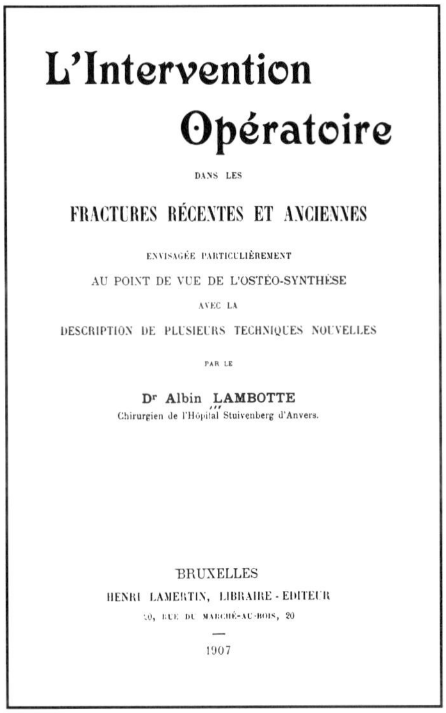
L'Intervention
Opératoire
DANS LES
FRACTURES RÉCENTES ET ANCIENNES
ENVISAGÉE PARTICULIÈREMENT
AU POINT DE VUE DE L'OSTÉO-SYNTHÈSE
AVEC LA
DESCRIPTION DE PLUSIEURS TECHNIQUES NOUVELLES
PAR LE
Dr Albin LAMBOTTE
Chirurgien de l'Hôpital Stuivenberg d'Anvers.
BRUXELLES
HENRI LAMERTIN, LIBRAIRE - EDITEUR
20, RUE DU MARCHÉ-AU-BOIS, 20
1907

Figure 5.15 Lambotte's book on the operative treatment of fractures, published in 1907 includes the first use of the term *osteosynthesis.*

Albin Lambotte (1866–1956) was born in Brussels, where his father was a professor of anatomy, biology, and chemistry at the university. His older brother, Elie, was a surgeon and became the greatest influence on his life. After his medical education, Albin Lambotte became a house officer on his brother's service at the hospital of Schaerbeck in suburban Brussels. There, Elie Lambotte enjoyed the reputation of a daring pioneer in abdominal surgery. His premature death was a great personal loss to his brother. Albin Lambotte obtained an appointment at the hospital of Stuyvenberg in Antwerp in 1890 and spent the rest of his professional life there. At Stuyvenberg he was a general surgeon who operated on patients with all sorts of diseases and injuries. However, the treatment of fractures remained his major interest. Slowly he began to develop his armamentarium and technique for the internal fixation of fractures and for external skeletal fixation. Lambotte had unusual artistic and manual skills as well. He was a talented artist, sculptor, lute maker, musician, and fisherman. He was perseverant and analytical, and his influence as a teacher was as a result both subtle and lasting.

Lambotte published his accumulated experience on the treatment of fractures by surgical methods in 1907, his subtitle introducing the term *osteosynthesis*[25] (figure 5.15). He reported on 187 patients with only two deaths due to infection. He believed that open reduction and internal fixation were indicated in cases of displaced, comminuted, and "puncture-compound" fractures as well as fractures complicated by arterial and nerve injuries. To fix the fractures, Lambotte used wire sutures and cerclage, screws, staples, plates, and external skeletal fixation. In patients with diaphyseal fractures, those that were transverse were fixed with a plate and screws or external skeletal fixation; those that were oblique, by cerclage or cerclage in combination with external skeletal fixation. Metaphyseal fractures were fixed with staples, screws, and plates. An integral part of Lambotte's treatment was the institution of early active, assisted motion. A second, expanded edition of his book appeared in 1913.[26]

Staples were added to the surgical armamentarium by Alberto Jacoel in 1901.[27] Originally designed to fix fractures of the patella, they became popular and were widely used to fix metaphyseal and even diaphyseal fractures. The shanks of these original staples were barbed to promote retention (figure 5.16). Other modifications were introduced rapidly (figure 5.17).

Cerclage was one of the oldest forms of internal fixation. Wire and wire tighteners of all types have been used. The wire has been secured by knots, twists, and even by drops of electrician's solder.[28] Robert Milne used flexible threaded pins and nuts[29] (figures 5.18a,b). In 1914 Vittorio Putti designed a narrow metal band,[30] and a similar system was devised two years later by Frederick William Parham and E. Denegre Martin[31] (figures 5.19, 5.20). Heavier and larger bands for cerclage were introduced by A. Collins and F. E. Hagie.[32] The possibilities of banding with increasingly larger apparatus found ultimate expression in the *manchon*, or muff, designed by Contremoulins[33] (figure 5.21). Paul Niehans introduced the use of long nails or pins for the fixation of fracture fragments in 1904[34] (figure 5.22).

In the United States, the open reduction and internal fixation of fractures continued to interest surgeons. Indeed, their role in the treatment of fractures was assessed accurately as early as 1900 by Scudder at the Massachusetts General Hospital:

> *In conclusion, the ideal result to be aimed at after a fracture is union of the fracture without impairment of the function of the limb, either immediately or remotely. The generally accepted methods of treating fractures do not give satisfactory results in many cases. There is a need for a radical departure in the treatment of closed fractures. Anesthesia and the X-ray afford the means of accurate diagnosis. Sepsis is practically abolished. From analogy in excisions and osteotomy, closed fractures of bone may safely be treated by open incision. The cases reported in the literature, expressing the opinions of many surgeons, demonstrate that the open method of treatment is satisfactory and an advance upon generally accepted methods.*
>
> *Under these circumstances, it is fair to state that closed fractures should be treated by open incision and internal fixation, when other methods fail to secure reduction and immobilization. The open method*

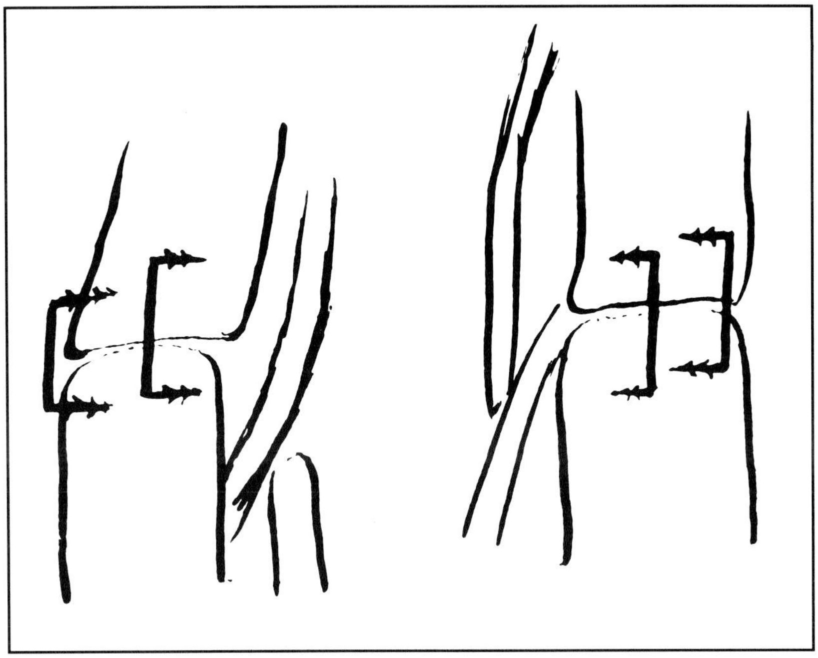

Figure 5.16 The first staples used for the internal fixation of fractures had barbs. From Jacoel, "Une agrafe pour sutures osseuses," *Presse méd* (December 25, 1901): 143.

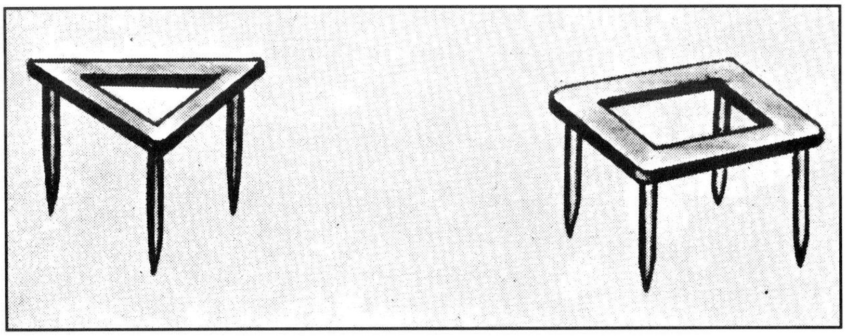

Figure 5.17 Lambotte's gold-plated staples. From W. S. Bickham, *Operative Surgery*, (Philadelphia: W. B. Saunders, 1924), 2:369.

will then be used more and more in oblique fractures of the diaphysis of long bones, in complicated fractures about joints; in all fractures associated with injury to nerve trunks, with injury to great blood-vessels, and associated with threatening gangrene.[35]

L. W. Steinbach reported on a series of patients with tibial fractures treated by internal fixation using silver plates and galvanized steel screws that same year.[36] In 1906 Edward Martin discussed the technical problems of internal fixation very extensively.[37] By 1912 Joseph A. Blake could report the results for 106 patients with fractures treated by operations using wires, nails, screws, dowels, pins, and plates.[38] Emil H. Beckman at the Mayo Clinic was an ardent follower of Lane and believed that plates were the preferred method

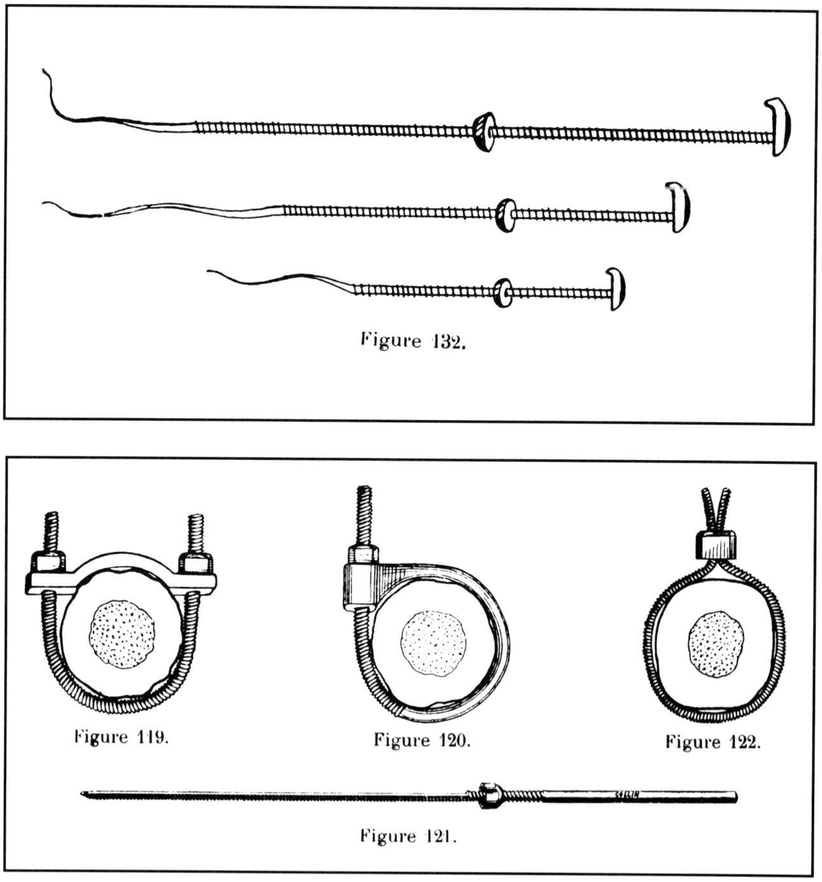

Figures 5.18a,b Cerclage with flexible threaded pins. From Milne, "Remarks," *Clin J. B. Murphy* 2(1913): 229–34.

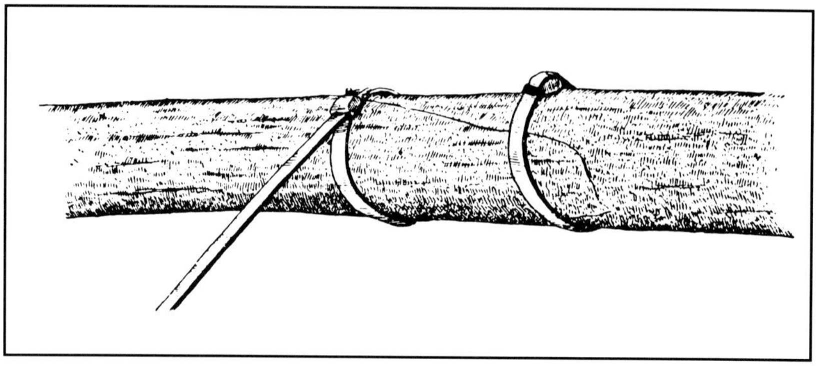

Figure 5.19 Putti's band. From F. W. Parham, "Circular Constriction in the Treatment of Fractures," *SGO* 23(1916): 541–44.

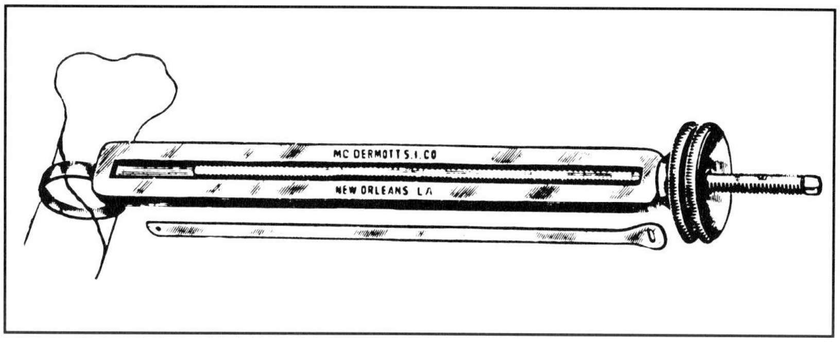

Figure 5.20 The Parham-Martin band. From Parham, "Circular Constriction in the Treatment of Fractures," *SGO* 23(1916): 541–44.

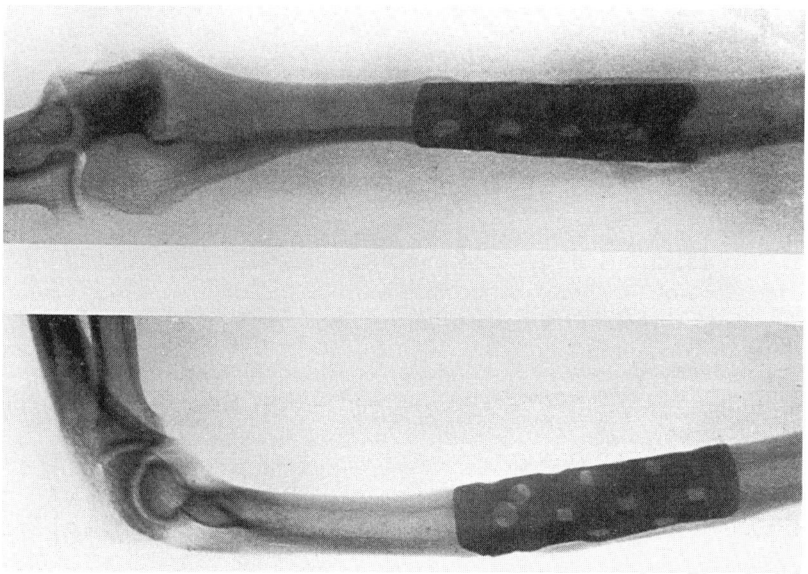

Figure 5.21 The "manchon" or muff of Contremoulins. From A. Moruzi, *Synthèse et prosthèse osseuses* (Paris: G. Doin, 1929), facing p. 82.

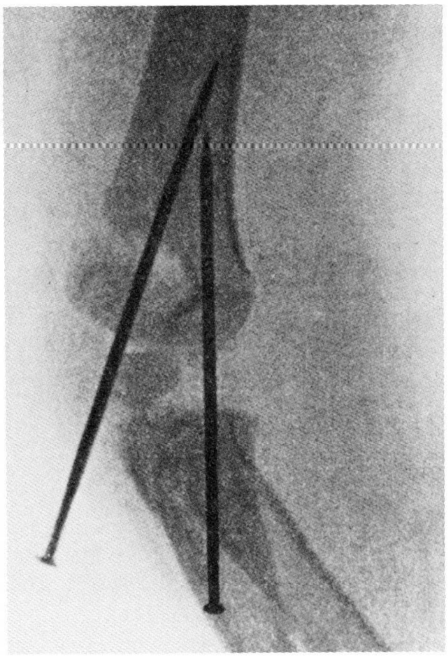

Figure 5.22 Closed reduction and pin fixation of a supracondylar fracture of the humerus. From Niehans, "Zur Fracturebehandlung durch temporare Annagelung," *Arch klin Chir* 73(1904): 167–78.

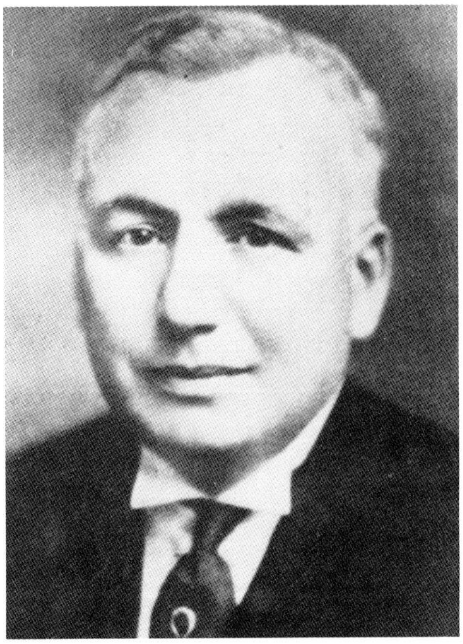

Figure 5.23 William O'Neill Sherman (1880-1979) did the most to popularize internal fixation in the United States. From C. S. Venable and W. G. Stuck, *The Internal Fixation of Fractures* (Springfield, Ill.: Charles C Thomas, 1947), 15.

of fixation for diaphyseal fractures.[39] Harry Mitchell Sherman and D. Tait studied screw fixation for articular fractures in dogs and cats and reported favorably on their experience with the method in treating articular and periarticular fractures in patients.[40]

William O'Neill Sherman (1880 1979), did the most to popularize internal fixation in the United States[41] (figure 5.23). His indications for operation included 1) closed fractures which could not be treated satisfactorily by means of splints, traction, etc. (including fractures of both bones of the forearm); 2) open fractures; 3) irreducible fractures; and 4) malunited fractures.[42] He favored the use of steel plates and screws because of their ease of application and the anatomical reduction that could be obtained. Operations were delayed until seven to ten days after injury because he believed that the local conditions at the fracture site were most favorable at that time. Postoperatively, the limbs were protected by splints. Passive and active assisted motion and massage began about three weeks after operation. Sherman was unhappy with the quality of the bone plates available because he had experienced breakage during the immediate postoperative period. As the surgeon for the Carnegie Steel Company of Pittsburgh, he was in an ideal position to experiment with better metal alloys and to use them in the manufacture of appliances whose design was based on engineering principles. He was able to devise plates made from a vanadium steel alloy and introduced self-tapping screws of the same material designed to fit into the holes of the plates[43] (figure 5.24). His search for improved metal alloys and his application of engineering principles in the design of the implants were major contributions.

Lane's successor among the English surgeons in the field of the operative treatment of fractures was Ernest W. Hey-Groves (1872–1944) (figure 5.25). He was trained at St. Bartholomew's Hospital, London, and practiced in Bristol, where he occupied the chair of surgery. In spite of a busy practice, he found time to perform anatomical and experimental studies of some importance. From the anatomical studies came his operation for the repair of the anterior cruciate ligament of the knee,[44] and from the experimental studies, which dealt with fracture healing, came improvement in fixation devices. He was a pioneer in the development of intramedullary fixation, interfragmentary fixation and the use of double onlay plates (figures 5.26, 5.27) He introduced the use of curved plates for better apposition to the diaphysis.[45] The holes in these plates were aligned in such a manner that the screws transfixed the bone on different radii for better fixation. His book *On Modern Methods of Treating Fractures* was based upon his experiments and his clinical experience and was prescient in some of its conclusions:[46]

The operative treatment of fractures should aim at completely counteracting this displacing force. It should not only accurately replace the fragments, but do so in such a mechanically efficient way that displace-

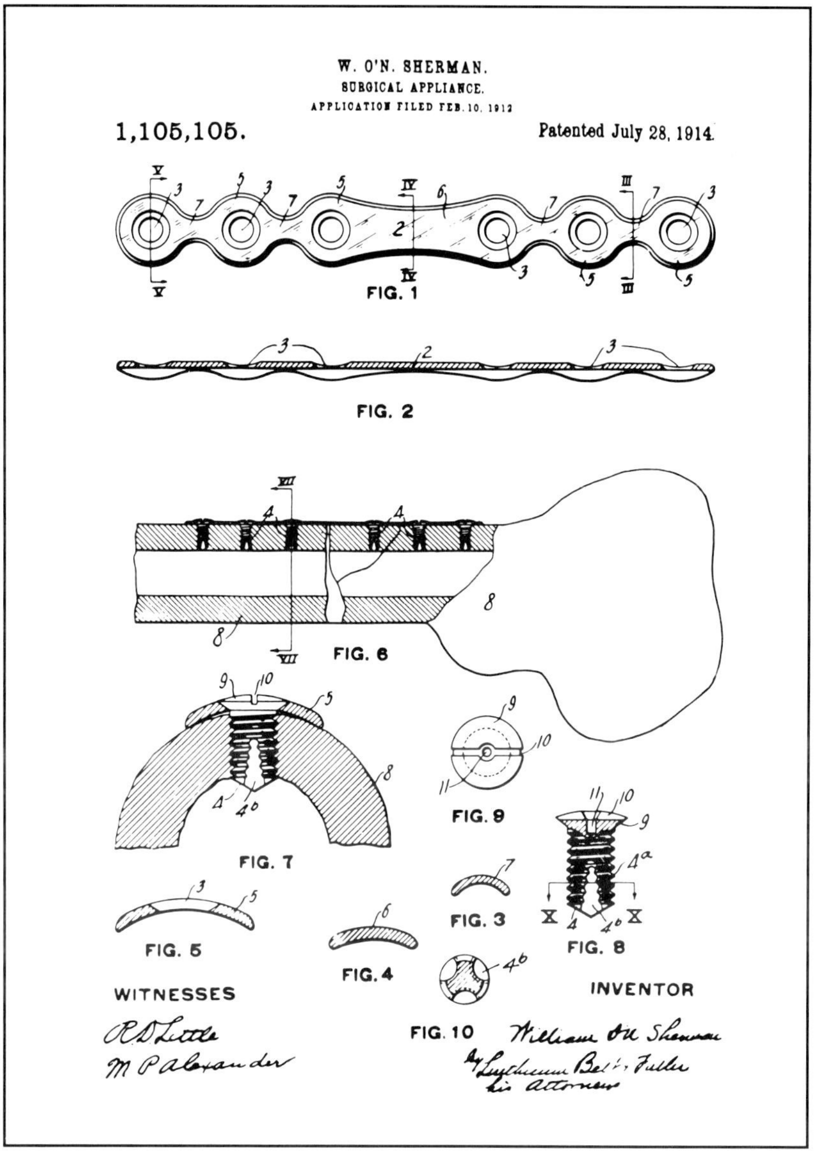

Figure 5.24 The Sherman plate and self-tapping screw. From Sherman, "Vanadium Steel Bone Plates and Screws," *SGO* 14(1912): 629.

ment cannot occur. The mere presence of an aseptic indifferent foreign body in the tissues has no effect on their healing, unless there is an interposition of its substance between structures which ought to unite. That the frictional grip between a bone and a screw will rapidly give way if subjected to too much tension owing to absorption of bone. Mechanical efficiency in the direct operative treatment of fractures can be obtained in two ways: a. by the use of long plates, pins, or bolts which transfix and hold the bone by some broad flanges or nut; and b. by the use of strong solid intramedullary pegs. Perfect anatomical union and normal function usually result from either of the above methods. Normal sound rapid repair is perfectly consistent with absolute rigidity.[47]

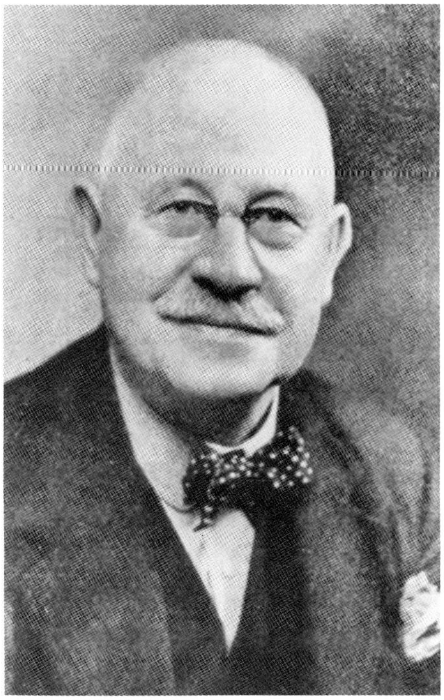

Figure 5.25 Ernest W. Hey-Groves (1872–1944). From "E. W. Hey-Groves," obituary, *J Bone Joint Surg* 27(1945): 340.

It is not surprising that closed methods of treating fractures would come under close scrutiny as a result of the double impact of the introduction of the X ray and surgical techniques for open reduction and internal fixation. At the annual meeting of the British Medical Association in 1910, a committee was appointed and charged "to report on the ultimate results obtained in the treatment of simple fractures with or without operation." More than 2,900 cases were reviewed, only 208 of which had been treated by surgical methods. The committee consulted with experts advocating a wide variety of approaches to the treatment of fractures including Lane, Lambotte, Fritz Steinmann, Bernhard Bardenheur, and Lucas-Championnière. Its report, published in 1912 contained some very interesting conclusions. For example:

> *It is possible either by non-operative or by operative treatment to obtain a high percentage of good results in children. In comparison with the non-operative results in children, the aggregate results of non-operative treatment in those past childhood are not satisfactory.*

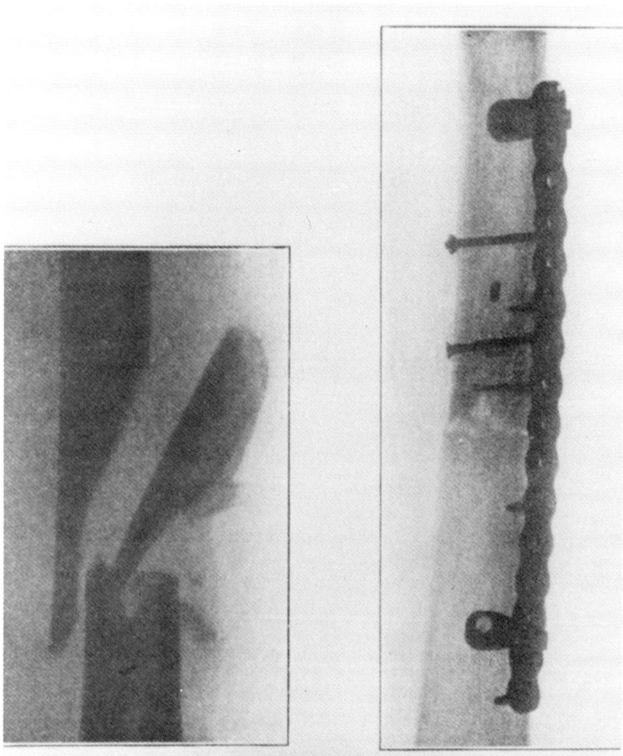

Figure 5.26 Interfragmentary fixation with neutralization plate. "Femur of Lt. Jones before operation. Same bone after operation. The large loose fragment was twisted round and had to be replaced. It was bolted to the upper fragment and this was then fixed to the lower by a clipped plate." From Hey-Groves, "Ununited Fractures," in *Orthopaedic Surgery of Injuries*, ed. Robert Jones (London: Oxford University Press, 1921), 1:139.

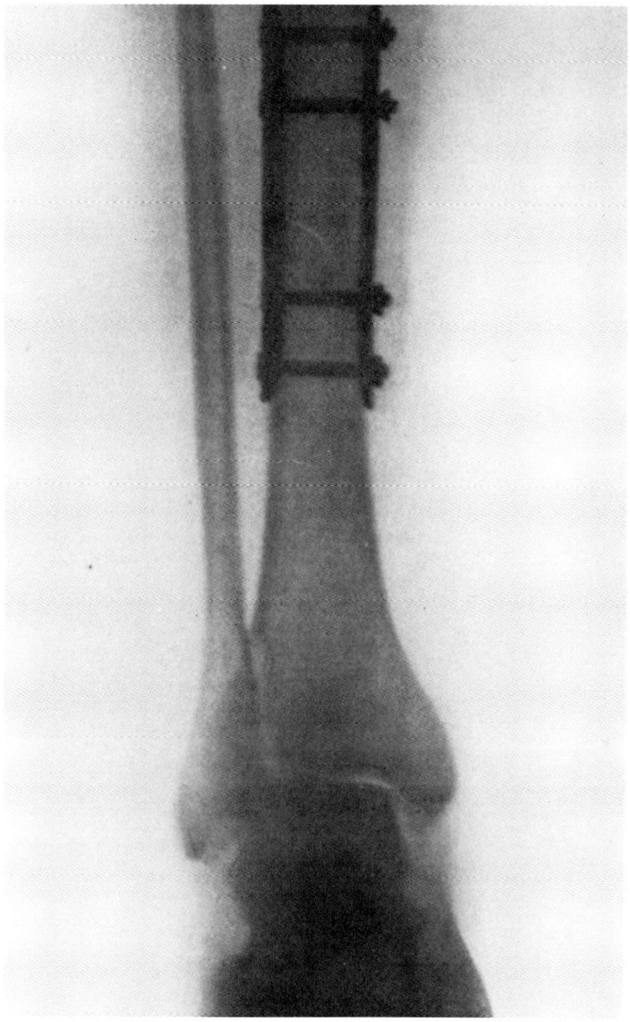

Figure 5.27 Double onlay plating. From Hey-Groves, *Modern Methods of Treating Fractures* (London: John Wright & Sons, 1916), 206.

In nearly all age groups, operative cases show a higher percentage of good results than non-operative cases.

Although the functional result may be good with an indifferent anatomical result, the most certain way to obtain a good functional result is to secure a good anatomical result. No method, whether non-operative or operative, which does not definitely promise a good anatomical result, should be accepted as the method of choice. For this reason mobilization and massage by themselves have not been found to secure a high percentage of good results. They are, however, valuable supplementary methods of treatment. Similarly, of operative methods, those which secure reposition and absolute fixation of the fragments yield better results than methods which fall short of this; imperfect fixation of the fragments by wire or other suture has been found to be an unsatisfactory procedure in the treatment of fractures of the long bones, with the exception of the olecranon process of the ulna.

Operative treatment should not be regarded as a method to be employed in consequence of the failure of non-operative measures, as the results of secondary operations compare very unfavorably with those of immediate operations.

In order to secure the most satisfactory results from operative treatment, it should be resorted to as soon as after the accident as practicable. It is necessary to insist that the operative treatment of fractures requires special skill and experience and such facilities and surroundings as will ensure asepsis. It is, therefore, not a method to be undertaken except by those who have constant practice and experience in such surgical procedures.[48]

Immediately following the publication of the committee's report, Robert Jones commented on it at considerable length, supporting the efficient use of non-operative "mechanical" methods of treatment where indicated:

The authors of the report call upon us to bear in mind, that the operative treatment of fractures is yet in its infancy . . . Non-operative treatment, on the other hand, is thoroughly established. This statement should be modified, for in a progressive science nothing ever is thoroughly established. Before we reach to new things we must ask ourselves if we have done the best by the old; and it is only by being critics of our own work that we can discover, each for himself, which procedure will in his own hands give the best results. We owe a debt of gratitude to Arbuthnot Lane. He has roused the surgical world from apathy on this question, and I feel assured that the reawakening will be to our common good, to the perfecting of our mechanical methods and the improvement of our operative technique.[49]

At the meeting of the American Surgical Assocation in 1912, it was resolved "That the president appoint a committee to prepare a statement of the relative value of the operative and non-operative treatment of fractures of the long bones (closed and open) to which shall be added an opinion as to the value of radiography in the determination of the choice of the method of treatment." Delayed by World War I, the final committee report did not appear until 1921.[50] Among its conclusions were that

neither the non-operative nor the operative method is to be recommended exclusively. Each has its indications and should be employed when required. Generally speaking the age period under fifteen years is the period in which non-operative methods are especially effectual. The open method when adopted should be employed early. It may be used at any age period, except in senile cases, whenever a skiagram [X-ray] shows a deformity or a position of the fragments which obviously cannot be reduced or when proper efforts at reduction and retention have proved unavailing. Some form of rigid plate applied directly to the bone seems to be the best fixation method in operative cases. Open operations for multiple fractures should be undertaken only by experienced surgeons who are thoroughly equipped by training and who have proper instruments and apparatus to meet all the possible indications of the operation.[51]

The reports of these two important committees clearly show that the operative treatment of fractures had become an established method of treatment. Why then was the further development of these methods delayed for so many years? The reports themselves acknowledged that the operative treatment required specially trained surgeons, operating under optimal conditions, with an expensive and complicated armamentarium. The battlefields of World War I could provide none of these. Instead, inadequate numbers of poorly trained surgeons provided care for enormous numbers of patients with fractures under less than optimal, even appalling, conditions. Only the simplest methods could be used safely. The disruption caused by World War I and the economic depression that followed arrested the momentum that was necessary for continued progress. When interest in the operative treatment of fractures gradually rekindled, new developments fell, generally, into four major areas; the treatment of hip fractures, intramedullary fixation, compression as an aid to fracture fixation, and the development of suitable metal alloys.

The successful application of surgical techniques in the treatment of hip fractures was delayed because of difficulties in arriving at an accurate diagnosis. Although pathologists at the autopsy table had observed that most extracapsular (lateral) fractures healed, albeit with deformity, and that most intracapsular (medial) fractures did not, clinicians at the bedside could not differentiate regularly between these two major categories. This ambiguity was not resolved until after the introduction of the hip X ray—and, in fact, much later, since adequate lateral X rays of the hip were not readily available until the 1930s. As a result, although there is extensive early literature dealing with the fixation of fresh and ununited hip fractures with metal nails and bone pegs, most of it is anecdotal in character[52] (figure 5.28).

Nicholas Senn of Milwaukee was the first surgeon to seriously consider the question of internal fixation in fractures of the neck of the femur. At the meeting of the American Surgical Association at Coney Island in 1882, he presented the specimen of a patient who had died two years following an impacted fracture of the neck of the femur. The fracture had solidly united.[53] The surgeons in the audience reacted with skepticism and disbelief. Returning to the attack at the next meeting of the same group the following year, Senn came prepared with a massive amount of data, including references to fifty-four cases of healed intracapsular hip fractures and a report of a large series of animal experiments.[54] Using cats and dogs, he had produced intracapsular hip fractures by drilling multiple small holes in the neck of the femur and breaking it through by manipulation. The animals

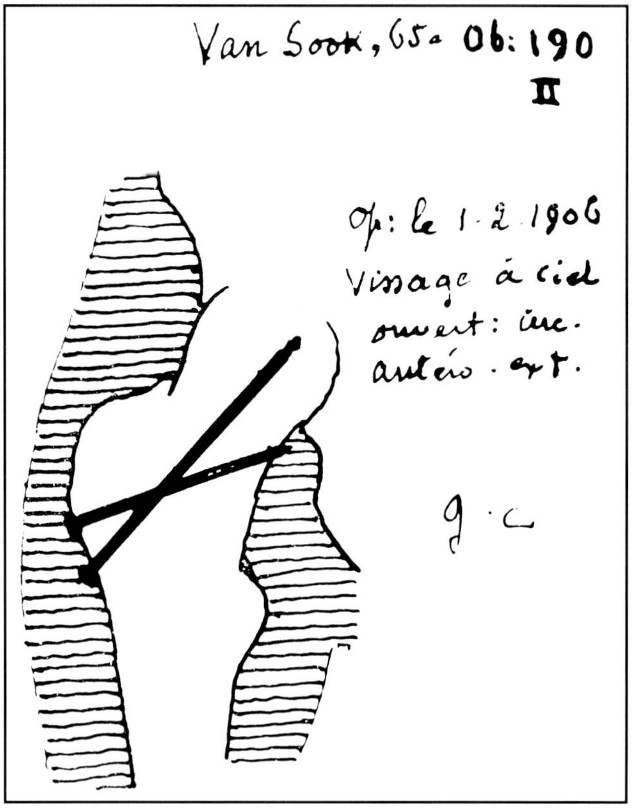

Figure 5.28 Lambotte's hip-nailing, 1906. From Lambotte, *Les débuts de l'ostéosynthèse*, (N.p.: n.p., n.d.), 108.

were divided into three different groups: 1) untreated; 2) treated by reduction and immobilization in a spica of plaster of paris; and 3) treated by reduction and pinning of the fractures with a nail of iron or pegs of ivory or bone. Of the eight animals in the third group, two became infected while six proceeded to solid union. On the basis of his experiments, Senn suggested that displaced fractures of the neck of the femur be treated by 1) immediate reduction of the fracture under anesthesia; 2) fixation in a plaster of paris spica; 3) lateral pressure over the greater trochanter (i.e., impaction); and 4) direct fixation of the fracture with a bone peg. Of the last step, he said, "The operation offers no great technical difficulties in its execution and, if done under strict antiseptic precautions, does not expose the patient to any additional risks." This paper was received much like its predecessor. During the heated discussion that followed its presentation, Senn is quoted as saying: ". . .any person who can hit the head of the femur in a cat will certainly not miss it in the operating room on the human subject." As a result of a flood of criticism, Senn did not attempt operative fixation in his patients, but contented himself with reduction, impaction, and fixation in a spica.[55]

In 1904 Royal Whitman revived and improved upon Senn's method.[56] In Europe this method was popularized by Otto Lofberg who, in a long-term follow-up of 306 patients with fractures of the neck of the femur, reported good osseous union in 67 percent.[57] Results obtained in the United States were not as satisfactory, however.[58] Frederic Jay Cotton had pointed out both the importance of slight over reduction of the fractures into a valgus position and the importance of impacting the fracture after reduction.[59] This experience with closed reduction and immobilization demonstrated that these difficult fractures would heal and challenged surgeons to develop effective methods of internal fixation. The technique of blind nailing or pegging through a small incision on the lateral aspect of the femur, even with the help of an anterior-posterior X ray, was not successful enough to be adopted widely. In 1912 Fred Houdlett Albee began to carry out an open reduction and bone-pegging through two incisions, one anterior and one lateral. This allowed him to reduce the fracture under direct vision and to ensure the proper placement of the peg in the neck and head of the femur[60] (figure 5.29). Hey-Groves utilized a similar method with pegs made of ivory, beef bone, or autogenous grafts.[61] Marius Nygaard Smith-Petersen devised a new approach to the hip joint, using one incision that gave full exposure anteriorly and laterally.[62] Using this incision, he reduced fractures of the neck of the femur and fixed them with a three-flanged nail.[63] He discarded the use of older style nails and pegs because of their bulk and their tendency to loosen:

> *To eliminate these two weak points, a flanged nail was devised which brought about absolute fixation in all directions and displaced a minimum amount of bone. Because of its flanges, the nail is gripped by the cortex of the bone so that there can be no rotation; because of its shape, the surface area is much greater than that of the ordinary nail and friction is proportionally increased; because of the minimum displacement of bone, there is less pressure necrosis surrounding it; consequently the fixation is sustained and complete, not temporary and partial*[64] [figure 5.30].

The open reduction and nailing of fractures of the neck of the femur rapidly gave way to closed reduction and nailing under X-ray control. This was the result of improvements in the fracture tables, which permitted good lateral X rays of the hip to be taken, better methods of closed reduction of the fractures, and the introduction of cannulated nails.[65] Although H. Heyward Wescott had introduced a technique for closed nailing under X-ray control using the original flanged nail, it was quickly superseded by Sven Johansson's method using a cannulated nail[66] (figure 5.31). Fluoroscopy was used to observe reduction and nail placement in some clinics.[67] By 1938 the methods of closed reduction and nailing of femoral neck fractures were well established.[68]

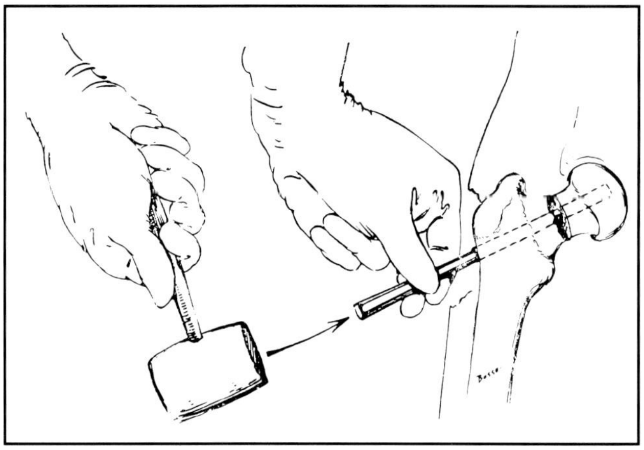

Figure 5.29 Hip-nailing by Albee's technique. From Albee, *Orthopedic and Reconstructive Surgery: Industrial and Civilian* (Philadelphia: W. B. Saunders, 1919), 609.

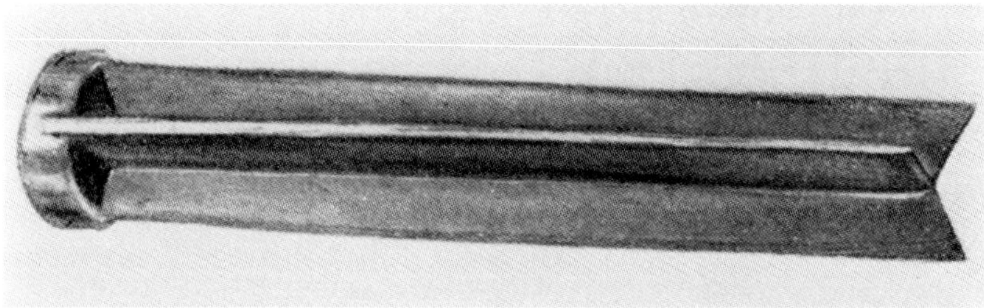

Figure 5.30 The Smith-Petersen nail. Note the absence of cannulation. From Smith-Petersen, et al., "Intracapsular Fractures of the Neck of the Femur," *AMA Arch Surg* 23(1931): 715–59.

Jacques Leveuf and Charles Girode present an excellent description of the technique used by Delbet for the closed reduction of hip fractures and fixation using only an anterior-posterior X ray.[69] Beginning in 1907, Delbet had developed this method using bone pegs and screws, singly or in combination (figures 5.32, 5.33). In the United States, Martin used the same approach, advocating fixation of the fractures with two wood screws.[70] The screw-bolt designed by Myron O. Henry was first inserted under direct vision using a pertrochanteric approach; percutaneous insertion under X-ray control was later adopted.[71] Robert K. Lippmann reviewed the subsequent evolution of Henry's screw-bolt in presenting his own[72] (figure 5.34). Further improvements in design were made by Danis (figure 5.35) and Charnley[73] (figure 5.36).

The use of multiple small pins for the fixation of the intracapsular hip fractures was introduced by D. R. Telson and N. S. Ransohoff.[74] Using local anesthesia, the fracture was reduced under X-ray control and fixed by the insertion of multiple pins. Further refinement of this method was carried out by F. J. Gaenslen[75] (figure 5.37). Specially designed pins for fixation were introduced by Knowles, Moore, and

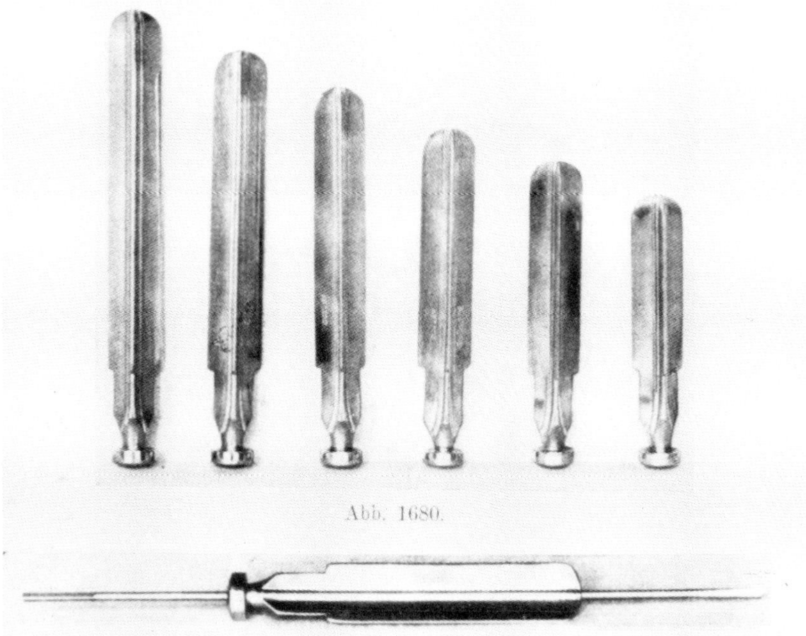

Figure 5.31 Böhler's modification of the triflanged nail. Note the wide flanges and the cannulation. From Lorenz Böhler, *Technik der Knochenbruchbehandlung im Frieden und im Kriege* (Vienna: W. Maudrich, 1943), 2:890.

Nystrom[76] (figures 5.38, 5.39). A very precise orientation of the pins that provided superior fixation of the fracture while at the same time allowing impaction of the fracture was achieved by William M. Deyerle[77] (figure 5.40).

The development of a prosthesis to replace the head of the femur in the treatment of fractures of the neck of the femur grew out of experience with resections and reconstructive operations for old injuries and diseases of the hip. In 1927 Hey-Groves described the use of a prosthesis made of ivory to replace the head of the femur[78] (figure 5.41). Austin T. Moore and Henry R. Bohlman used a metal prosthesis to replace the upper end of the femur in a patient with a giant cell tumor.[79] The technique of prosthetic replacement of the head of the femur was given impetus immediately following World War II by brothers Robert and Jean Judet in France, who designed a prosthesis made of methacrylate with a stem similar to that used by Hey-Groves[80] (figure 5.42). Modifications of this stemmed prosthesis were introduced in the United States by Earl McBride and J. E. M. Thomson .[81] It soon became apparent that the fixation of such prostheses in the femoral neck and greater trochanter was inadequate, and that support from a point further distally was essential. L. T. Peterson attempted to accomplish this by placing the ball on the end of a combination nail-plate screwed to the side of the femoral shaft.[82] Lippmann supported his stemmed prosthesis with an intramedullary nail.[83] However, the best devices were those designed by Moore and Frederick R. Thompson.[84] Made in one piece, the stems were seated in the medullary canal of the upper end of the femur (figure 5.43).

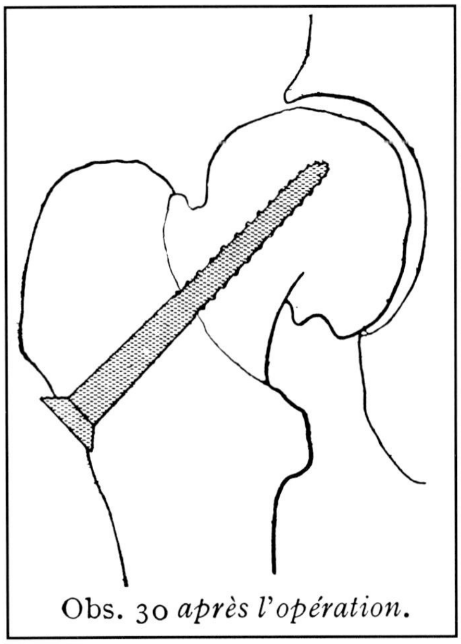

Figure 5.32 Delbet's hip screw. From Leveuf and Girode, *Le Traitement des fractures du col du fémur par la méthode du professeur Pierre Delbet* (Paris: Masson, 1927).

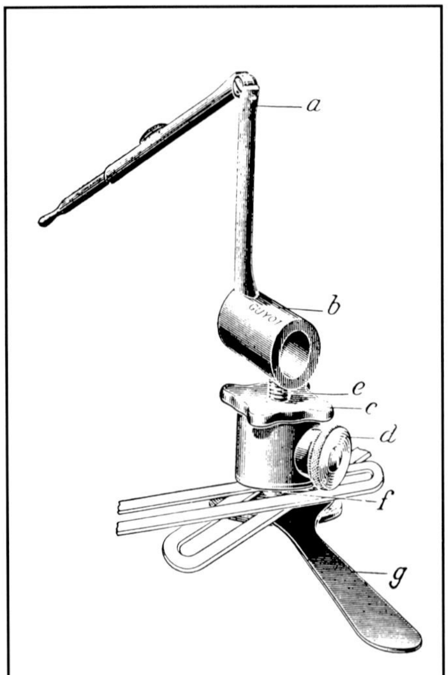

Figure 5.33 The "cannon of Delbet," the device used to direct the hip screw in the absence of a lateral X ray. From Leveuf and Girode, *Le Traitement des fractures.*

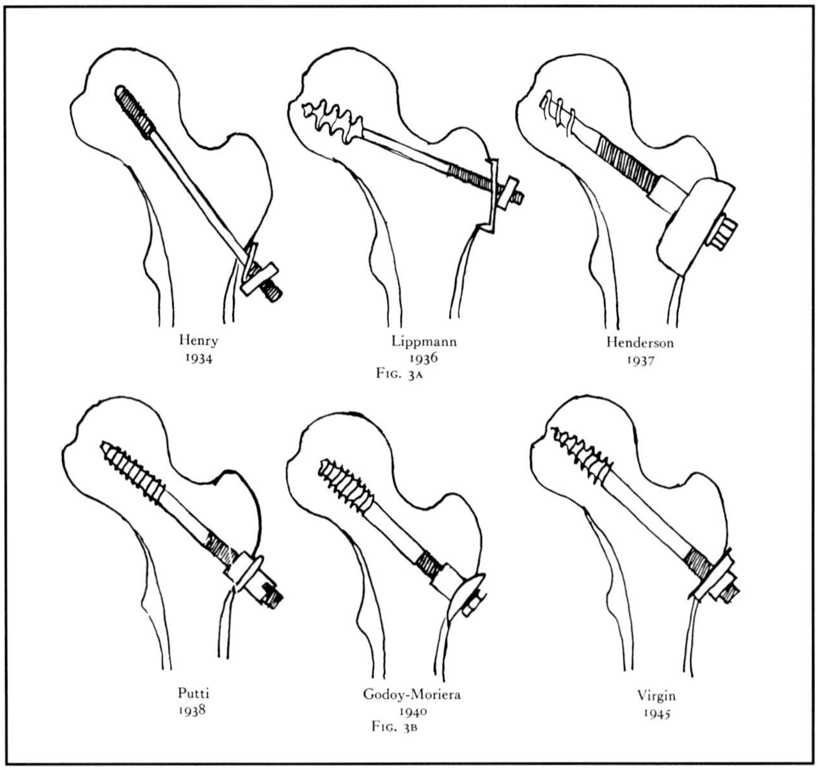

Figure 5.34 The evolution of the hip screw, showing the devices of Henry, Lippman, Henderson, Putti, Godoy-Morira, and Virgin. From R. K. Lipmann, "Recent Experiences with the Corkscrew Bolt in Fractures of the Hip," *Am J Surg* 78(1949): 54–64.

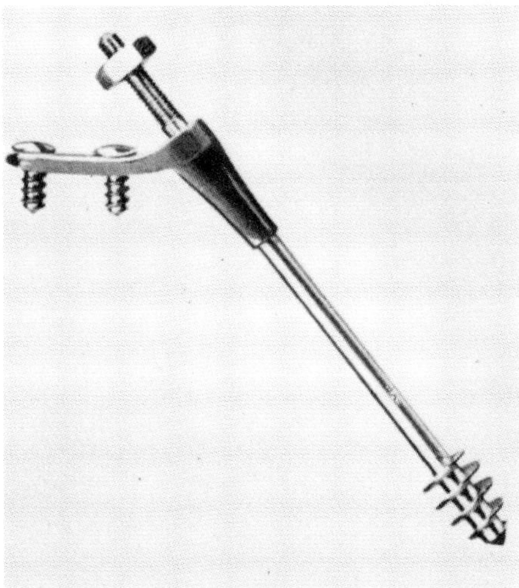

Figure 5.35 The compression hip screw of Danis. From Robert Danis, *Théorie et pratique de l'ostéosynthèse* (Paris: Masson, 1949).

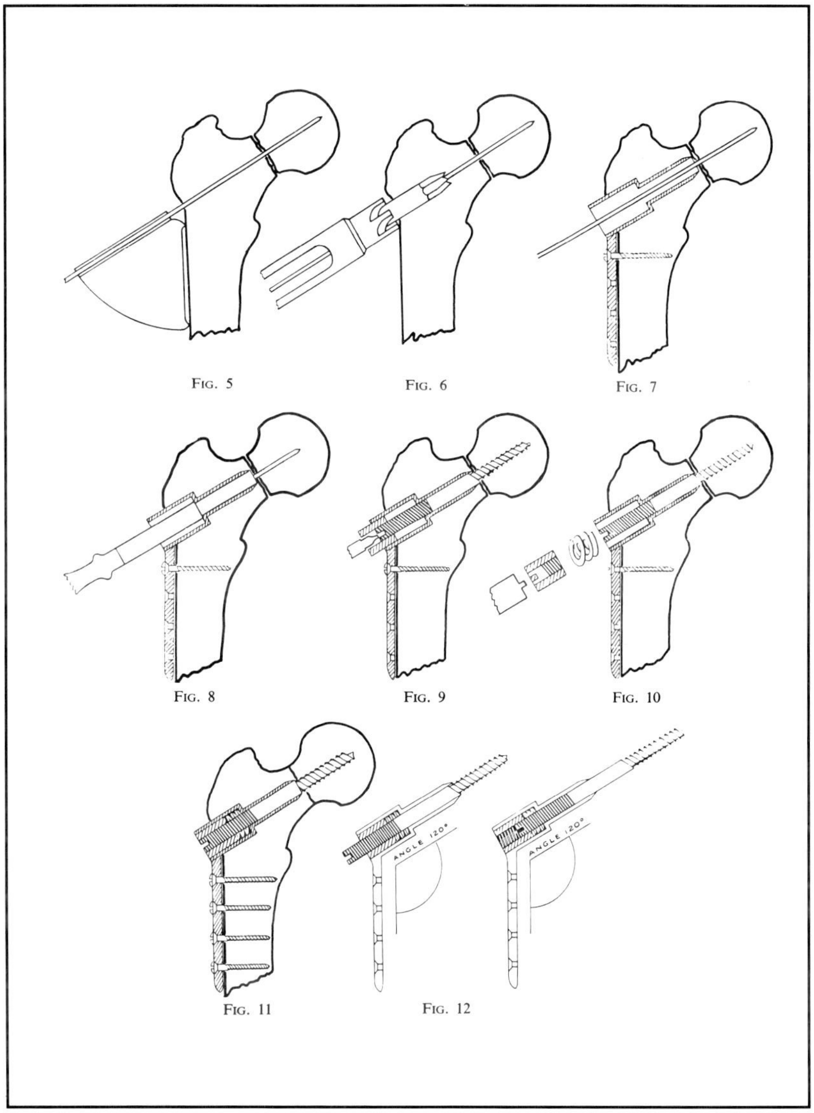

Figure 5.36 Charnley's compression hip screw. From John Charnley et al., "The Treatment of Displaced Fractures of the Neck of the Femur," *J Bone Joint Surg* 39B(1957): 45–65.

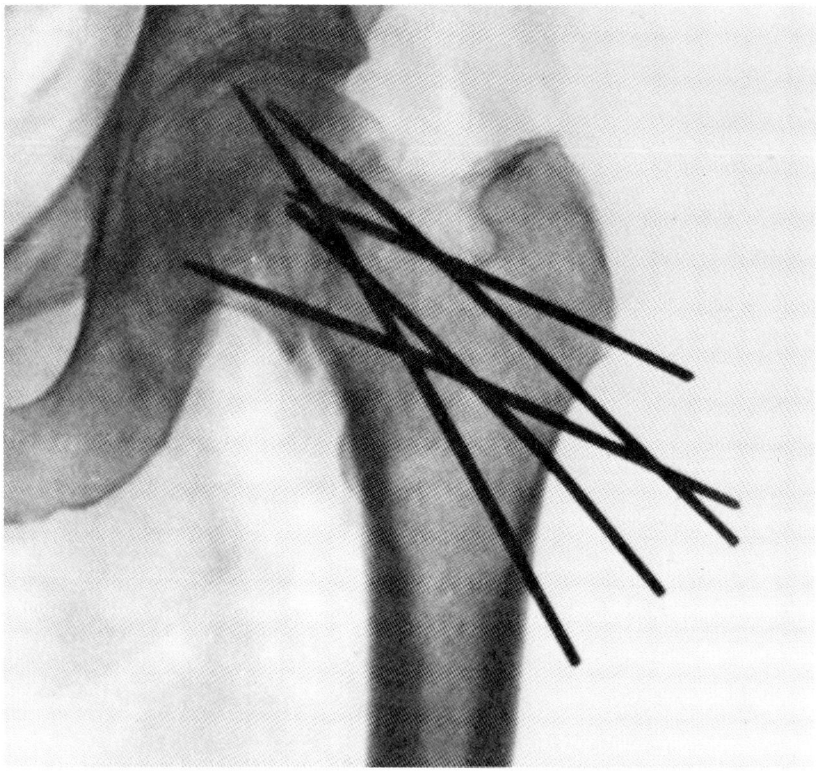

Figure 5.37 Fixation of an intracapsular hip fracture by means of multiple small pins. From Gaenslen, "Subcutaneous Spike Fixation of Fresh Fractures of the Neck of the Femur," *J Bone Joint Surg* 17(1935): 739–48.

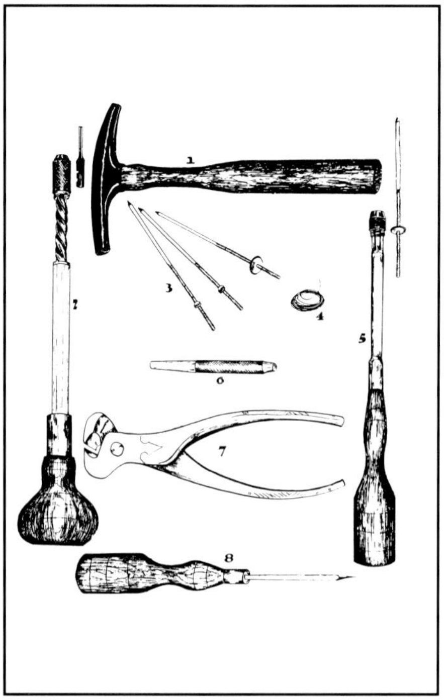

Figure 5.38 The armamentarium of Moore. From Austin Moore, "Fractures of the Hip Joint: Treatment by Extra-Articular Fixation with Adjustable Nails," *SGO* 64(1937): 420–36.

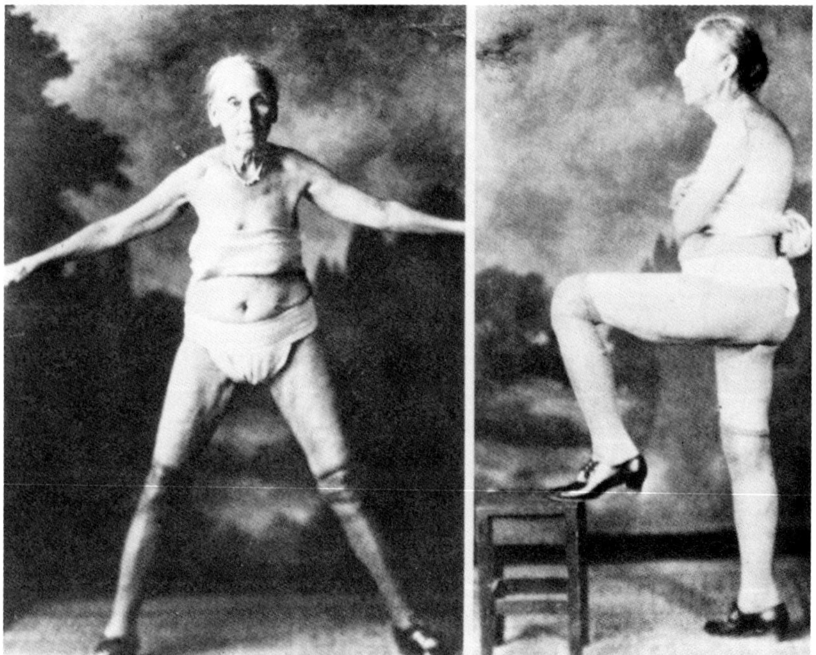

Figure 5.39 One of Moore's good results. From Moore, "Fractures of the Hip Joint," 420–36.

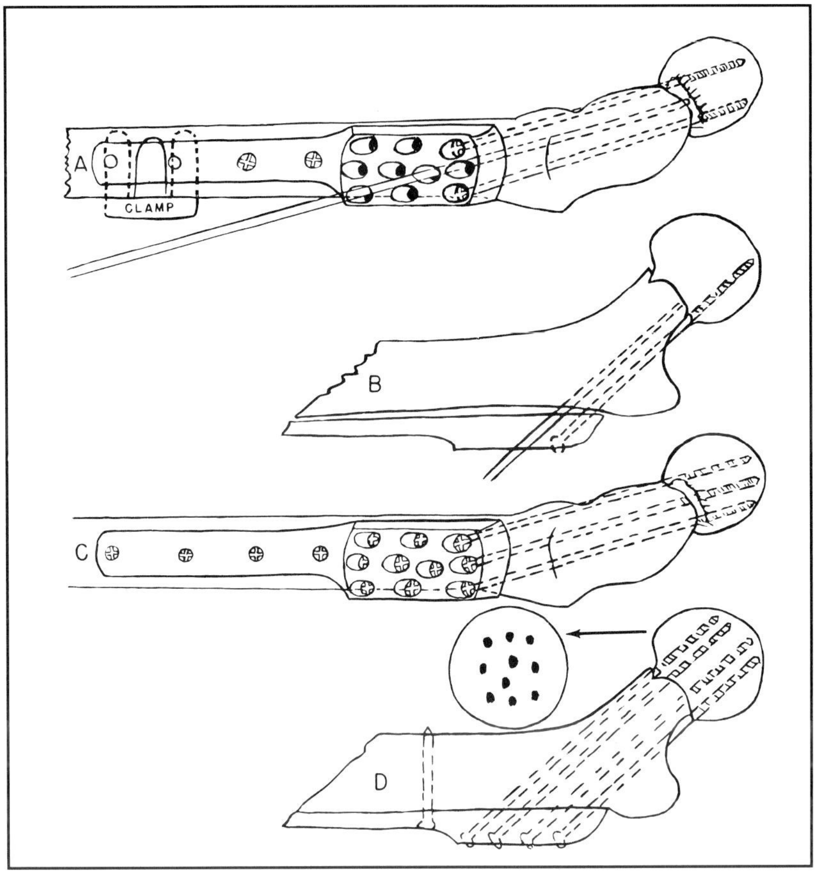

Figure 5.40 The Deyerle system for hip-pinning. From Deyerle, "Absolute Fixation with Contact Compression in Hip Fractures," *Clin Orthop* 13(1959): 279–97.

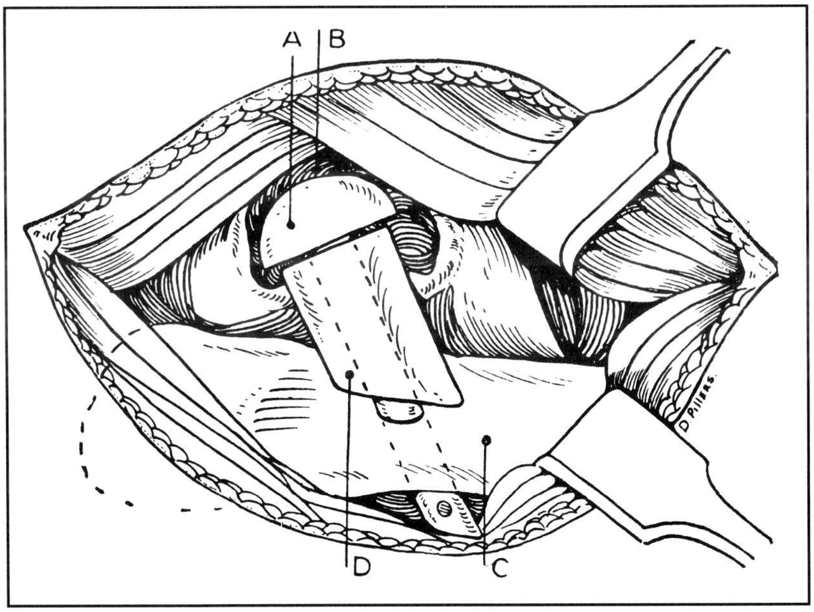

Figure 5.41 A femoral head prosthesis made of ivory used by Hey-Groves. From Hey-Groves, "Some Contributions to the Reconstructive Surgery of the Hip," *Brit J Surg* 14(1926–27): 486–517.

As early as 1914 it was appreciated that fixation with a peg, nail, or screw was insufficient to prevent varus displacement for extracapsular (lateral) fractures of the hip, and M. E. Preston introduced a nail with a side-plate (figure 5.44). Further improvements were delayed for many years, however. In 1934 Lawson Thornton began to use a Smith-Petersen nail to which a side-plate could be bolted[85]. E. L. Jewett described the combination of a Smith-Petersen nail welded onto a Hawley plate (figure 5.45),[86] while Alonzo J. Neufeld used a light nail-plate combination made of one piece of metal[87] (figure 5.46). Initial problems of breakage with these devices led to improvements in design and fabrication. Nail-plate combinations permitting impaction and settling were the work of Ernst Pohl (figure 5.47), W. A. Pugh (figure 5.48), and William K. Massie.[88]

The idea of stabilizing diaphyseal fractures by inserting a device into the medullary canal is an old one. It can be discerned dimly in the *enclavement* of Bérenger-Féraud.[89] Early proponents of the idea were Senn and H. Bircher.[90] There were, however, two basic problems to be solved before the method could become useful: finding the best material for the device, and developing the technique of insertion. When short pegs were used, ivory, bone, and horn served the purpose (figure 5.49). As the length of the pegs increased, these brittle materials gave way to metal rods. These, too, had limitations until suitable metal alloys and designs were developed. The technical problems of inserting the devices across the fracture line were difficult.

In 1913 Georg Schone described his method of internally fixing fractures of the radius and ulna using a long, flexible silver pin, 2.8 to 4.0 mm in diameter, introduced into the medullary canal at a distance from the fracture site.[91] Under fluoroscopic control, the fracture was reduced and the pin was advanced across the fracture into the other fragment (figure 5.50). Opening the fracture was necessary only in cases of distal radius fracture and in old fractures. Schone emphasized that the pin should be sufficiently long and should fit snugly into the medullary cavity.

The year previously, Hey-Groves had reported his results from animal experiments and with human patients using pegs made of bone and metal. Some of the pegs had a small cross-piece in the middle to keep them from slipping too far into the medullary canal. Others had a wire sling attached to them that allowed them to be inserted completely into one fragment and then drawn up into the second fragment after the fracture was reduced. He concluded:

The advantages of the intra-medullary peg method in the operative treatment of fractures may be summarized as follows:

1) *It can be easily and quickly performed.*

2) *It requires a very much smaller incision and less exposure of the soft parts.*

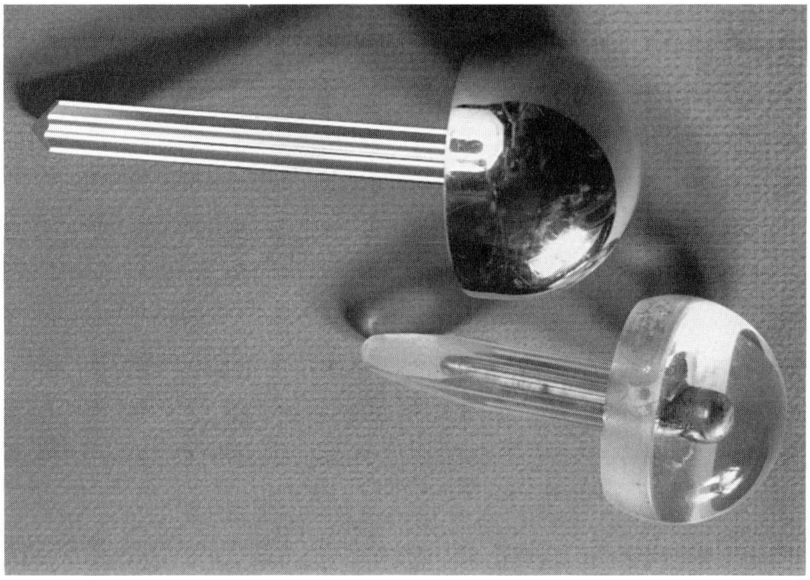

Figure 5.42 The acrylic stemmed hip prosthesis of the Judet brothers (bottom) and a later metallic counterpart.

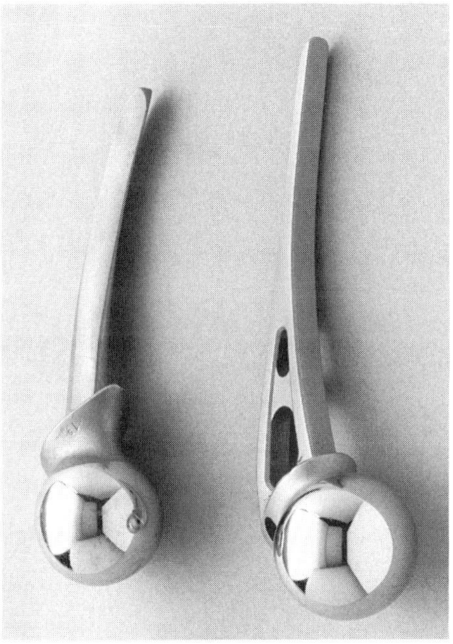

Figure 5.43 The intramedullary stemmed hip prostheses of Thompson (left) and Moore (right).

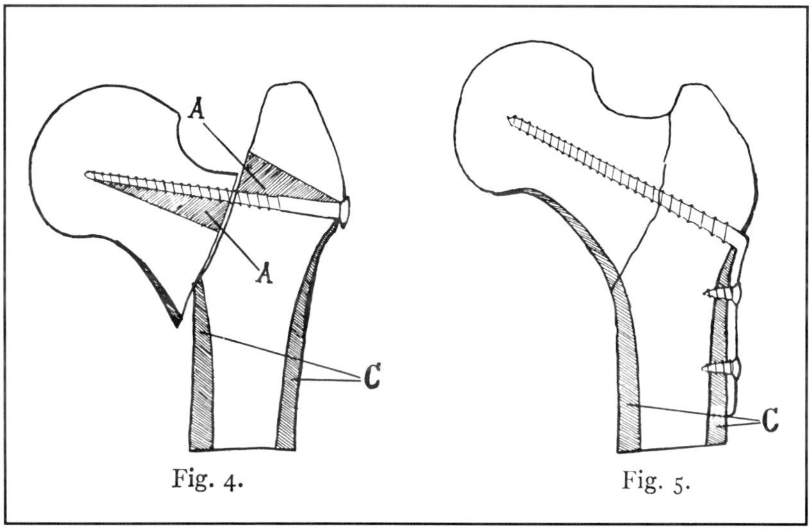

Figure 5.44 The nail-plate combination of Preston. From Preston, "New Appliance for the Internal Fixation of Fractures of the Femoral Neck," *SGO* 18(1914): 260–61.

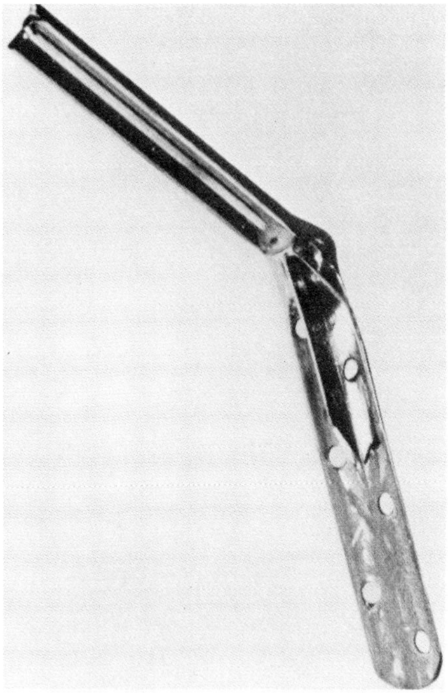

Figure 5.45 The Jewett nail-plate combination, which consisted initially of a three-flanged nail welded to a Hawley plate. From Jewett, "One-Piece Angle Nail for Trochanteric Fractures," *J Bone Joint Surg* 23(1941): 803–10.

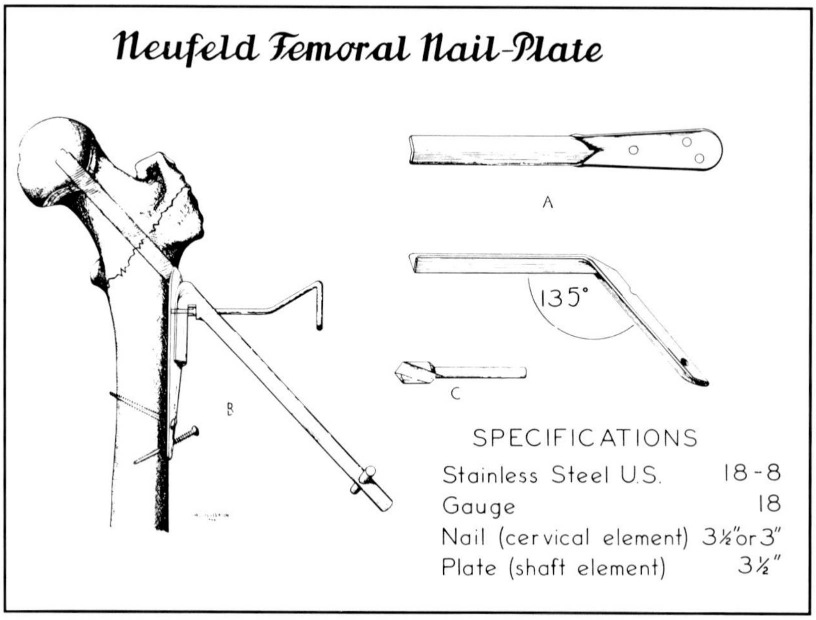

Figure 5.46 The one-piece nail-plate combination of Neufeld. From G. M. Taylor et al., "Internal Fixation for Intertrochanteric Fractures," *J Bone Joint Surg* 26(1944): 707–12.

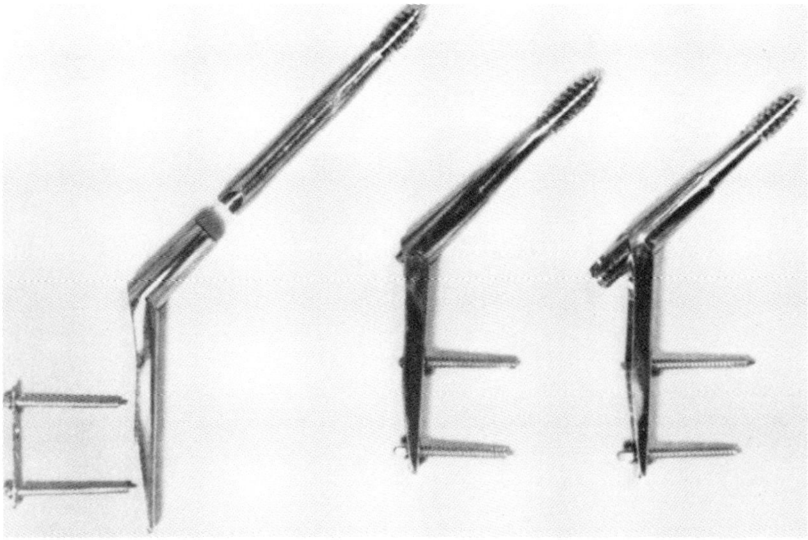

Figure 5.47 The sliding hip screw designed by Ernst Pohl of Kiel. From W. Schumpelick and P. N. Jantzen, "A New Principle in the Operative Treatment of Trochanteric Fractures of the Femur," *J Bone Joint Surg* 37A(1955): 693–98.

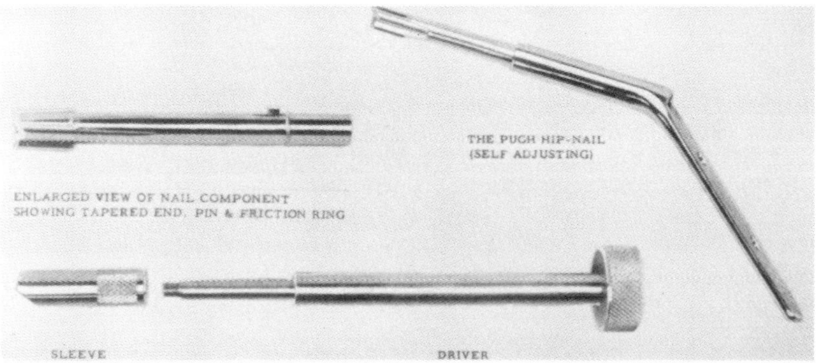

Figure 5.48 The sliding hip nail designed by Pugh. From Pugh, "A Self-Adjusting Nail-Plate for Fractures about the Hip Joint," *J Bone Joint Surg* 37A(1955): 1085–93.

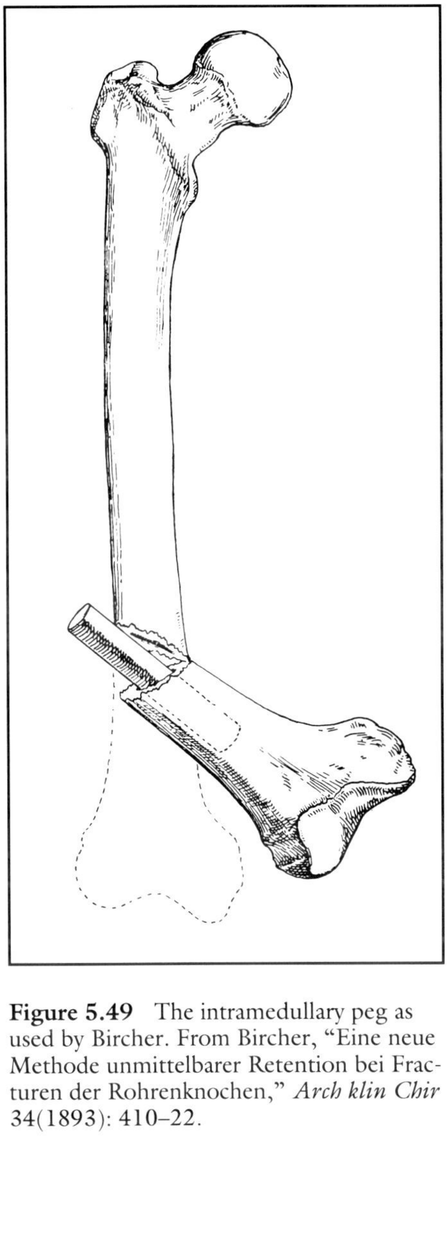

Figure 5.49 The intramedullary peg as used by Bircher. From Bircher, "Eine neue Methode unmittelbarer Retention bei Fracturen der Rohrenknochen," *Arch klin Chir* 34(1893): 410–22.

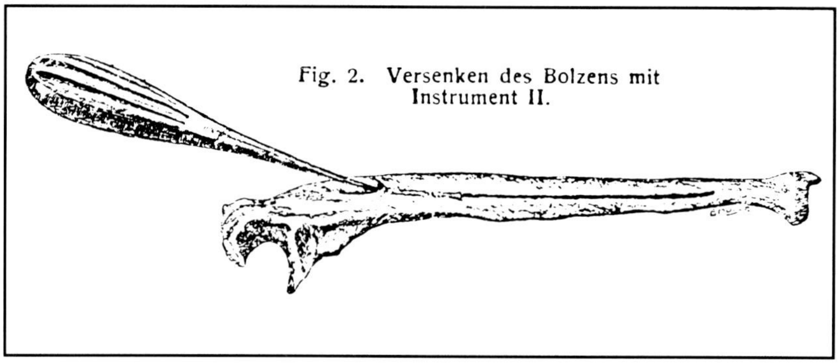

Figure 5.50 Closed intramedullary nailing of the ulna under fluoroscopic control. From Schone, "Zur Behandlung von Vorderarmfrakturen mit Bolzung," *Münch med Wschr* 60(1913): 2327–28.

> 3) *It involves a minimum of injury to the periosteum.*
>
> 4) *It adjusts the bone in the correct position.*
>
> 5) *It allows slight movements between the fragments which is beneficial for rapid union.*
>
> 6) *It makes the use of external splints unnecessary after operation and massage and movements are thus rendered possible as soon as the wound has healed.*[92]

Intramedullary bone pegs were also used to fix fractures in the United States, but, as in Britain, did not enjoy wide popularity.[93] Hey-Groves's technique for inserting pegs into the femur continued to evolve. By the end of World War I he had given up short pegs and was using long, solid metal rods or fenestrated metal tubes to fix complicated fractures[94] (figures 5.51, 5.52).

In spite of this promising start, the development of intramedullary fixation was slow. Lambotte described the use of intramedullary pins to fix metacarpal fractures in 1925[95]. However, interest in the use of bone pegs persisted.[96] It was not until the late 1930s that the use of intramedullary pins became firmly established.

In Meridian, Mississippi, in 1936, two brothers, Leslie V. and H. Lowry Rush, were challenged by the problem posed by a complicated Monteggia fracture. They responded by stabilizing it with a Steinmann pin inserted into the medullary canal of the ulna[97] (figure 5.53). The success of this initial case stimulated them to develop an intramedullary pinning system using flexible pins with "sled runner" points.[98] The stability of the fixation depended upon the dynamics of the prebent pins rather than tight fit in the medullary canal.[99] (figure 5.54). Fixation with these Rush pins was far superior to that obtained by C. Lambrinudi's and Gordon Murray's methods of using inramedullary Kirschner wires, while the intramedullary nails designed by F. P. Sage for use in the radius and ulna were never popular.[100] In addition to using single pins for intramedullary fixa-

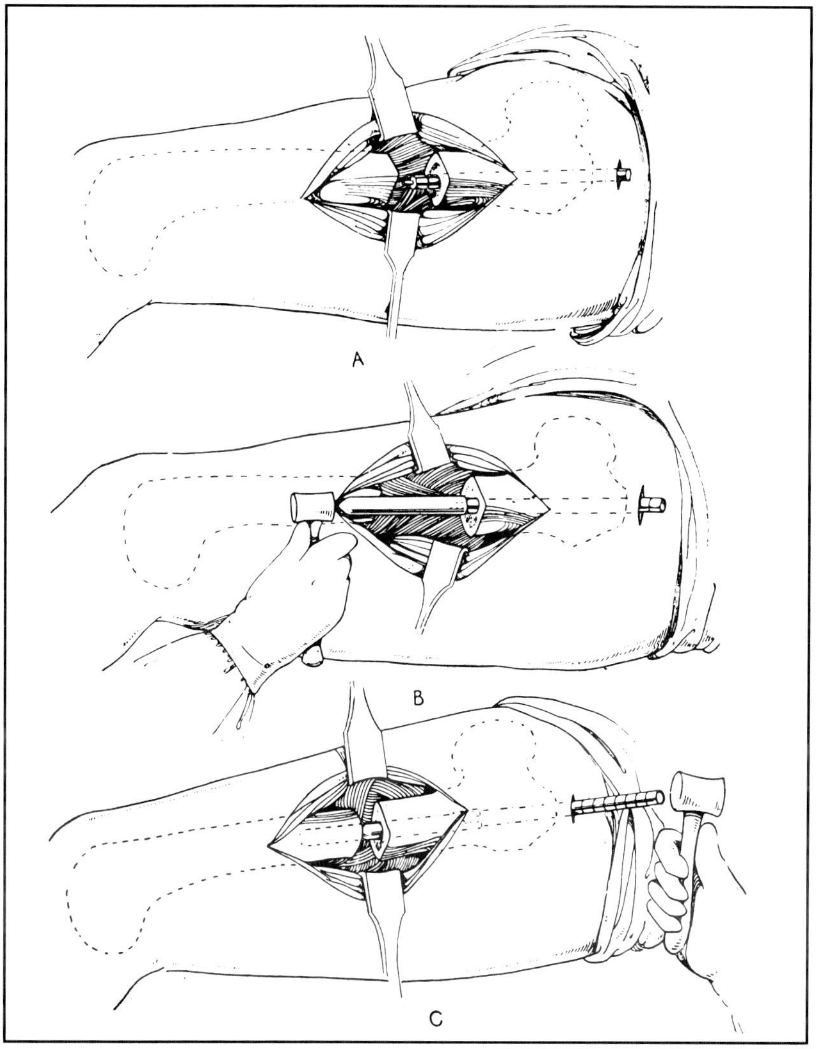

Figure 5.51 Hey-Groves's method of open retrograde intramedullary nailing of fractures of the shaft of the femur. From R. Watson-Jones, "Medullary Nailing of Fractures after 50 Years," *J Bone Joint Surg* 32B(1950): 694–729.

tion, the Rush brothers also used multiple pins, particularly in a technique for the fixation of supracondylar fractures of the femur.

At the same time that the Rush brothers were working out their methods of intramedullary fixation, Gerhard Kuntscher (1900-1972) was arriving independently at his own solution to the problem (figure 5.55). Kuntscher studied the biomechanics of the hip and the treatment of hip fractures in the clinic of the University of Kiel.[101] He concluded that the operation of hip-nailing for the fixation of intracapsular hip fractures was ideal. It was done through a small incision with a minimal risk of infection, the fracture site was not opened, and fixation was secure enough so that no external fixation was required. Why couldn't these principles be applied to other fractures?

Kuntscher's animal experiments convinced him that the endosteum was not important in fracture healing and that disruption of

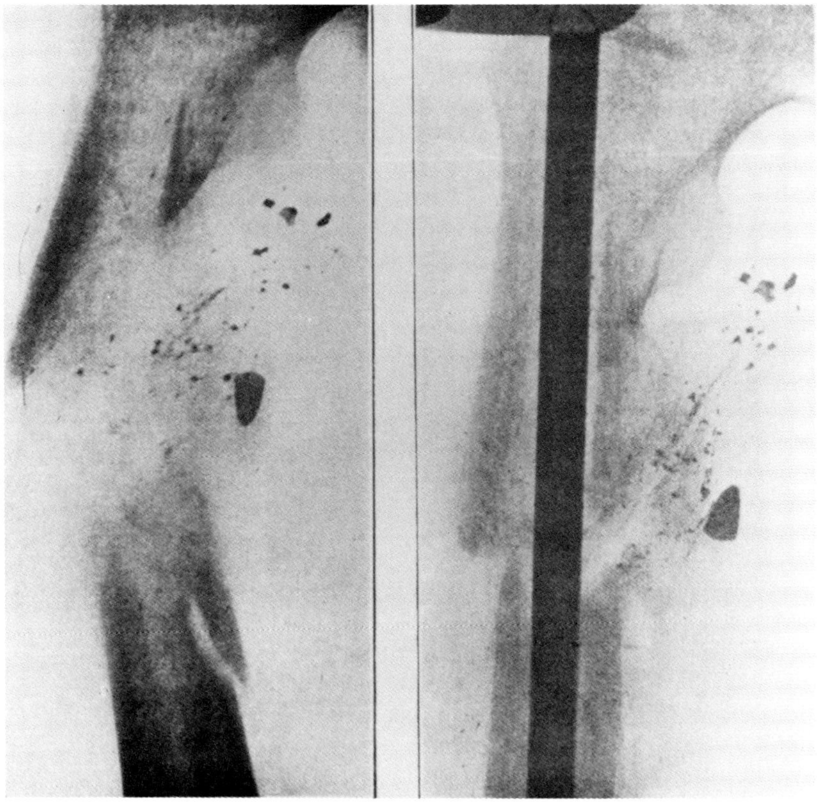

Figure 5.52 Intramedullary nailing of a gunshot fracture of the femur. From Hey-Groves, "Ununited Fractures," in *Orthopaedic Surgery*, ed. Jones (London: Oxford University Press, 1921), 1:154.

the endosteum with an intramedullary nail should not interfere with fracture healing. He established these conditions for a satisfactory method of intramedullary fixation:

> 1) *The fixation must be such, i.e., like a hip pinning, that function of the limb is not impaired.*
>
> 2) *The fixation should be accomplished without opening the fracture site through an incision as far from the fracture site as possible.*
>
> 3) *The fixation must provide satisfactory biomechanical conditions for callus formation.*[102]

By 1940 his technique for the intramedullary nailing of femoral shaft fractures had been perfected, and he reported the results in twelve patients (nine fractures, one pathological fracture, and two osteotomies) using nails of his own design made of V^2A steel. By the end of World War II, he had multiplied his techniques to include a wide variety of methods of intramedullary fixation that could be applied to all of the long bones.[103] An examination of his book, *Technik der Marknagelung* (figure 5.56), reveals that Kuntscher's concepts in addition to embracing intramedullary nailing with a

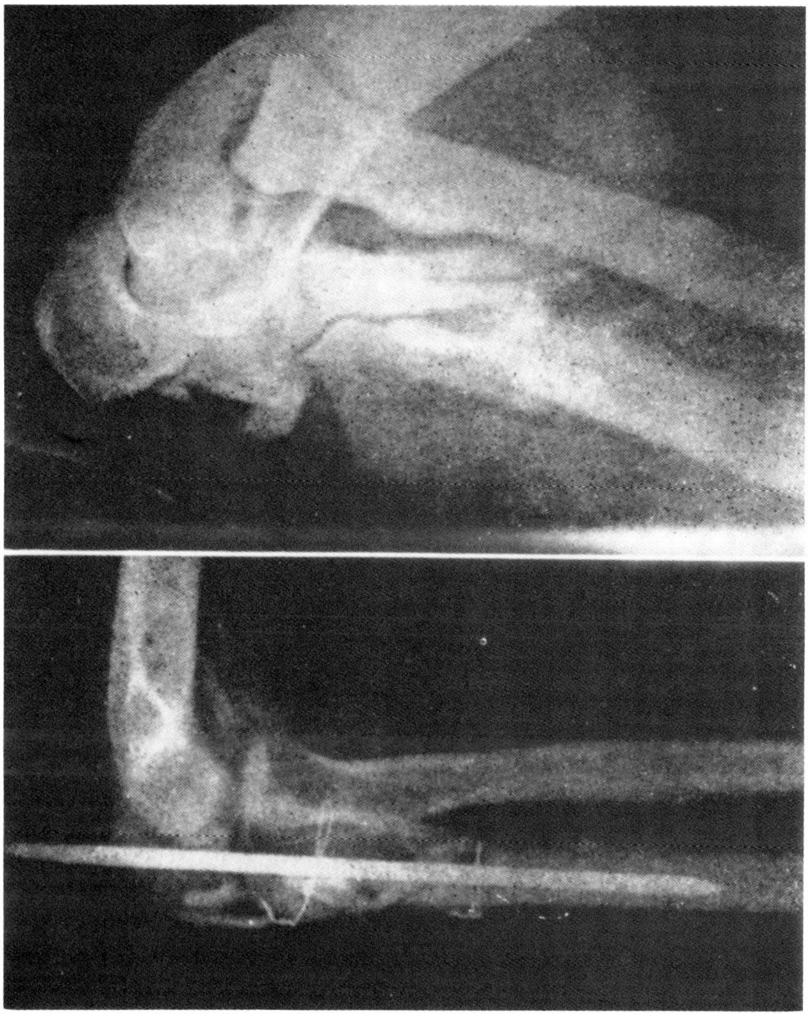

Figure 5.53 The first case treated by the Rush brothers by intramedullary pinning. From L. V. Rush, *Atlas of Rush Pin Techniques*, 2d ed. (Meridian, Miss.: Berivon, 1976), 1.

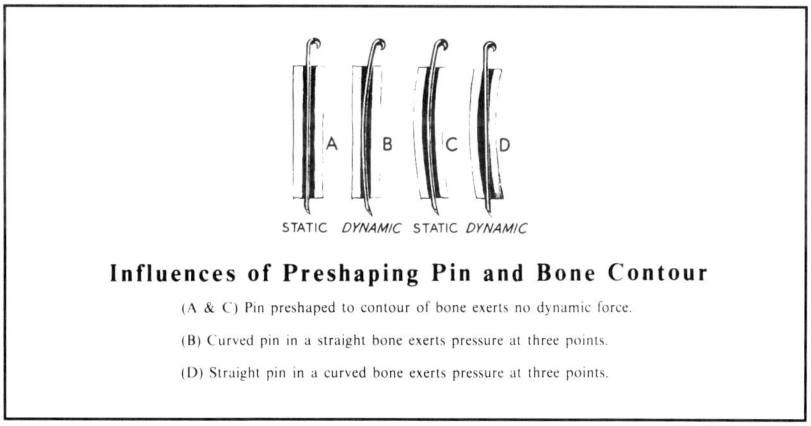

Figure 5.54 The principle of three-point fixation in intramedullary pinning of straight and curved bones. From Rush, *Atlas*, 32.

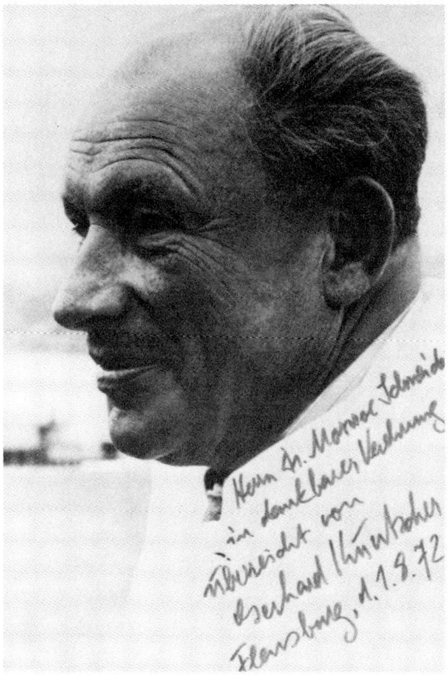

Figure 5.55 Gerhard Kuntscher (1900–1972). From "Gerhard Kuntscher," obituary, *J Bone Joint Surg* 56A(1974): 208–9.

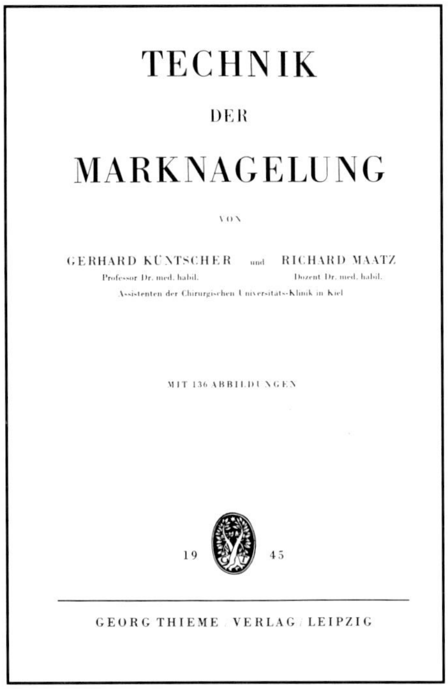

TECHNIK

DER

MARKNAGELUNG

VON

GERHARD KÜNTSCHER und RICHARD MAATZ

Professor Dr. med. habil. Dozent Dr. med. habil.

Assistenten der Chirurgischen Universitäts-Klinik in Kiel

MIT 136 ABBILDUNGEN

19 45

GEORG THIEME VERLAG LEIPZIG

Figure 5.56 The first major work on intramedullary nailing.

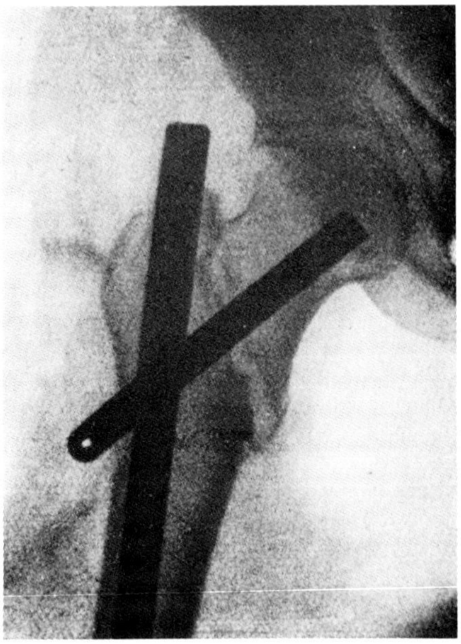

Figure 5.57 The "Y-nailing" for trochanteric and subtrochanteric fractures of the femur. From G. Kuntscher and R. Maatz, *Technik der Marknagelung* (Leipzig: Georg Thieme, 1945), figure 121.

cloverleaf nail, also included "Y nailing" (figure 5.57) and the use of multiple, small intramedullary nails (figure 5.58). This latter technique has been further developed by K. H. Hackethal and J. Ender.[104] The experience with civilian and military trauma during World War II provided a test of Kuntscher's methods, and they rapidly gained advocates. [105] The first notice of Kuntscher's methods in the United States was in the medical section of the weekly news magazine *Time* (March 12, 1945), which printed a photograph of a femoral shaft fracture treated by an intramedullary nail in an American prisoner of war. The first experience with Kuntscher's method in the United States was reported by William Russell MacAusland in 1947.[106] In the United States, Dana Street and Otto Lottes quickly introduced their own nail designs and techniques.[107] There is no question, however, that these methods, as well as others, are based upon the pioneering work of the Rush brothers and Gerhard Kuntscher.

The use of compression as an aid to fracture fixation grew out of a method described by J. Albert Key for the fusion of a tuberculous knee.[108] The operation consisted of a synovectomy and debridement of the joint followed by excision of the articular surfaces of the distal femur and proximal tibia. The two sawcuts exposed large flat surfaces of cancellous bone, which, when approximated, provided a large area for healing. Two large pins were inserted through the distal femur and proximal tibia. These pins were then attached together on either side by turnbuckles, which were tightened to provide compression. A plaster of paris splint was added for further fixation. This method of compression arthrodesis was popularized by Charnley.[109] In discussing his operation, Key noted:

> *It is based upon the belief, that, other things being equal, two bones will most readily unite if they are placed in contact and absolutely immobilized until union by bone has occurred. . . .if two broad surfaces of cancellous bone be continually pressed together and the limb supported in a plaster cast, the immobilization will be practically absolute. Whether or not the positive pressure also stimulates osteogenesis and union between the bones I do not know. I have attempted to answer this question in the laboratory, but as yet the results are inconclusive.*[110]

A. Glucksmann studied the effects of pressure on the growth of osteoblasts in tissue culture and demonstrated that the multiplying cells did react directly to mechanical stresses, but his experiments were otherwise inconclusive.[111]

In 1943, E. Townsend and C. Gilfillian introduced a new type of bone plate, 20 cm long, which could be stacked and staggered, one plate upon another, to strengthen and extend the length to be covered.[112] A feature of these plates was their oval holes, which allowed the plates to be applied across the fracture line with the screws not completely tightened. When all was in place, the fracture's surfaces were manually impacted to obtain maximum apposition and the screws quickly snugged up. A heavier plate with oval holes was introduced by Collison in 1950.[113] A modified bone plate with oval holes to allow the bone ends to approximate after the initial phase of absorption had earlier been described by Henry Stuart MacLean in 1914.[114]

In the meantime, George W. N. Eggers began using an "internal contact plate" for the treatment of diaphyseal fractures.[115] This device consisted of a slotted plate held in place by screws that were tightened sufficiently to maintain position but loosely enough to allow them to slide in the plate permitting compression of the fracture site by muscular contraction and weight bearing (figure 5.59). Eggers based his design on experiments he had performed on the calvaria of rats, which indicated that pressure or compression, within limits, promoted fracture healing.[116] Unfortunately, Eggers's technique provided neither reliable compression or fixation.

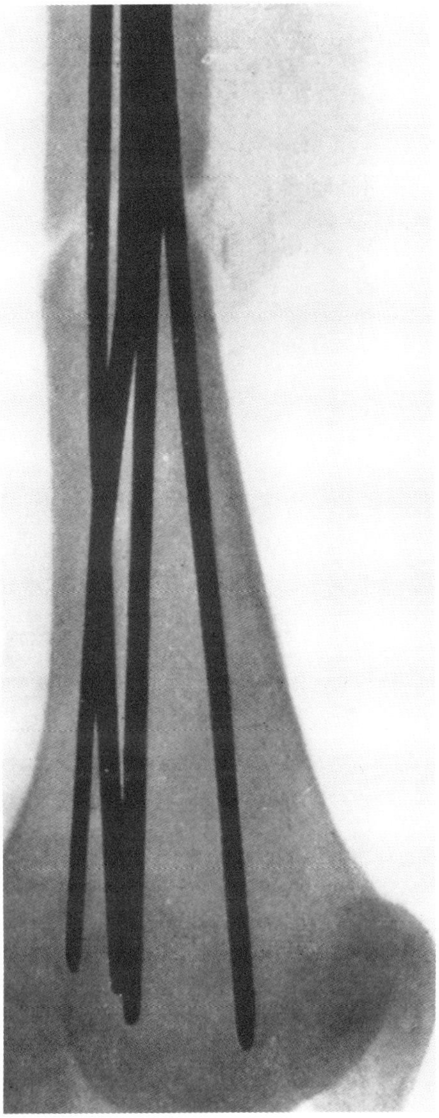

Figure 5.58 Medullary pinning with multiple small flexible pins. From Kuntscher, *Practice of Intramedullary Nailing* (Springfield, Ill.: Charles C Thomas, 1967), 241.

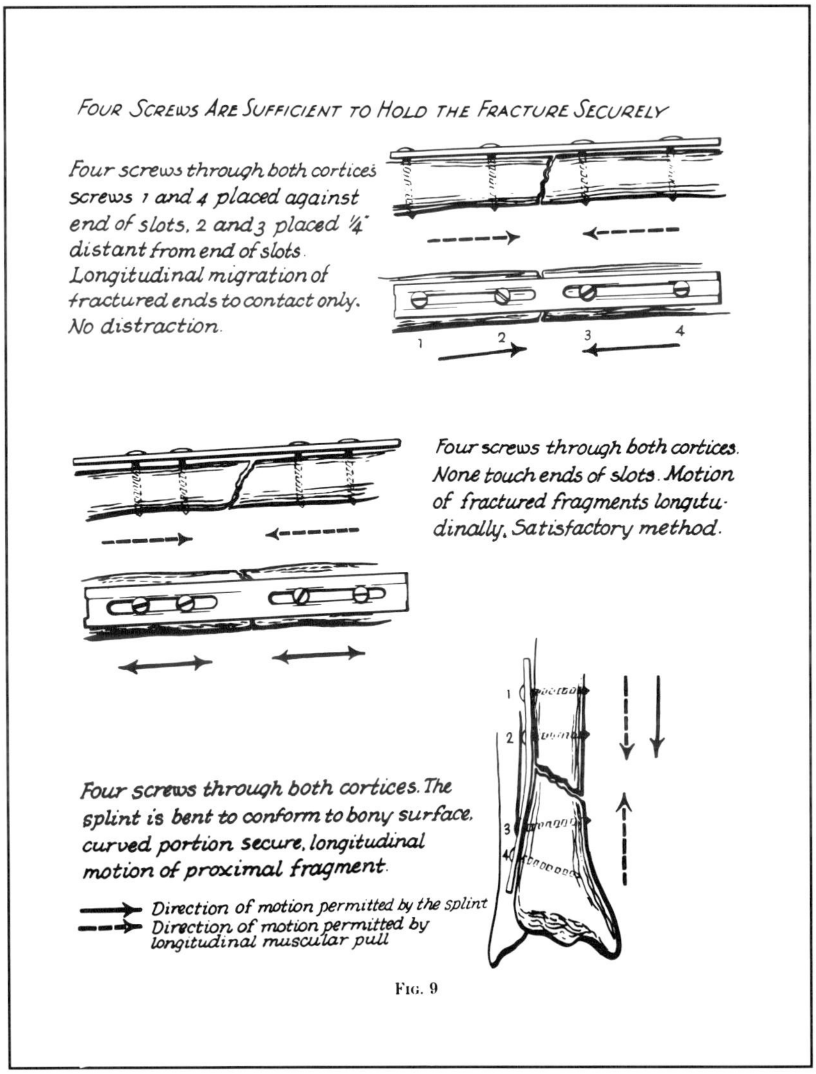

Figure 5.59 Eggers's plates. From Eggers, "Internal Contact Splint," *J Bone Joint Surg* 30A(1948): 47.

At the same time, Peterson was reviewing the status of internal fixation with plates and screws on behalf of the Office of the Surgeon General. He concluded that the deficiencies in the plates were due to improper design, variations in the hardness of the metal, improper manufacture, and poor quality control. The screws did not always fit the plates; the design of the heads was unsatisfactory, and the threads were cut poorly. The drill points were too brittle, and sizing was not consistent. He urged that the plates, screws, and drill points all be made of the same metal alloy. He promoted a more precise technique using a drill guide to center the hole, a power drill, and screws whose heads accurately fit the holes. He used a tap to cut threads in the bone for the screws, but abandoned this technique as too time-consuming. He also used interfragmentary compression and double-onlay plates for femoral shaft fractures.[117] Increased precision in technique was promoted by the introduction of a simple device for determining the length of the screws required[118] (figure 5.60).

In 1949 Robert Danis (1880–1962) (figure 5.61) published his book, *Théories et pratique de l'ostéosynthèse* (figure 5.62), in which he stated these objectives:

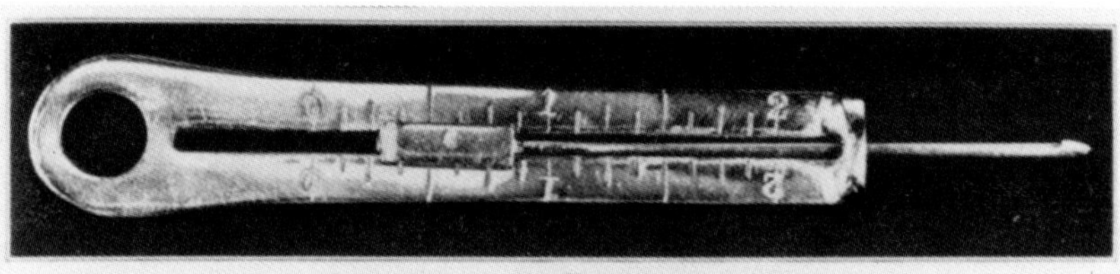

Fig. 1
Instrument open.

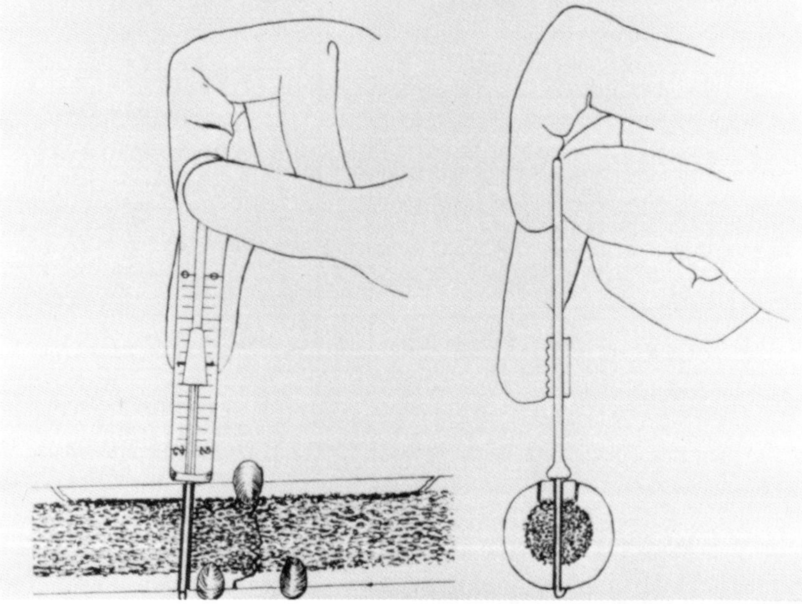

Figure 5.60 The depth gauge. From J. J. Flanagan, "Instrument for Accurate Measurement of Bone Screws," *J Bone Joint Surg* 27(1945): 723.

Osteosynthesis is not entirely satisfactory unless it attains the following three objectives:

—the capability of immediate mobilization and activity of the muscles in the region and in the neighboring joints.

—the restoration of the bone in its original form.

—the union, per primum (soudure autogène), of the bony fragments without apparent callus formation.[119]

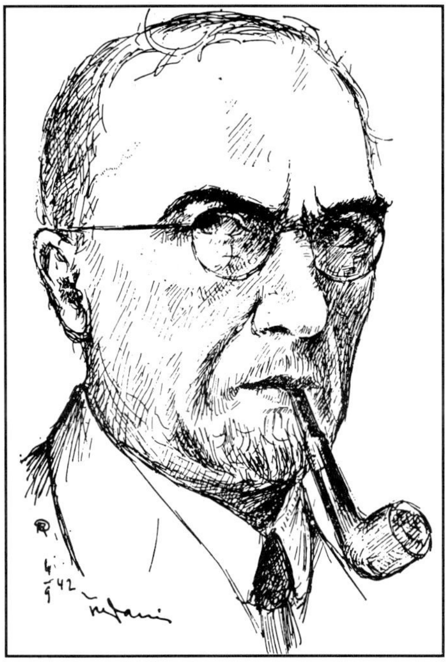

Figure 5.61 Robert Danis (1880–1962). From "Nécrologie: Dr. Robert Danis," *Rev chir orthopéd réparatrice l'appareil moteur* 48(1962): 764–65.

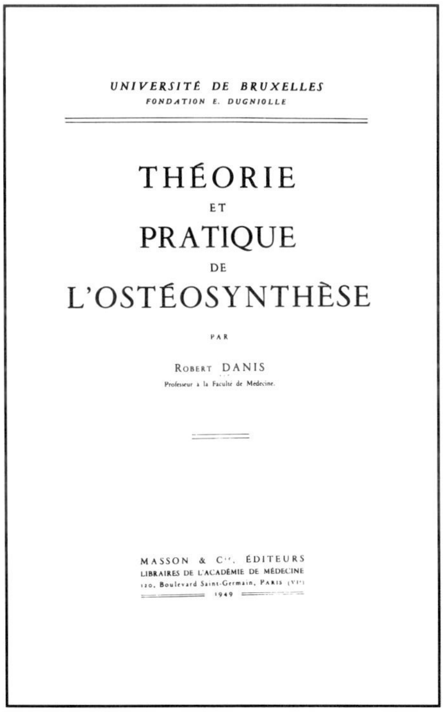

UNIVERSITÉ DE BRUXELLES
FONDATION E. DUGNIOLLE

THÉORIE
ET
PRATIQUE
DE
L'OSTÉOSYNTHÈSE

PAR

ROBERT DANIS
Professeur à la Faculté de Médecine.

MASSON & Cie, ÉDITEURS
LIBRAIRES DE L'ACADÉMIE DE MÉDECINE
120, Boulevard Saint-Germain, PARIS (VIe)
1949

Figure 5.62 Danis's book of internal fixation.

These objectives were to be reached by the use of rigorous asepsis and appliances made from compatible metals designed to provide solid fixation employing axial compression. The *coapteurs* of Danis (figure 5.63) were the first plates designed for the internal fixation of diaphyseal fractures that combined the principles of compression and rigid fixation. To go with these plates he also designed a system of cortical and cancellous screws (figure 5.64).

Danis, like Lambotte, was a surgeon of broad interests, initially in vascular surgery and later in osteosynthesis. He approached the latter problem from both a biological and a mechanical point of view. He was able to demonstrate that fracture fragments could heal without external callus formation, and he achieved this goal in patients.

In 1951 Charles Scott Venable improved upon the design of the *coapteur* of Danis with the introduction of an "inboard" compression plate (figure 5.65). A more cumbersome double-plating system using compression was presented by Jacques Boreau and P. Hermann[120] (figure 5.66). The animal experiments carried by Zachary B. Friedenberg and George French (figure 5.67) indicated that the optimum pressure across a diaphyseal fracture was twelve to eighteen pounds; pressures greater than thirty pounds produced necrosis.[121] They concluded that the enhanced healing associated with compression was due primarily to more secure fixation and impaction rather than to the compression itself.

In 1956 George W. Bagby (b. 1923) (figure 5.68), of the Mayo Clinic, described a compression plate system based on the geometry of the oval hole of the Collison plate and the shape of the head of the screw[122]. The hole in the bone was eccentrically located in the oval hole in the plate, and as the screw was tightened down into place the plate shifted slightly, producing compression at the fracture site (figure 5.69). In animal experiments, he demonstrated that compression did not stimulate osteogenesis, but it did increase approximation and immobilization at the fracture site.[123] As another important contribution to the technique of plating, Bagby described how the shape of the plate could be used to produce a dynamic impacting force[124] (figure 5.70). The "outboard" compression plate device was described by Maurice E. Müller of St. Gallen, Switzerland in 1961[125] (figure 5.71).

The results of open reduction and internal fixation were not always favorable. In 1928 Roscoe N. Gray, a medical referee for Aetna Insurance Company, after a review of 34,753 compensation files from northern California, concluded that

It is questionable if open bone surgery should ever be done except by highly trained men, with highly trained assistants, in highly trained hospitals; otherwise disaster is likely to result.[126]

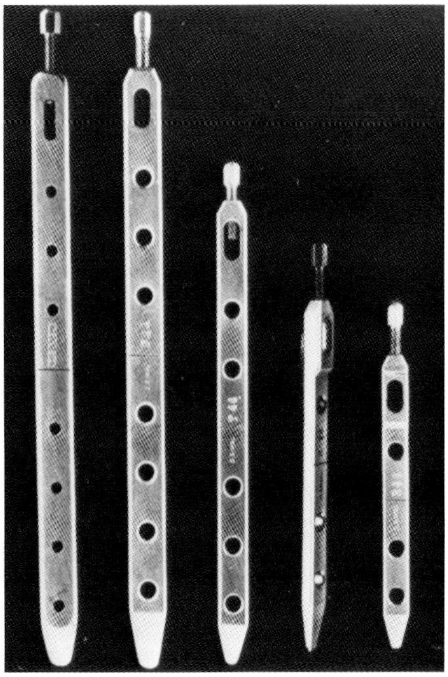

Figure 5.63 The "coapteurs" or compression plates of Danis. From Danis, *Théorie et pratique*, (Paris: Masson, 1949).

Thirty years later, Müller met with a group of fifteen Swiss surgeons and orthopedists to form the Arbeitsgemeinschaft für Osteosynthesefragen (AO), the Association for the Study of Internal Fixation[127] (figure 5.72). A student of Danis, Müller had become disenchanted with the results of both the operative and nonoperative methods of treatment being used in his community. From this meeting came a consensus that effective treatment of fractures should include anatomical reduction, rigid internal fixation, atraumatic technique, and early active mobilization of the injured extremity during the first ten days following operation. The AO set as its goals the performance of appropriate animal experiments, the development of a comprehensive technical armamentarium, and a thorough and complete follow-up and evaluation of all patients treated by their members. One of the first fruits of this enterprise was the publication of the members' initial experience. The *Technik der Operativen Frakturenbehandlung* (figure 5.73) was a comprehensive monograph on the principles of the internal fixation of fractures.[128] Having established for themselves the value of this approach, the AO carried out an educational program of monumental proportions. As a result, both the principles and the procedures espoused by the AO are used throughout the world.

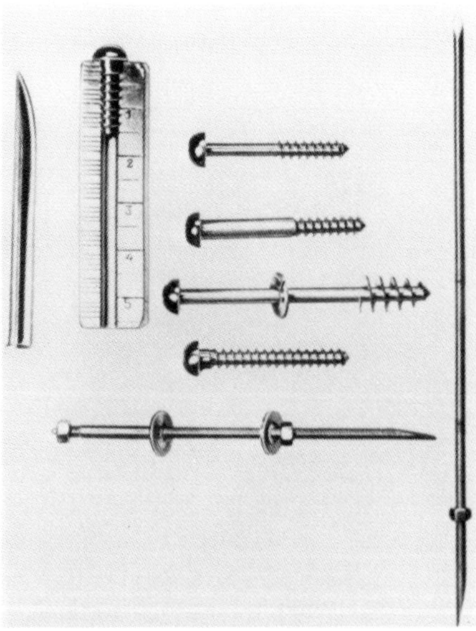

Figure 5.64 Cortical and cancellous screws and other devices of Danis. From Danis, *Théorie et pratique*,

Tension band-wiring (*Zügurtungsosteosynthese*) is a form of internal fixation for fractures through cancellous bone that provides rigid fixation by means of pins; it prevents shear, and a tension band provides compression. The technique invokes those engineering principles embodied in prestressed concrete beams and girders. Friedrick Pauwels illustrated this principle in 1935 (figure 5.74), but it remained for B. G. Weber to demonstrate the wide applicability of this technique.[129]

Along with the development of suitable designs for implants to be used for the internal fixation of fractures was a continuing search for the best materials from which to fabricate them. Surgeons tended to use materials easily at hand. Those of biologic origin—bone, ivory, horn, etc.— were used in the hope that they might absorb or be incorporated into the healing bone with a minimal reaction. Metal nails, screws, pins, and plates initially were of the quality that could be found in any hardware store. Sometimes devices made of one metal were plated with another, and it was common to use plates made of one metal with screws made of a second. The use of all these

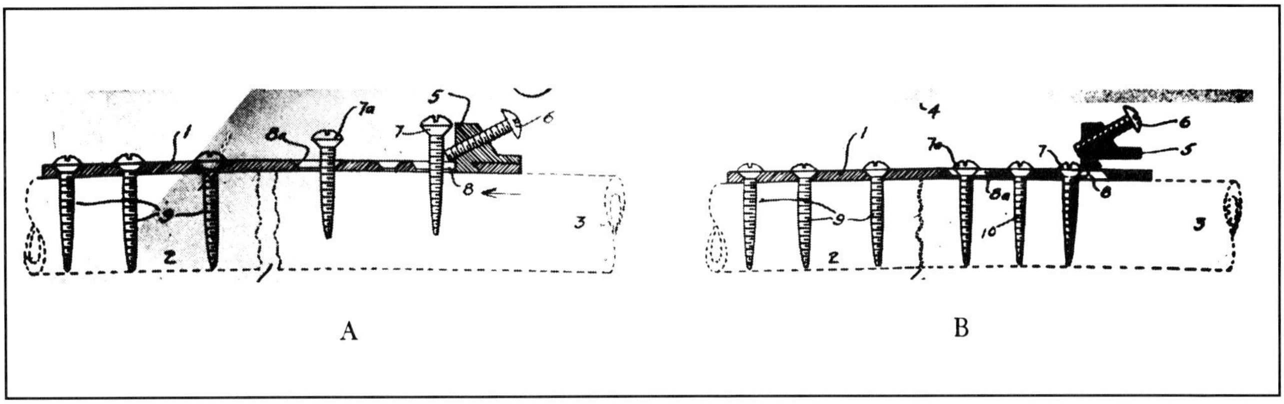

Figure 5.65 The "inboard" compression device of Venable. From Venable, "An Impacting Bone Plate to Attain Closed Coaptation," *Ann Surg* 133(1951): 808–12.

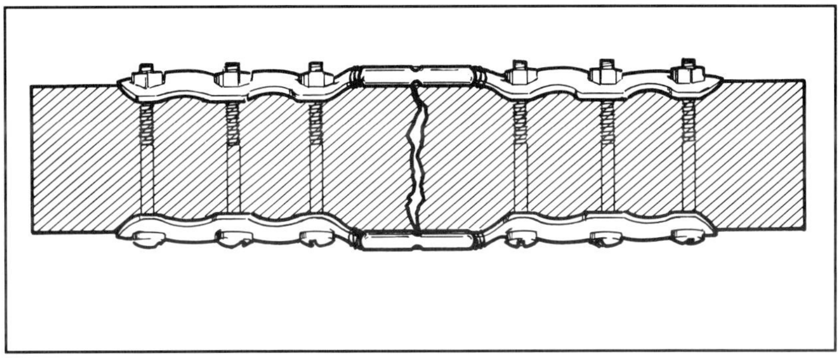

Figure 5.66 The compression device of Boreau and Hermann. From Boreau and Hermann, "Plaque d'ostéosynthèse permettant l'impaction des fragments," *Presse méd* 60(1952): 356.

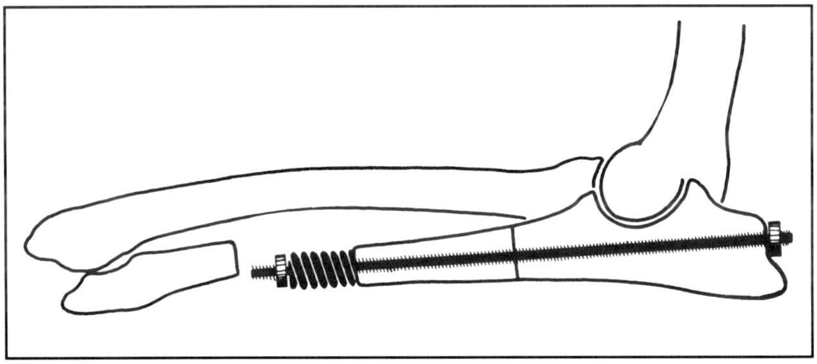

Figure 5.67 The experimental design used by Friedenberg and French to study the effect of compression on fracture healing. From Friedenburg and French, "The Effects of Known Compression Forces on Fracture Healing," *SGO* 94(1952): 743–48.

materials produced many failures due to nonunion, severe soft tissue reactions, and breakage and corrosion of the implants.

In Germany, internal fixation found a strong advocate in Fritz Konig.[130] He favored the use of implants made of ivory because he had observed adverse reactions to metallic devices buried in tissues. E. J. Brougham and A. C. Eeke manufactured plates and screws of ox bone:

> *All the methods (utilizing ivory, human, and animal bone) have their origin in the effort to procure the use of a probable absorbable material, and so dispense with the metallic fixation material which frequently causes a great deal of trouble*[131] [figure 5.75].

The persistence of the use of ivory and bone pegs well into this century is an indication that metals suitable for implants are a recent development.[132] Lane equated the "rarefying osteitis" associated with a reaction between the bone and the metallic implant with infection and denied that it occurred in his patients.[133] However, Erling Dahl-Iverson estimated in 1928 that this complication occurred in 35 percent of patients with fractures of the long bones treated by internal fixation.[134] On the basis of their study of fifteen

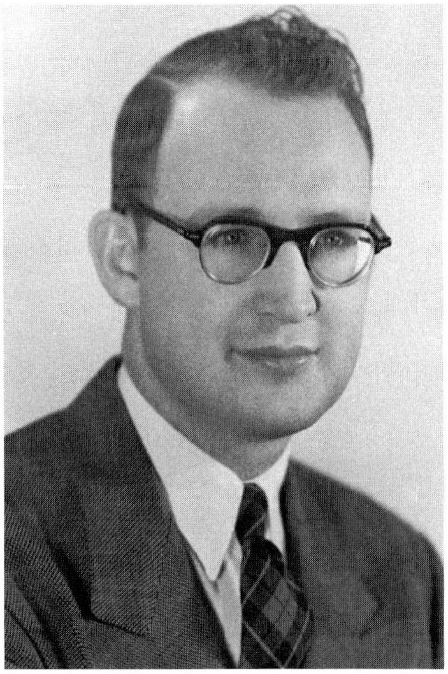

Figure 5.68 George W. Bagby (b. 1923)

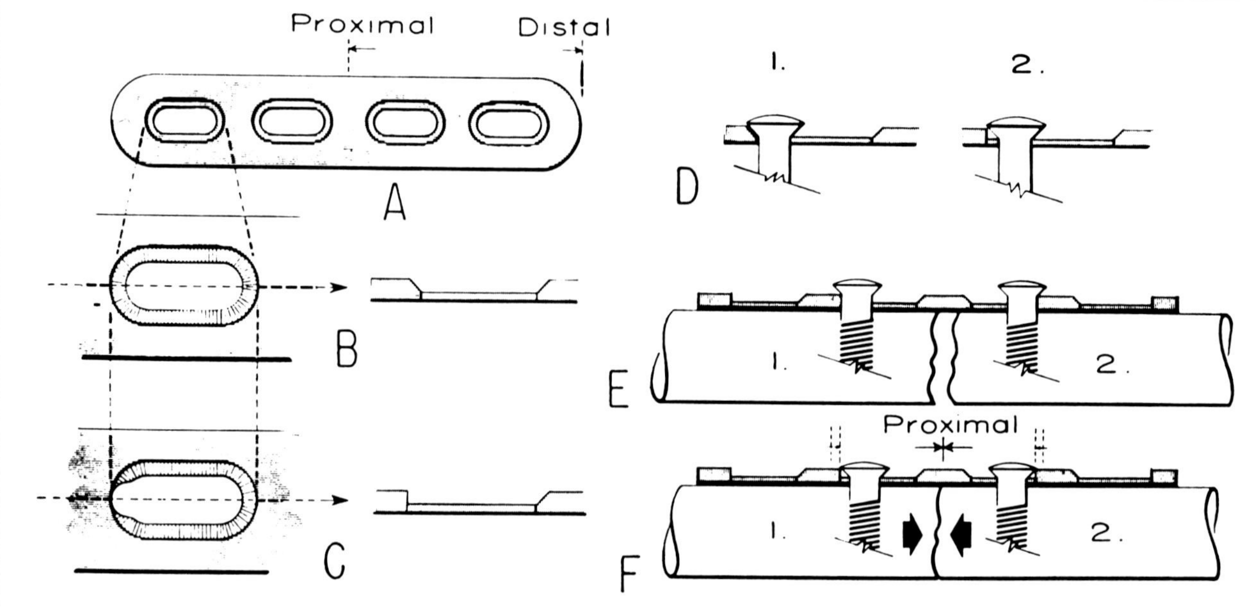

FIG. 1. Use of a modified Collison bone plate to apply compressing force. A, unaltered Collison plate .B, views of Collison plate in longitudinal section. C, views of modified Collison plate. The distal slanted end of the slot has been made vertical. D, this shows (1) the relationship of a screw in the slot of an unmodified plate and (2) the relationship in a modified plate. E, screws in position in a modified plate. At least two screws must be brought to this position before completely turning them down to create the impacting force. F, screws have been turned down and the fragments have become more closely approximated.

Figure 5.69 The Bagby plate. From Bagby, and J. M. Janes, "The Effect of Compression on the Rate of Fracture Healing Using a Special Plate," *Am J Surg* 95(1958): 761–71.

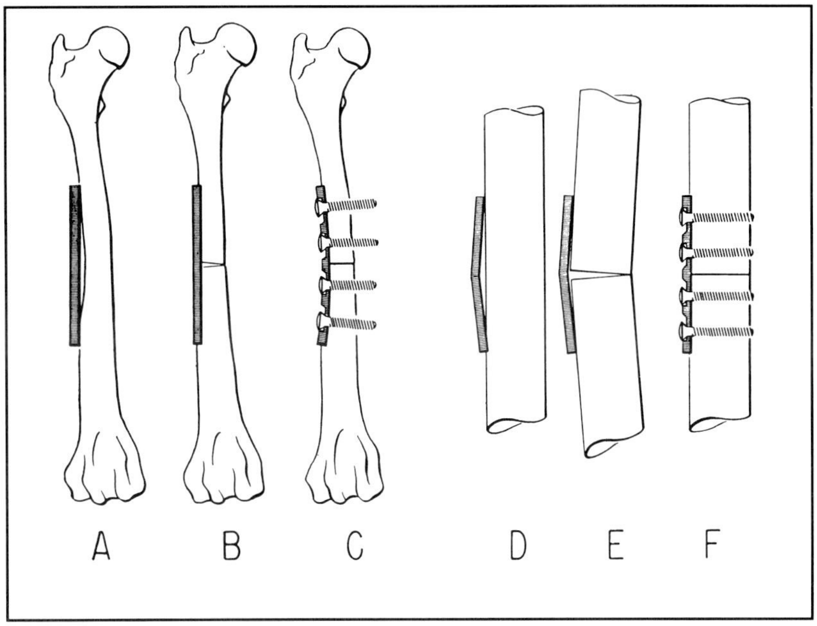

Figure 5.70 Bagby's principles of the application of the plates to straight and to curved bones. From Bagby and Janes, "An Impacting Bone Plate," *Mayo Clin Proc* 32(1957): 55–57.

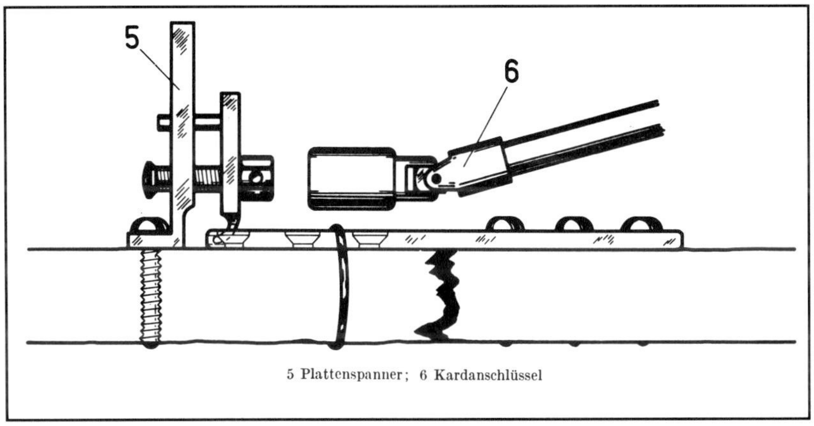

Figure 5.71 Müller's "outboard" compression device. From Müller et al., *Technik der Operativen Fracture Behandlung* (Berlin: Springer Verlag, 1963), 56.

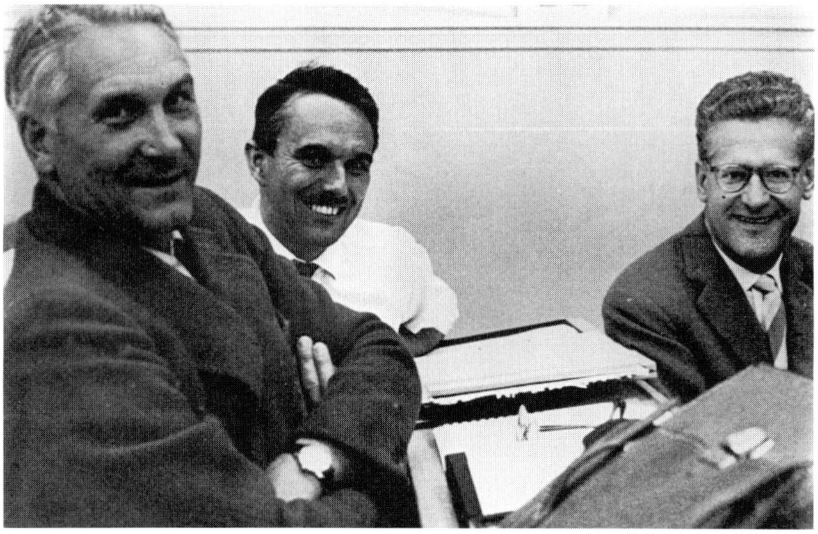

Figure 5.72 The leaders in founding the Arbeitsgemeinschaft für Osteosynthesefragen, or AO: H. Willneger, M. E. Müller, and M. Allgower.

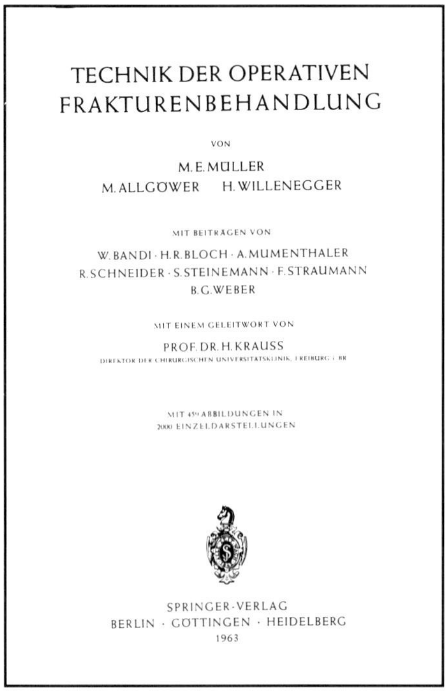

TECHNIK DER OPERATIVEN
FRAKTURENBEHANDLUNG

VON

M. E. MÜLLER
M. ALLGÖWER H. WILLENEGGER

MIT BEITRÄGEN VON

W. BANDI · H. R. BLOCH · A. MUMENTHALER
R. SCHNEIDER · S. STEINEMANN · F. STRAUMANN
B. G. WEBER

MIT EINEM GELEITWORT VON

PROF. DR. H. KRAUSS
DIREKTOR DER CHIRURGISCHEN UNIVERSITÄTSKLINIK, FREIBURG I. BR

MIT 459 ABBILDUNGEN IN
2000 EINZELDARSTELLUNGEN

SPRINGER-VERLAG
BERLIN · GÖTTINGEN · HEIDELBERG
1963

Figure 5.73 The book that first fully set forth the principles of fracture treatment espoused by the AO.

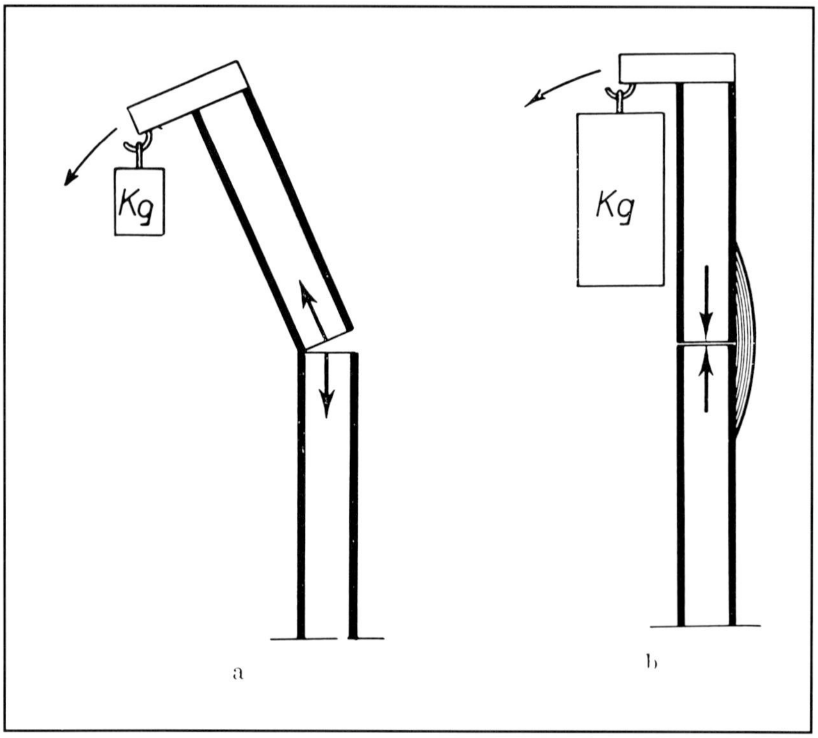

Figure 5.74 The principle of tension band-wiring. From Pauwels, *Der Schenkelhalsbruch: ein mechanisches Problem* (Stuttgart: Ferdinand Enke, 1935), 9.

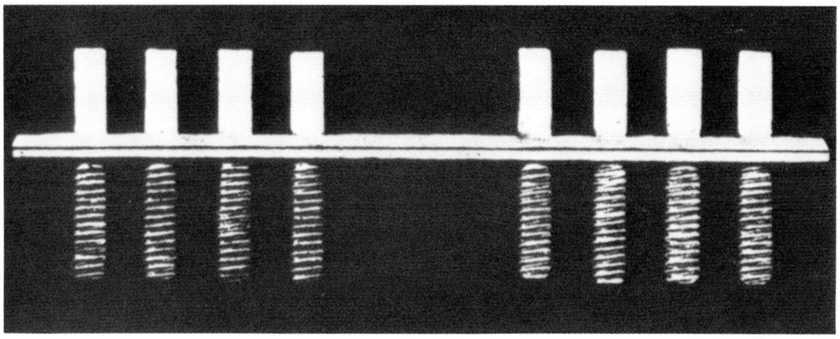

Figure 5.75 The ox bone plate of Eeke-Brougham. From William Williams Keen, *Surgery, Its Principles and Practice* (Philadelphia: W. B. Saunders, 1921), 7:422.

patients, René Leriche and A. Policard concluded that the plates used by Lambotte inhibited fracture healing and new bone formation because of the deposition of iron salts in the local tissues.[135] They stressed the advantage of using plates made of more nonreactive metals such as gold, silver, magnesium, and aluminum. The extensive literature on the reaction of tissues, especially bone, to the implantation of metals that accumulated during the nineteenth century has been reviewed by Georges Menegaux and Donatien Odiette and by Venable and Stuck.[136] L. G. Gazziotti, in 1923, and Arthur Adalbert Zierold, in 1924, reported animal experiments describing the reaction of bone to the implantation of a wide variety of metals.[137] They concluded that while different metals produced varying degrees of reaction, none were inert. In 1932 Menegaux and Odiette of the Institute du Cancer in Paris began their study of the cytotoxicity of metals. The results of their experiments were collected in an important monograph, *L'ostéosynthèse au point de vue biologique*, published in 1936.[138] A major portion of their work was done with tissue cultures of fibroblasts from chicken embryos and human osteoblasts. Into these cultures they placed individual discs (1.5 mm in diameter) of twelve pure metals, eight alloys of alumnium, two alloys of magnesium, and twenty-one different types of steel. The discs of copper, magnesium, the alloys of magnesium, aluminum-bronze, and two of the steels gave evidence of a high degree of toxicity. Only the discs of gold, alumnium, lead, and three of the steels (V^2A Extra, nickel, and Platinostainless) showed no toxicity. In other experiments, two discs of different metals were placed in tissue cultures together. In these cultures, the toxicity of a metal was neither enhanced nor inhibited by the presence of another, although they noted the presence of local electrolytic couples.

Menegaux and Odiette also studied the formation of salts of calcium and phosphorus in tissue culture and found that this was inhibited by all pure metals, alumnium alloys, and most steels except V^2A, Inchal, and Platinostainless. It is interesting that there was no correlation between cytotoxicity and salt inhibition. In other experiments, metal discs were implanted subperiosteally and within the bones of rats, rabbits, and dogs.

On the basis of this work they reached the following conclusions:

1. *The tissue reaction to the metal is a general nonspecific one.*
2. *The use of metal implants in patients involves important problems of cytotoxicity.*
3. *It is the nature of the implants themselves that is responsible for* l'osteiten rarefiante *or* maladie metallique du cal, *complications that accompany osteosynthesis.*
4. *Only gold, aluminum, lead, and the steels,* V^2A *Extra, Nickel, and Platinostainless, showed no toxicity.*

In order for osteosynthesis to take its hoped for place in surgery, we believe that it is necessary to find a rigid metal, easy to work and to manipulate, which behaves in the healing bone tissues as a completely inert material.[139]

L. Jones and B. A. Lieberman in the United States, working at the same time, emphasized the importance of knowing the exact composition of any metal used in osteosynthesis.[140]

While Menegaux and Odiette published their monograph on the cytotoxicity of metals, Venable and Stuck were beginning their experiments on the electrolytic activity of metallic implants. They implanted screws made from various metals into the tibiae of dogs and made the following observations:

1. *After a period of weeks, metallic ions could be found in the soft tissue about the screws.*
2. *There was evidence of migration of metallic ions of one metal to the region of a screw of another metal.*
3. *These migrations were related to the electromotive forces between the metals.*
4. *Metals that corroded rapidly produced the most damage to bone.*
5. *The application of a micro-ammeter to the screws demonstrated the presence of small electric currents.*

In vitro experiments followed in which "batteries" were constructed by immersing implants of different metals in Ringer's solution and measuring the current generated between them. As a result of their experiments, they believed that they had conclusively proved "that the cause of failure of previous metal appliances in bone surgery was due to electrolytic reactions about the appliances in the presence of blood serum." In other words, if we remember constantly that electrolytic action is the root of all evil in internal fixation and has never produced conditions favorable to it, there will be no trouble from use of metal appliances.[141] In their experiments, Stuck and Venable identified an alloy of cobalt (65 percent), chromium (30 percent), and molybdenum (5 percent), later called Vitallium, as being totally inert and possessing some of the other properties desirable for the fabrication of devices for internal fixation.

The work of Menegaux and Odiette on cytotoxicity and of Stuck and Venable on electrolytic reactions provided some understanding of certain types of implant failure and established some criteria for the choice of metals for implants. The nonferrous alloys of cobalt, chromium, and molybdenum, as well as some special steels, became the favored materials. Titanium has since been added to this list.[142] However, the search for the ideal metal or alloy continues, and the standards which that it must meet grow more stringent with each decade.[143]

A completely anomalous approach to internal fixation of fractures was proposed in 1958 by Michael P. Mandarino and Joseph E. Salvatore, who used a rigid form of polyurethane which was polymerized at the time of application to the bone.[144] The material was injected into the medullary cavity, commonly in association with groups of small reinforcing rods, and the reaction was controlled to limit exothermic heat. The polymer became almost completely solid in twenty to thirty minutes and was fully cured within twenty-four to forty-eight hours. The technique was used in the treatment of diaphyseal fractures, particularly of the tibia, and pathological fractures.[145] This method did not gain acceptance. However, the concept was a good one and was revived in 1972 for use in the treatment of pathological fractures using methylmethacrylate in association with metallic fixation devices.[146]

Notes

1. P. E. L. Evans, "Cerclage Fixation of a Fractured Humerus in 1775: Fact or Fiction," *Clin Orthop* 174(1983): 138–42.

2. L. J. B. Bérenger-Féraud, *Traité de l'immobilisation directe des fragments osseux dans les fractures* (Paris: Adrien Delahaye, 1870).

3. E. Gourniou, "L. J. B. Bérenger-Féraud (1832–1900), Médecine générale du service de santé de la marine," *Arch méd pharm nav* 128(1938): 297–312.

4. Bérenger-Féraud, *Des fractures en V au point de vue de leur gravité et de leur traitement* (Paris: Henneuyer et Fils, 1864).

5. Bérenger-Féraud, "De l'immobilisation directe des fragments dans les fractures compliquées," *Bull Acad Méd Paris* 30(1864–65): 83–87.

6. Bérenger-Féraud and Trouette, "Note sur la composition de l'urine de la fièvre bilieuse dite hématurique," *Gaz hôp civ milit* 45(1872): 1155–56; id., *De la fièvre bilieuse mélanurique des pays chaud comparée avec le fièvre jaune* (Paris: Adrien Delahaye,1874); J. W. W. Stephens, *Blackwater Fever: A Historical Summary and Summary of Observations Made over a Century* (London: University Press of Liverpool, Hodder & Stoughton, 1937).

7. Bérenger-Féraud, *Traité de l'immobilisation.*

8. Ibid., 9.

9. Joseph Lister, "An Address on the Treatment of Fracture of the Patella," *Brit Med J* 2(1883): 855.

10. Samuel Cooper, "Treatment of Fractured Patella by Malgaigne's Hooks," *San Fran Med Press* 2(1861): 13–16.

11. M. Ravitch, *A Century of Surgery: The History of the American Surgical Association* (Philadelphia: Lippincott, 1981), 2: 340.

12. Charles A. Powers, "The Question of Operative Interference in Recent Simple Fractures of the Patella," *Trans Am Surg Assoc* 16(1898): 53–103.

13. Hansmann, "Eine neue Methode der Fixierung der Fragmente bei complicirten Fracturen," *Dtsch Ges Chir* 15(1886): 134–37.

14. J. Dollinger, "Knochennaht ohne Durch bohrung des Knochens," *Zentralbl Chir* 20(1883): 25–26; V. Willie, "Eine Verbessrung der Technik der Knochensutur," *Zentralbl Chir* 19(1892): 945–50.

15. H. Bircher, "Eine neue Methode unmittelbarer Retention bei Fracturen der Rohrenknochen," *Arch klin Chir* 34(1893): 410–422.

16. Nicholas Senn, "A New Method of Direct Fixation of the Fragments in Compound and Ununited Fractures," *Trans Am Surg Assoc* 11(1893): 125–51.

17. J. Ransohoff, "The Operative Treatment of Irreducible Subcutaneous Fractures," *Trans Am Surg Assoc* 15(1897): 203–13.

18. W. E. Tanner, *Sir W. Arbuthnot Lane, His Life and Work* (Baltimore: Williams and Wilkins, 1946).

19. W. Arbuthnot Lane, "Some Clinical Observations on the Principles Involved in the Surgery of Fractures," *Clin J* 5(1894): 392–400.

20. Lane, *The Operative Treatment of Fractures* (London: Medical Publishing Co., 1905), 32–33.

21. Lane, "On the Advantage of the Steel Screws in the Treatment of Ununited Fractures," *Lancet* 2(1893): 1500–1501; id., "A Method of Treating Simple Oblique Fractures of the Tibia and Fibula More Efficient Than Those in Common Use," *Trans Clin Soc London* 27(1893–94): 167–75.

22. Lane, "Some Clinical Observations on the Principles Involved in the Surgery of Fractures," *Clin J* 5(1894): 392–400.

23. Lane, *Operative Treatment of Fractures.*

24. Lane, "Clinical Remarks on the Operative Treatment of Fractures," *Brit Med J* 1(1907): 1037–38.

25. Albin Lambotte, *L'intervention opératoire dans les fractures récentes et anciennes envisagée particulièrement au point de vue de l'ostéo-synthèse* (Brussels: Lamertin, 1907).

26. Lambotte, *Chirurgie opératoire des fractures* (Paris: Masson, 1913).

27. A. Jacoel, "Une agrafe pour sutures osseuses," *Presse méd* (25 Dec. 1901): 143; id., *Traitement des fractures par les agrafes osseuses* (Paris: Henri Jouve, 1903).

28. J. Nicolaysen, "Lidt om Diagnosen og Behandlingen af Fr. colli femoris," *Nord med Ark* 30(1897): 1–18.

29. R. Milne, "Remarks," *Clin J. B. Murphy* 2(1913): 229–34.

30. V. Putti, "Un nuovo metodo di osteosintesi," *Clinica chir* 22(1914): 1021–24.

31. F. W. Parham, "Circular Constriction in the Treatment of Fractures of the Long Bones," *SGO* 23(1916): 541–44.

32. A Collins, "A New Fracture Band," *JAMA* 74(1920): 950–51; F. E. Hagie, "Bone Band and Band Introducer," *JAMA* 86(1926): 840.

33. A. Moruzi, *Synthèse et prothèse osseuses* (Paris: G. Doin, 1929), 59–90.

34. P. Niehans, "Zur Fracturebehandlung durch temporare Annagelung," *Arch klin Chir* 73(1904): 167–78.

35. C. L. Scudder, "The Open or Operative Treatment of Fresh Fractures: Is It Ever Justified?" *Boston Med Surg J* 142(1900): 289–93.

36. L. W. Steinbach, "On the Use of Fixation Plates in the Treatment of Fractures of the Leg," *Ann Surg* 31(1900): 436–42.

37. E. Martin, "The Open Treatment of Fractures," *SGO* 3(1906): 258–71.

38. J. A. Blake, "The Operative Treatment of Fractures," *SGO* 14(1912): 338–45.

39. E. H. Beckman, "Repair of Fractures with Steel Splints," *SGO* 14(1912): 71–76.

40. H. M. Sherman and D. Tait, "Fractures near Joints and Fractures into Joints," *SGO* 19(1914): 131–41.

41. T. L. Hazlett and W. W. Hummel, *Industrial Medicine in Western Pennsylvania, 1850–1950* (Pittsburgh: University of Pittsburgh Press, 1957).

42. W. O. Sherman, "Vanadium Steel Bone Plates and Screws," *SGO* 14(1912): 629–34.

43. Ibid., 629–34.

44. E. W. Hey-Groves, "Operation for the Repair of the Crucial Ligaments," *Lancet* 2(1917): 274–75.

45. Hey-Groves, "Demonstration: Notes on Some Appliances," *Brit Med J* 2(1914): 835–36.

46. Hey-Groves, *On Modern Methods of Treating Fractures* (Bristol: John Wright and Sons, 1916).

47. Ibid., 157–159.

48. "Report of the Committee on Treatment of Simple Fractures," *Brit Med J* (30 Nov. 1912): 1505–41.

49. R. Jones, "Presidential Address on the Present Position of Treatment of Fractures," *Brit Med J* 2(1912): 1589–94.

50. J. F. Binnie et al., *Treatment of Fractures: Reports of the Committee on Fractures of the American Surgical Association for 1913, 1914, 1915, 1916, 1917, 1918, 1921* (American Surgical Association, 1922), iii.

51. Ibid., 82.

52. Uno Lindgren, "The Treatment of Fractures of the Neck of the Femur," *Acta chir scand* 57(1924): 55; Nicolaysen, "Lidt om Diagnosen," 1–18.

53. Senn, "A Case of Bony Union after Impacted Intra-Capsular Fracture of the Neck of the Femur," *Trans Am Surg Assoc* 1(1883): 167–70.

54. Senn, "Fractures of the Neck of the Femur," *Trans Am Surg Assoc* 1(1883): 333–452.

55. Senn, "The Treatment of Fractures of the Neck of the Femur by Immediate Reduction and Permanent Fixation," *JAMA* 13(1889): 150–59.

56. Royal Whitman, "A New Treatment for Fractures of the Neck of the Femur," *Med Record (NY)* 65(1904): 441–47; id., "The Abduction Treatment of Fracture of the Neck of the Femur," *J Bone Joint Surg* 7(1925): 374–91.

57. Otto Lofberg, "The Treatment of Fractures of the Neck of the Femur," *Acta chir scand* 57(1924): 504–32.

58. "Report of a Commission Appointed by the American Orthopedic Association to Study the End Results of Intra-Capsular Fractures of the Neck of the Femur," *J Bone Joint Surg* 12(1930): 966–79.

59. F. J. Cotton, "Artificial Impaction in Hip Fracture," *Am J Orthop Surg* 9(1911): 680–86; Cotton and G. M. Morrison, "Hip Fractures: Valgus Position—Accidental or Engineered?" *J Bone Joint Surg* 20(1938): 461–68.

60. F. H. Albee, *Bone Graft Surgery* (Philadelphia: W. B. Saunders, 1917).

61. Hey-Groves, "Treatment of Fractured Neck of the Femur with Especial Regard to the Results," *J Bone Joint Surg* 12(1930): 1–11.

62. M. N. Smith-Petersen, "New Approach to the Hip Joint," *Am J Orthop* 15(1917): 592.

63. Smith-Petersen et al., "Intracapsular Fractures of the Neck of the Femur," *AMA Arch Surg* 23(1931): 715–59.

64. Ibid., 715.

65. G. W. Hawley, "A New Fracture, X-ray and Orthopedic Table," *Am J Surg* 18(1932): 19–25; G. W. Leadbetter, "A Treatment for Fractures of the Neck of the Femur," *J Bone Joint Surg* 15(1933): 931–40; id., "Closed Reduction of Fractures of the Neck of the Femur," *J Bone Joint Surg* 20(1938): 109–13.

66. Sven Johansson, "On the Operative Treatment of Medial Fractures of the Neck of the Femur," *Acta orthop scand* 3(1932): 362–92; H. H. Wescott, "A

Method for the Internal Fixation of Transcervical Fractures of the Femur," *J Bone Joint Surg* 6(1934): 372.

67. Thomas King, "Recent Intracapsular Fractures of the Neck of the Femur," *Med J Australia* 1(1934): 5–15.

68. W. W. Plummer, "Comments on Lateral Fixation in Fresh Fractures of the Neck of the Femur," *J Bone Joint Surg* 20(1938): 97–107.

69. J. Leveuf and C. Girode, *Le traitement des fractures du col du fémur par la méthode du professeur Pierre Delbet* (Paris: Masson, 1927).

70. E. D. Martin and A. C. King, "Preliminary Report of a New Method of Treating Fractures of the Neck of the Femur," *New Orl Med Surg J* 75(1923): 710–15.

71. M. O. Henry, "Proximal Osteosynthesis in Intracapsular Fracture of the Hip: An Experimental Study," *J Bone Joint Surg* 13(1931): 530–37; id., "Intracapsular Fracture of the Hip: A New Device for Lateral Osteosynthesis," *J Bone Joint Surg* 16(1934): 168–72; id., "Lateral Introduction of the Screw-Bolt in Intracapsular Fracture of the Hip," *J Bone Joint Surg* 20(1938): 400–404.

72. R. K. Lippmann, "Recent Experiences with the Corkscrew Bolt in Fractures of the Hip," *Am J Surg* 78(1949): 54–64.

73. J. C. Charnley et al., "The Treatment of Displaced Fractures of the Neck of the Femur by Compression," *J Bone Joint Surg* 39B(1957): 45–65; Robert Danis, *Théorie et pratique de l'ostéosynthèse* (Paris: Masson, 1949).

74. D. R. Telson and N. S. Ransohoff, "Treatment of Fractured Neck of the Femur by Axial Fixation with Steel Plates," *J Bone Joint Surg* 17(1935): 727–38.

75. F. J. Gaenslen, "Subcutaneous Spike Fixation of Fresh Fractures of the Neck of the Femur," *J Bone Joint Surg* 17(1935): 739–48.

76. F. L. Knowles, "Fractures of the Neck of the Femur," *Wis Med J* 35(1936): 106–8; Austin Moore, "Fractures of the Hip Joint: Treatment by Extra-Articular Fixation with Adjustable Nails," *SGO* 64(1937): 420–36; Gunnar Nystrom, "Osteosynthesis of Medial Fractures of the Femoral Neck with the Aids of Three Nails (Multiple Nailing)," *Acta chir scand* 91(1944): 449–71.

77. W. M. Deyerle, "Absolute Fixation with Constant Compression in Hip Fractures," *Clin Orthop* 13(1959): 279–97.

78. Hey-Groves, "Some Contributions to the Reconstructive Surgery of the Hip," *Brit J Surg*, 14(1927): 486–517.

79. A. T. Moore and H. R. Bohlman, "Metal Hip Joint: A Case Report," *J Bone Joint Surg* 25(1943): 688–92.

80. Robert Judet and Jean Judet, "Essais de reconstruction prosthétique de la hanche après résection de la tête fémorale," *J chir* 65(1949): 17–24.

81. Earl D. McBride, "A Femoral Head Prosthesis for the Hip Joint," *J Bone Joint Surg* 34A(1952): 989–96; J. E. M. Thomson, "A Prosthesis for the Femoral Head," *J Bone Joint Surg* 34A(1952): 175–82.

82. L. T. Peterson, "The Use of a Metallic Femoral Head," *J Bone Joint Surg* 33A(1951): 65–73.

83. R. K. Lippmann, "The Transfixion Hip Prosthesis," *J Bone Joint Surg* 39A(1957): 759–85.

84. Moore, "Metal Hip Joint: A New Self-Locking Vitallium Prosthesis," *Southern Med J* 45(1952): 1015–18; id., "The Self-Locking Metal Hip Prosthesis," *J Bone Joint Surg* 39A(1957): 811–27; F. R. Thompson, "Vitallium Intramedullary Hip Prosthesis," *NY Med J* 52(1952): 3011–18; id., "Two and a Half Years' Experience with a Vitallium Intramedullary Prosthesis," *J Bone Joint Surg* 36A(1954): 489–500.

85. L. Thornton, "The Treatment of Trochanteric Fractures: Two New Methods," *Piedmont Hosp Bull* 10(1937): 21–28.

86. E. L. Jewett, "One-Piece Angle Nail for Trochanteric Fractures," *J Bone Joint Surg* 23(1941): 803–810.

87. G. M. Taylor, A. J. Neufield, and J. Janzen, "Internal Fixation for Intertrochanteric Fractures," *J Bone Joint Surg* 26(1944): 707–712.

88. W. K. Massie, "Functional Fixation of Femoral Neck Fractures: Telescoping Nail Technique," *Clin Orthop* 12(1958): 230–55; W. Pugh, "A Self-Adjusting Nail-Plate for Fractures about the Hip Joint," *J Bone Joint Surg* 37A(1955):

1085–93; W. Schumpelick and P. M. Jantzen, "A New Principle in the Operative Treatment of Trochanteric Fractures of the Femur," *J Bone Joint Surg* 37A(1955): 693–98.

89. Bérenger-Féraud, *Traité de l'immobilisation*, 244.

90. Senn, "A New Method of Direct Fixation of the Fragments in Compound and Ununited Fractures," *Trans Am Surg Assoc* 11(1893): 125–51; H. Bircher, "Eine neue Methode unmittlebarer Retention bei Fracturen der Rohrenknochen," *Arch klin Chir* 34(1893): 410–22.

91. Georg Schone, "Zur Behandlung von Vorderarmfrakturen mit Bolzung," *Münch med Wschr* 60(1913): 2327–28.

92. Hey-Groves, "Some Clinical and Experimental Observations on the Operative Treatment of Fractures with Special Reference to the Use of Intermedullary Pegs," *Brit Med J* 2(1912): 102–105.

93. E. Hoaglund, "New Method of Applying Autogenous Intramedullary Bone Transplants and of Making Autogenous Bone Screws," *SGO* 24(1917): 243–46.

94. Hey-Groves, "Ununited Fractures, with Special Reference to Gunshot Injuries and the Use of Bone Grafting," *Brit J Surg* 6(1918–19): 203–47.

95. Lambotte, "L'ostéosynthèse par clouage transarticulaire dans les fractures juxtaarticulaires," *Paris chir*, (1925), 145–48.

96. P. L. Chigot, *L'enchevillement central des fractures diaphysaires* (Paris: Masson, 1937); Müller and Meernach, "Die Bolzang der Bruche der langen Rohrenknochen," *Zentralbl Chir* 60(1933): 1718–23.

97. L. V. Rush and H. L. Rush, "A Reconstructive Operation for Comminuted Fractures of the Upper Third of the Ulna," *Am J Surg* 38(1937): 332–33.

98. Ibid., 332–33; id., "A Technique for Longitudinal Pin Fixation of Certain Fractures of the Ulna and Femur," *Am J Surg* 21(1939): 619–626; id., "Evolution of Medullary Fixation of Fractures by the Longitudinal Pin," *Am J Surg* 78(1949): 324–33.

99. L. V. Rush, "Dynamic Factors in Medullary Pinning of Fractures," *Am Surg* 17(1951): 803–808.

100. C. Lambrinudi, "Intramedullary Kirschner Wires in the Treatment of Fractures," *Proc Roy Soc Med* 33(1940): 153–57; Nicolaysen, "Lidt om Diagnosen," 1–18; Schone, "Zur Behandlung von Vorderarmfrakturen mit Bolzung," *Münch med Wschr* 60(1913): 2327–28; H. Smith and F. P. Sage, "Medullary Fixation of Forearm Fractures," *J Bone Joint Surg* 39A(1957): 91–98.

101. Gerhard Kuntscher, "Die Spannungsverteilung am Schenkelhals," *Arch klin Chir* 185(1935): 302–19; id., "Über das Wesen der mechanisch bedingten Knochen und Gelenkerkrankungen," *Arch klin Chir* 193(1938): 665–68; id., "Ergebnisse und Indikation der Schenkelhalsnagelung," *Arch Orthop Unfall-Chir* 40(1939): 282–84.

102. Kuntscher, "Die Marknagelung von Knochenbruchen," *Klin Wschr* 19(1940): 6–10.

103. Kuntscher and R. Maatz, *Technik der Marknagelung* (Leipzig: Georg Thieme Verlag, 1945).

104. J. Ender and R. Simon-Weidner, "Die Fixierung der trochanteren Bruche mit runden elastichen Condylengeln," *Acta chir austrica* 2(1970): 40–42; K. H. Hackethal, *Die Bundel-Nagelung, experimentelle und klinische Studie uber eine neurtige Methode der Markraum-Schienung langer Rohrenknochen; Leitfaden der Technik* (Berlin: Springer Verlag, 1961).

105. L. Böhler, *Technik der Knochenbruchbehandlung im Frieden um im Krieg, vol. 3 die Marknagelung nach Kuntscher* (Vienna: Wilhelm Maudrich, 1944); C. Habler, *Die Stabile Osteosynthese (Marknagelung nach Kuntscher)* (Munich: J. F. Lehmanns Verlag, 1944); E. J. Moeys, *Osetosynthesis with a Long Intramedullary Metal Pin (Kuntscher's Method)* (Utrecht: Kemink en Zoon, 1948); R. Soeur, *L'ostéosynthèse au clou* (Paris: Masson, 1946).

106. W. R. MacAusland, "Medullary Nailing of Fractures of the Long Bones," *SGO* 84(1947): 85–89.

107. D. M. Street, "Medullary Nailing of the Femur," *JAMA* 143(1950): 709–14; id., "One Hundred Fractures of the Femur Treated by Means of the Diamond-Shaped Medullary Ball," *J Bone Joint Surg* 33A(1951): 659–69; Street et al., "The Medullary Nail: Presentation of a New Type and Report of a Case,"

AMA Arch Surg 55(1947): 423–32; J. O. Lottes, "Intramedullary Fixation for Fractures of the Shaft of the Tibia," *South Med J* 45(1952): 407–414; id., "Blind Nailing Techniques for Insertion of the Triflange Medullary Nail," *JAMA* 155(1954): 1039–42; Lottes et al., "Closed Reduction, Plate Fixation and Medullary Nailing of Fractures of Both Bones of the Leg," *J Bone Joint Surg* 34A(1952): 861–77.

108. J. Albert Key, "Positive Pressure in Arthrodesis for Tuberculosis of the Knee Joint," *South Med J* 25(1932): 909–15.

109. Charnley, "Positive Pressure in Arthrodesis of the Knee Joint," *J Bone Joint Surg* 30B(1948): 478–86.

110. Key, "Positive Pressure," 909–15.

111. A. Glucksmann, "Studies on Bone Mechanics in Vitro: Influence of Pressure on Orientation of Structure," *Anat Rec* 72(1938): 97–113.

112. K. Townsend and C. Gilfillian, "A New Type of Bone Plate and Screws," *SGO* 77(1943): 595–97.

113. G. W. Bagby, "Compression Bone-Plating: Historical Consideration," *J Bone Joint Surg* 59A(1977): 625–31.

114. H. S. MacLean, "A Modification of Lane's Plates," *Trans South Surg Assoc* 27(1914): 99–109.; H. J. Warthin, Jr., "Henry Stuart MacLean (1873–1954)," *Trans South Surg Assoc* 65(1953): 418–19.

115. G. W. N. Eggers, "Internal Contact Splint," *J Bone Joint Surg* 30A(1948): 40–51; Eggers and H. P. Roosth, "Contact Splint Survey," *Ann Surg* 149(1959): 21–29.

116. Eggers et al., "The Influence of the Contact-Compression Factor on Osteogenesis in Surgical Fractures," *J Bone Joint Surg* 31A(1949) 693–716.

117. L. T. Peterson and O. S. Reeder, "Dual Slotted Plates in Fixation of Fractures of the Femoral Shaft," *J Bone Joint Surg* 32A(1950): 532–541.

118. J. J. Flanagan, "Instrument for Accurate Measurement of Bone Screws," *J Bone Joint Surg* 27(1945): 723.

119. Danis, *Théorie et pratique*, n.p.

120. J. Boreau and P. Hermann, "Plaque d'ostéosynthèse permettant l'impaction des fragments," *Presse méd* 60(1952): 356.

121. Z. B. Friedenberg and G. French, "The Effects of Known Compression Forces on Fracture Healing," *SGO* 94(1952): 743–48.

122. Bagby, "The Effect of Compression on the Rate of Fracture Healing Using a Special Plate" (Master's Thesis, Mayo Clinic, 1956); Bagby and J. W. Janes, "An Impacting Bone Plate," *Mayo Clin Proc* 32(1957): 55–57.

123. Bagby and Janes, "The Effect of Compression on the Rate of Fracture Healing Using a Special Plate," *Am J Surg* 95(1958): 761–71.

124. Bagby and Janes, "Impacting Bone Plate," 55–57.

125. M. E. Müller, "Principes d'ostéosynthèse," *Helv chir acta* 28(1961): 196–206.

126. R. N. Gray, "Disability and Cost of Industrial Fractures," *J Bone Joint Surg* 10(1928): 27–38.

127. M. Allgower and P. G. Spiegel, "Internal Fixation of Fractures: Evolution of Concepts," *Clin Orthop* 138(1979): 26–29.

128. Müller et al., *Technik der Operativen Frakturenbehandlung* (Berlin: Springer Verlag, 1963).

129. F. Pauwels, *Der Schenkelhalsbruch: ein mechanisches Problem* (Stuttgart: Ferdinand Enke Verlag, 1935); B. G. Weber, "Grundlagen und Moglichkeiten der Zuggurtungs-osteosynthese," *Chirugia* 35(1964): 81–86.

130. Fritz Konig, "Ueber die Berechtigung fruhzeitiger blutiger Eingriffe bei subcutanen Knochenbruchen," *Arch klin Chir* 85(1905): 725–77; id., "Ueber die Implantation von Elfenbein zum Ersatz von Knochen und Gelenkenden," *Beitr klin chir* 85(1913): 91–114.

131. E. J. Brougham and A. C. Eeke, "A Preliminary Report of Treatment of Fractures by Fixation with Animal Bone Plates and Bone Screws," *SGO* 18(1914): 637–40.

132. M. S. Henderson, "The Use of Beef-Bone Screws in Fractures and Bone Transplantation," *JAMA* 74(1920): 715–17.

133. Lane, "The Operative Treatment of Simple Fractures," *SGO* 8(1909): 344–54.

134. E. Dahl-Iverson, "Sur la fréquence et la durée de l'ostéite après l'osteosynthèse, d'après l'examen de deux cent soixante-quatorze cas et l'examen ultérieur de fractures operées," *Lyon chir* 25(1928): 513–25.

135. R. Leriche and A. Policard, "Recherches biologiques sur l'ostéosynthèse à la plaque de Lambotte," *Bull mém soc chir Paris* 44(1918): 1145–48.

136. G. Menegaux and D. Odiette, *L'ostéosynthèse au point de vue biologique* (Paris: Masson, 1936); C. S. Venable and W. G. Stuck, *The Internal Fixation of Fractures* (Springfield: Charles C Thomas, 1947).

137. L. G. Gazzotti, "La osteogenesi in rapporto all azione chimica di alcuni metalli," *Chir org mov* 7(1923): 311–328; A. A. Zierold, "Reaction of Bone to Various Metals," *AMA Arch Surg* 9(1924): 365–412.

138. Menegaux and Odiette, *L'ostéosynthèse.*

139. Ibid., 164–65.

140. L. Jones and B. A. Lieberman, "Interaction of Bone and Various Metals," *AMA Arch Surg* 32(1936): 990–1006.

141. Venable and Stuck, *Internal Fixation of Fractures*, 63.

142. G. S. Leventhal, "Titanium: A Metal for Surgery," *J Bone Joint Surg* 33A(1951): 473–74.

143. J. Brettle, "A Survey of the Literature on Metallic Surgical Implants," *Injury* 2(1970): 26–39.

144. M. P. Mandarino and J. E. Salvatore, "Polyurethane Polymer (Ostamer): Its Use in Fractured and Diseased Bones," *Surg Forum* 9(1958): 762–65.

145. M. P. Mandarino, *Chemical Osteosynthesis in Orthopedic Surgery* (Springfield, Ill.: Charles C Thomas, 1960); Mandarino and Salvatore, "Polyurethane Polymer: Its Use in Fractured and Diseased Bones," *Am J Surg* 97(1959): 442–46; id., "Polyurethane Polymer: Its Use in Osseous Lesions," *Ann Surg* 149(1959): 107–109.

146. K. D. Harrington et al., "The Use of Methylmethacrylate as an Adjunct in the Internal Fixation of Malignant Neoplastic Fractures," *J Bone Joint Surg* 54A(1972): 1665–76.

CHAPTER SIX

The Treatment of Fractures by Traction

Ad pendum ligo plumbi traneundo chordam super parvem polegean; itaque tenebit tibiam in sua longitudine.

—Guy de Chauliac

MALGAIGNE CREDITS GUY de Chauliac with the introduction of continuous isotonic traction in the treatment of fractures.[1] This was accomplished by suspending a weight attached to the leg by a cord over a pulley at the foot of the patient's bed. Despite the attractiveness of this idea, practical considerations sharply limited its application. The technique was virtually unchanged five hundred years later in the nineteenth century, when continuous isotonic traction was applied more widely in treating fractures of the leg[2] (figure 6.1). The crux of the problem lay in the attachment of the traction device to the limb. The gaiter and the handkerchief are representative of the methods then generally used[3] (figure 6.2). While these methods might suffice for some isometric traction splints used for fractures of the shaft of the femur, they were inadequate when continuous isotonic traction was necessary. Two solutions to this problem were developed. The first applied traction to a splint firmly bound to the limb, and the second applied traction directly to the limb itself.

Both Mathias Louis Mayor and Johann Nepomuk Sauter had described the use of balanced suspended splints by which the lower limbs were supported but in which the element of traction was minimal or absent.[4] Suspension and traction were combined by Nathan Smith (1762–1829), one of the most distinguished surgeons and teachers in New England.[5] He wholeheartedly agreed with Pott's ideas and believed that the usual method of treatment of fractures of the femur was an abomination. He devised a gutter splint in the form of an inclined plane for the treatment of fractures of the femur. The fractured limb was bound into the well-padded splint. If there was shortening, continuous traction was applied to the leg by

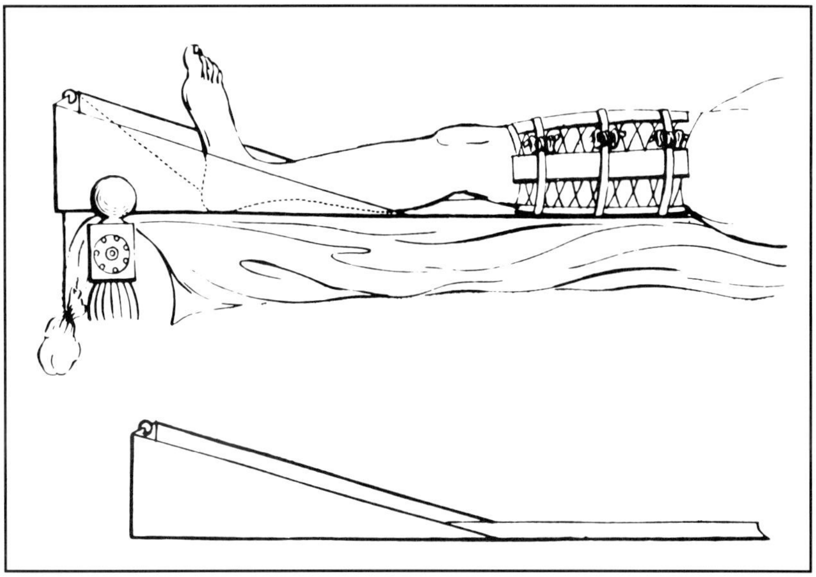

Figure 6.1 Apparatus for applying isotonic traction for treatment of a fracture of the shaft of the femur used by William C. Daniell of Savannah, Georgia, in 1829. The traction was attached to the ankle by means of silk handkerchief. From Daniell, "Method of Treating Fracture of the Thigh Bone," *Am J Med Sci* 4(1829): 330–33.

attaching a cord to the splint: the cord passed through a pulley and was fastened to a weight. The line of traction was the axis of the shaft of the femur (figure 6.3). "The weight of the body makes the counterextension which may be increased if necessary by raising a little the foot of the bed."[6]

Nathan Rhyno Smith (1797–1877), the second son of Nathan Smith, and himself a professor of surgery in Baltimore, improved upon his father's method.[7] He treated fractures of the shaft of the femur by means of a splint bound to the ventral side of the limb (figure 6.4). Both suspension and traction were maintained by means of cords attached to the splint. This method was particularly desirable when open, draining wounds were present, since it allowed access to the wound without removing the splint and provided for dependent drainage.

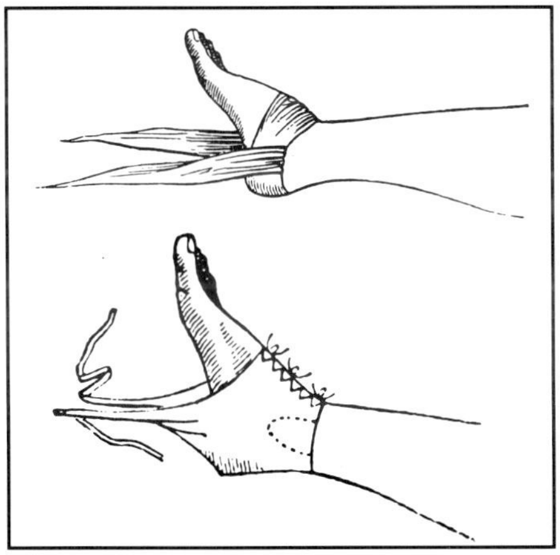

Figure 6.2 The handkerchief and the gaiter were the usual methods of applying traction to the legs. From F. W. Sargent, *On Bandaging and Other Operations of Minor Surgery* (Philadelphia: Lea & Blanchard, 1848).

This system of suspended traction was improved still further by John T. Hodgen of St. Louis. His splint was a modification of Nathan Rhyno Smith's apparatus and was designed specifically for the treatment of gunshot fractures of the femur[8] (figure 6.5). Hodgen's system was strongly recommended by Hamilton and was used extensively during the American Civil War.[9] This splint was introduced into England by Hodgen himself during a visit to St. Bartholomew's Hospital and was the method of choice for treating femoral shaft fractures on the wards of James Paget in 1867.[10] The Hodgen splint was widely used by military and civilian surgeons and saw considerable service in World War I.[11]

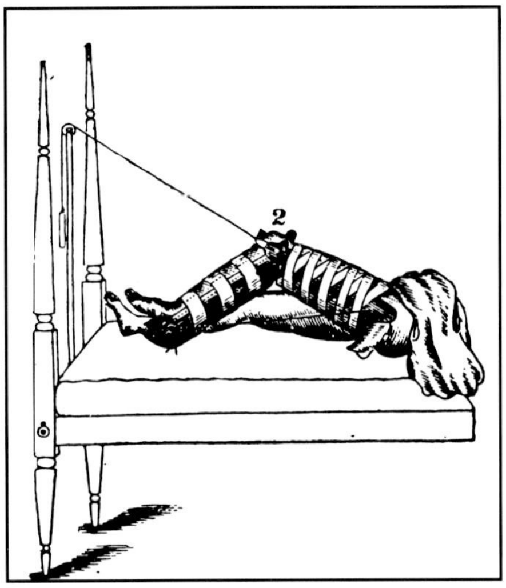

Figure 6.3 Nathan Smith's apparatus which allowed traction to be applied to a double-inclined plane. From Smith, *Observations on Fractures of the Femur, with an Account of a New Splint; Medical and Surgical Memoirs,* edited with addenda by N. R. Smith (Baltimore: W. A. Francis, 1831).

The application of adhesive plaster to the skin of the leg for the purpose of applying traction was introduced into surgical practice early in the nineteenth century by several surgeons. J. H. James began using such a system in England in 1828[12] (figure 6.6). At the same time, Joseph K. Swift, a student of John S. Dorsey, was using the same method in Philadelphia.[13] The technique was described by Samuel D. Gross in 1830:

> *In complicated fractures of the leg, it not unfrequently happens that the soft parts about the ankle are so much contused, or otherwise injured, as to render it impossible to employ the usual extending bands. When this is found to be the case, the difficulty can usually be remedied by applying to each side of the leg, as high up as the seat of the fracture will admit, a piece of strong muslin, about two feet and a half in length, two inches and a half in width, and spread at one of its extremities with adhesive plaster. The part which is applied upon the limb should be confined by three of four circular strips, so as to keep it firmly in its place and equalize the extending power. The free extremities of the extending bands should then be tied under the sole of the foot, and be secured to the block or bar which connects with the lower ends of the splints.*[14]

Josiah Crosby promoted the use of this method of traction in New England[15] (figure 6.7).

In addition to the treatment of fractures, skin traction was used for the treatment of other conditions. H. G. Davis of New York employed it in the treatment of tuberculosis of the hip *(morbus coaxarius)*. It was this application that caught the attention of

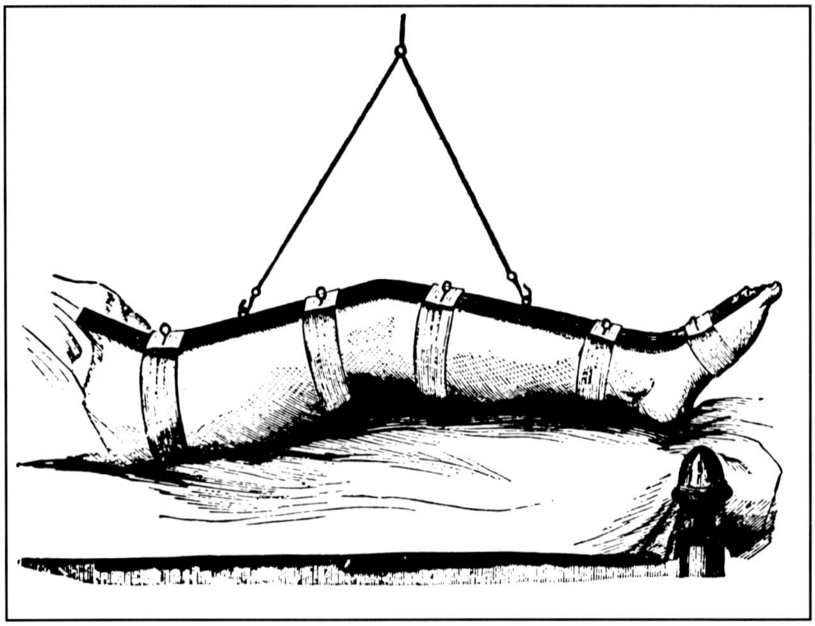

Figure 6.4 The suspension traction splint of Nathan Rhyno Smith. From Smith, *Treatment of Fractures of the Lower Extremity by Use of the Anterior Suspensory Apparatus* (Baltimore: Kelly & Piet, 1867), 15.

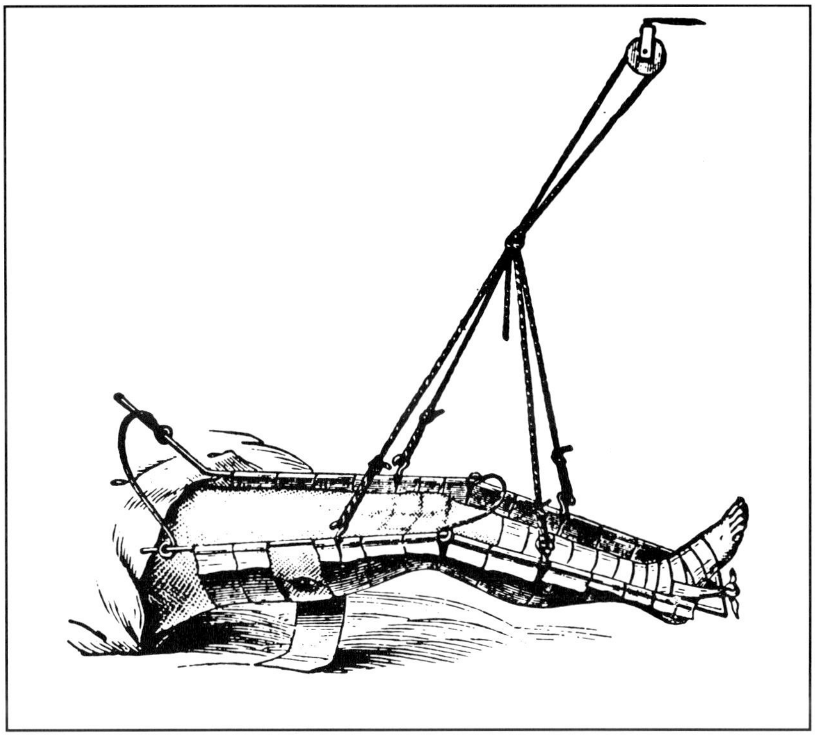

Figure 6.5 Hodgen's splint. From Frank Hastings Hamilton, *A Treatise on Military Surgery and Hygiene* (New York: Bailliere Brothers, 1865), 412.

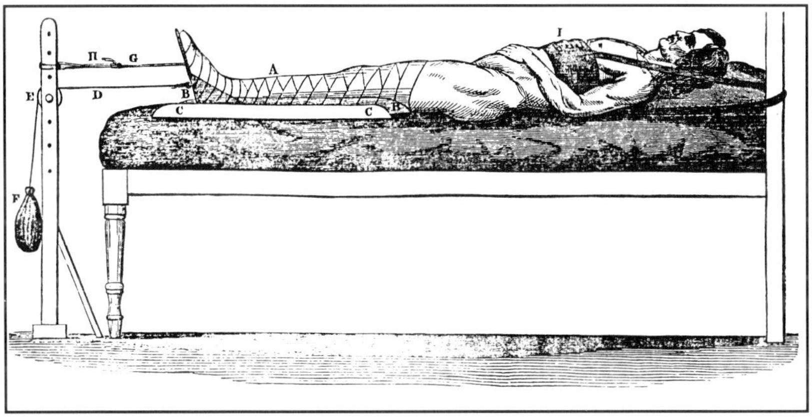

Figure 6.6 Isotonic traction applied by adhesive plaster according to the technique of James. From James, *The Retrospective Address in Surgery from July 1836 to July 1839* (Worcester: Henry Deighton, 1839).

Gurdon Buck, who then used it for the treatment of fractures of the femur. In 1861 he reported his experience with the use of the method in the treatment of twenty-one patients[16] (figure 6.8). During the American Civil War, skin traction was used extensively in the treatment of fractures, and the method became known as Buck's extension. The method was carried abroad, where it became

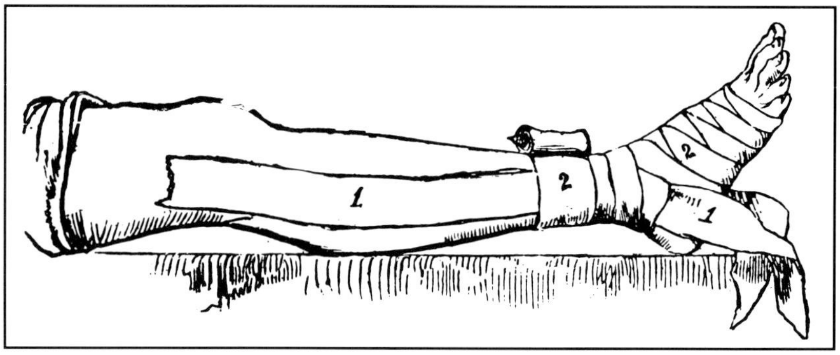

Figure 6.7 The application of adhesive traction to the skin as described by Crosby. From Hamilton, *Treatise*, 404.

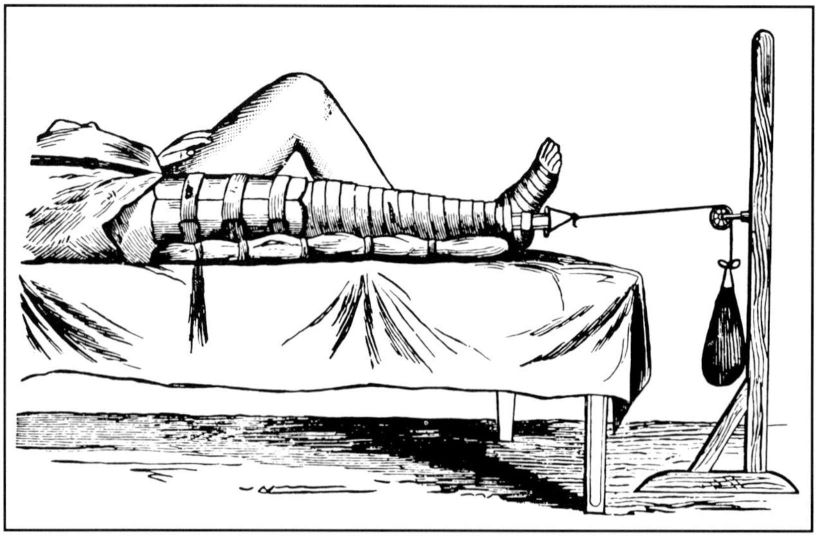

Figure 6.8 Buck's extension for treatment of fractures of the femur. From *The Medical and Surgical History of the War of Rebellion* (Washington, D.C.: Government Printing Office, 1883), pt. 3, 2:348.

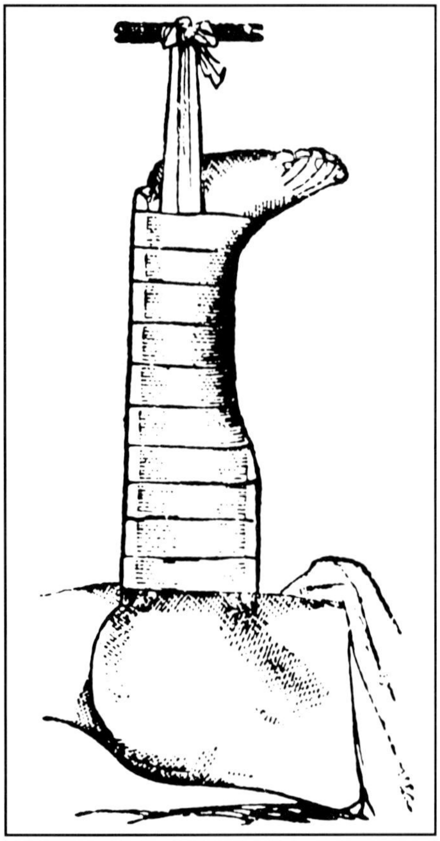

Figure 6.9 Bryant's traction for the treatment of fractures of the shaft of the femur in children. From Bryant, *The Practice of Surgery: A Manual* (London: J. & A. Churchill, 1872), 984.

known as the American method,[17] being introduced into France by Nélaton and into Germany by Richard Volkmann.[18]

The treatment of fractures of the shaft of the femur in small children in the middle of the nineteenth century consisted almost entirely of a program of studied neglect. "If all apparatus be dispensed with, and the child be only laid on a firm bed, with little or no head pillow, and with the broken limb, after setting it, bent at the hip and knee, and laid on its outer sides there it will remain."[19] Thomas Bryant, of Guy's Hospital, was not happy with the results:

I do not recommend this practice, but would advise instead that the injured limb of the child, together with the sound one, be flexed at a right angle with the pelvis, fixed by some light splint and hoisted upward to a cradle or bar above the bed. By these means, the weight of the body acts as a constant counter-extending force, the child can be well looked

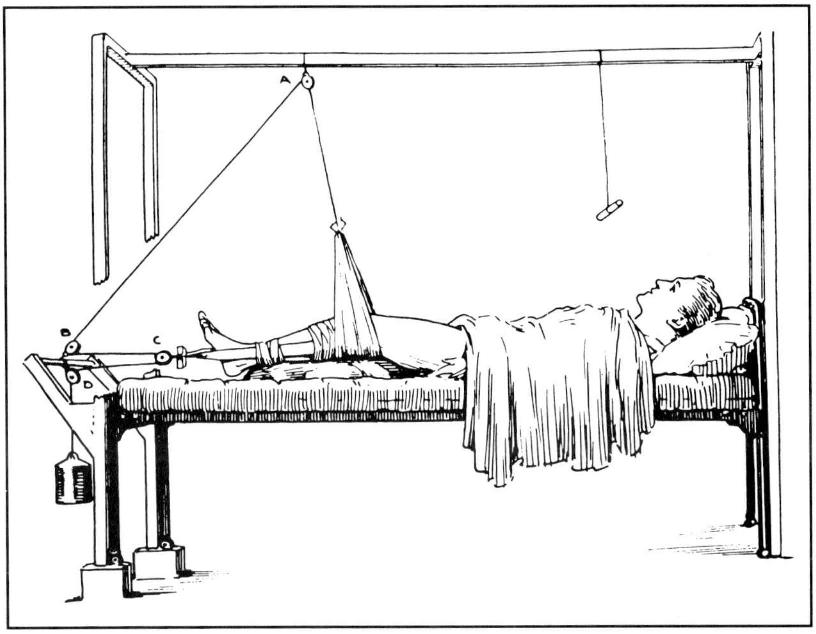

Figure 6.10 Russell's traction; note the flexion of the hip and knee. From Russell, "Fractures of the Femur: A Clinical Study," *Brit J Surg* 11(1924): 491–502.

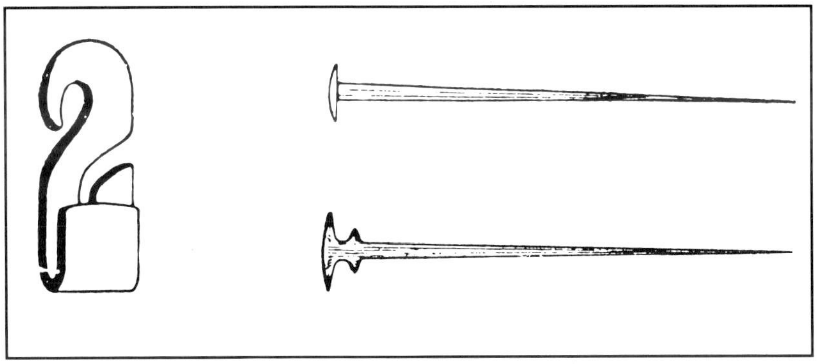

Figure 6.11 Steinmann's original pins and traction hooks. From Steinmann, "Eine neue Extensionsmethode in der Frakturenbehandlung," *Zentralbl Chir* 34(1907): 938–42.

to for the purposes of cleanliness, and a good result may be expected. At Guy's we have had excellent results from this practice[20] [figure 6.9].

In his text, *The Practice of Surgery*, Bryant describes putting both legs in traction, although his illustration shows only one. This sort of ambivalence still prevails, with some surgeons using traction on the injured limb only, and others on both. Bryant's traction quickly became popular; in Germany, it became known as Max Schede's method.[21]

Skin traction was adapted for the treatment of a wide variety of fractures in both the upper and lower extremities.[22] It was not until 1921, however, that an Australian surgeon, R. Hamilton Russell, one of Lister's last house officers, devised a method of utilizing skin

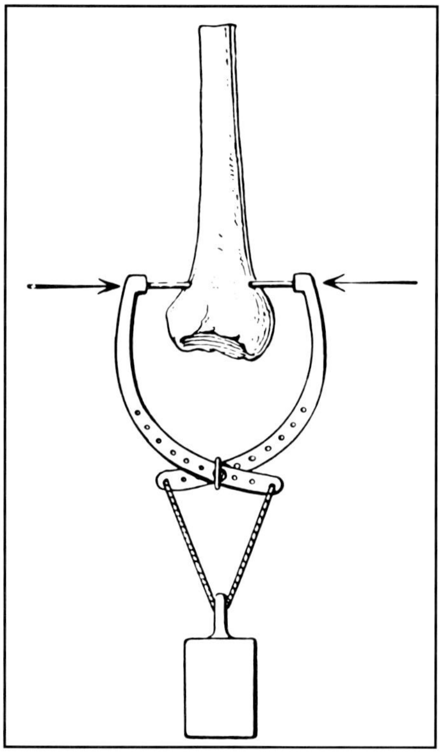

Figure 6.12 Steinmann's modified pin and bail. From Steinmann, "Die Nagelextension," *Ergeb Chir Orthop* 9(1916): 520–60.

traction in such a way that the advantages of the flexed position of the knee and hip could be enjoyed[23] (figure 6.10). Russell's traction has been used since its introduction for the closed treatment of fractures of the shaft of the femur and extracapsular hip fractures.

Malgaigne had demonstrated with his hooks for the treatment of patellar fractures and his point for the treatment of tibial fractures that mechanical forces, both pressure and tension, could be applied directly to the skeleton.[24] These methods were not used extensively before the introduction of sterile techniques, and even then further innovations were slow in coming. Carlos Ottolenghi, whose book *Tracción esqueletica* is a mine of historical information, credits Giuliano Vanghetti for reviving interest in skeletal traction.[25] In his experimental studies on kineplasty, Vanghetti made use of wires and pins inserted through muscles and tendons into bone.[26] In 1903 Alessandro Codivilla of the Rizzoli Institute of Bologna used skeletal traction applied by means of a pin placed through the *os calcis* in the treatment of malunited fractures and other deformities.[27] After correcting the deformity, the pin was incorporated into a plaster of paris dressing to provide isometric traction. In 1907 Fritz Steinmann of Bern described a method of applying isotonic skeletal traction by means of pins driven into the femoral condyles[28] (figure 6.11). He progressed from this initial attempt to the use of the through-and-through pin technique which bears his name[29] (figure 6.12). Codivilla and Steinmann carried on a polemic regarding their claims to priority in introducing skeletal traction.[30] Codivilla was interested in late problems of malunion and delayed union, and his traction was essentially isometric. Steinmann was interested in the treatment of fresh fractures, and his traction was primarily isotonic. Skeletal traction by means of simple screws, cup hooks, and other

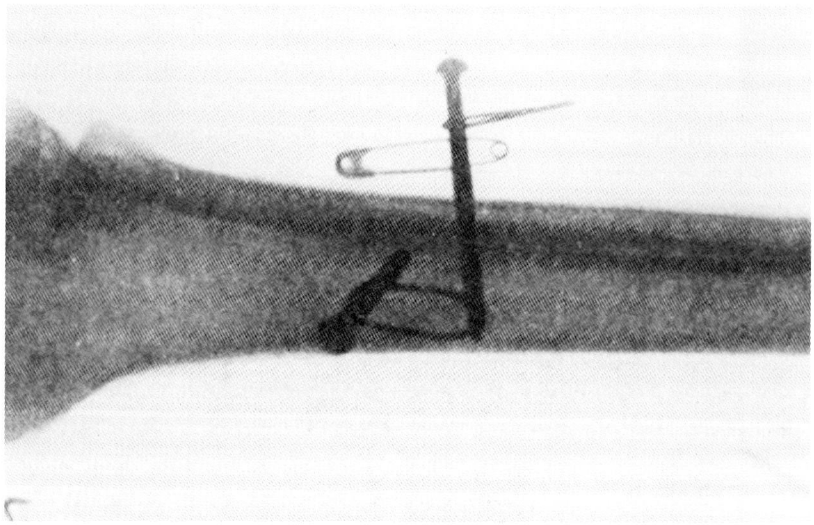

Figure 6.13 The use of hardware for skeletal traction. From M. Sinclair, *The Thomas Splint and its Modifications* (London: Oxford University Press, 1927), 32.

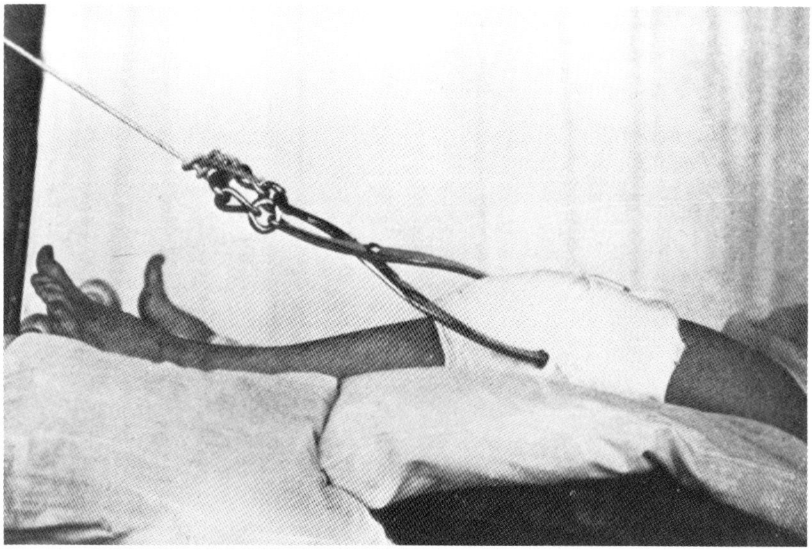

Figure 6.14 Ice tongs used for skeletal traction. From J. Ransohoff, "Ice Tongs Extension for Simple Fractures of the Femur," *Trans Am Surg Assoc* 30(1912): 706.

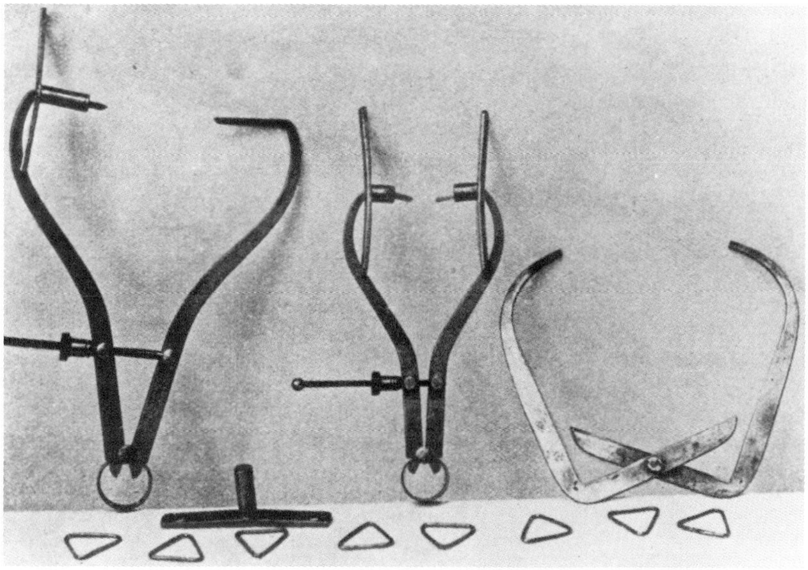

Figure 6.15 Tongs modified for medical use in treating fractures in World War I. From *Orthopaedic Surgery of Injuries*, ed. Robert Jones (London: Hodder & Stoughton, 1921), 127.

hardware has been used for many years[31] (figure 6.13).

In the surgical clinic in Erlangen in 1900, Walter Hermann Heinecke used a set of tongs of his own design to apply traction to the *os calcis* for the purpose of reducing fractures of the tibia and holding them in place during the application of a plaster of paris dressing.[32] Joseph Ransohoff applied ice tongs to the femoral condyles and used them to obtain traction for the treatment of femoral shaft fractures[33] (figure 6.14). Because of the ubiquity of tongs and

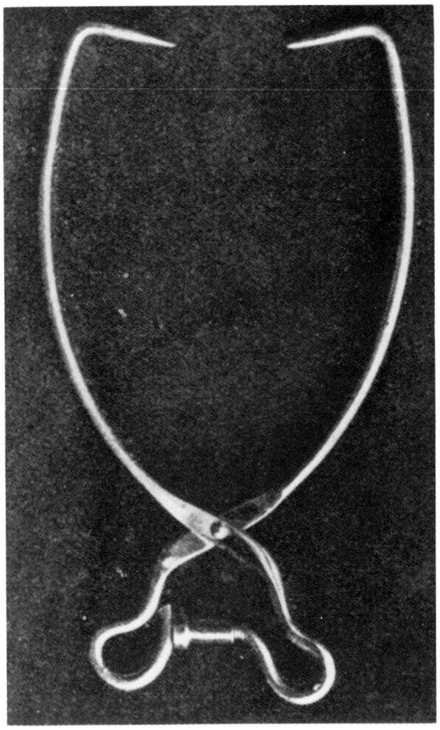

Figure 6.16 Major Pearson's ice-tong caliper. From *Orthopaedic Surgery*, ed. Jones, 129.

calipers and the ease with which they could be adapted for use in patients, tongs were used extensively for skeletal traction during World War I (figure 6.15). The most popular design in the Allied armies was that of Maurice G. Pearson, who also designed the attachment for the Thomas splint to permit knee flexion[34] (figures 6.16, 6.17). The popularity of tongs gradually diminished because of the complications, particularly infection, associated with their use.[35] Today, tongs remain in our armamentarium only in their special application for skull traction.

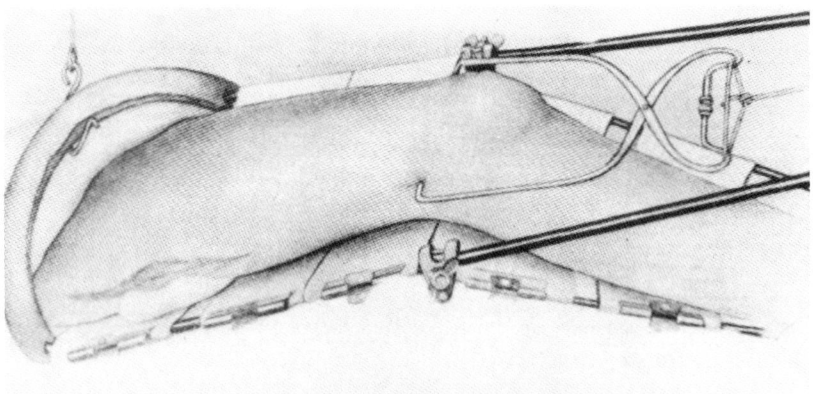

Figure 6.17 Pearson's tongs and Pearson's attachment used with a Thomas splint for the treatment of the shaft of the femur by skeletal traction with the hip and knee bent. From Pearson and J. Drummond, *Fractured Femurs: Their Treatment by Caliper Extensions* (London: Oxford University Press, 1919).

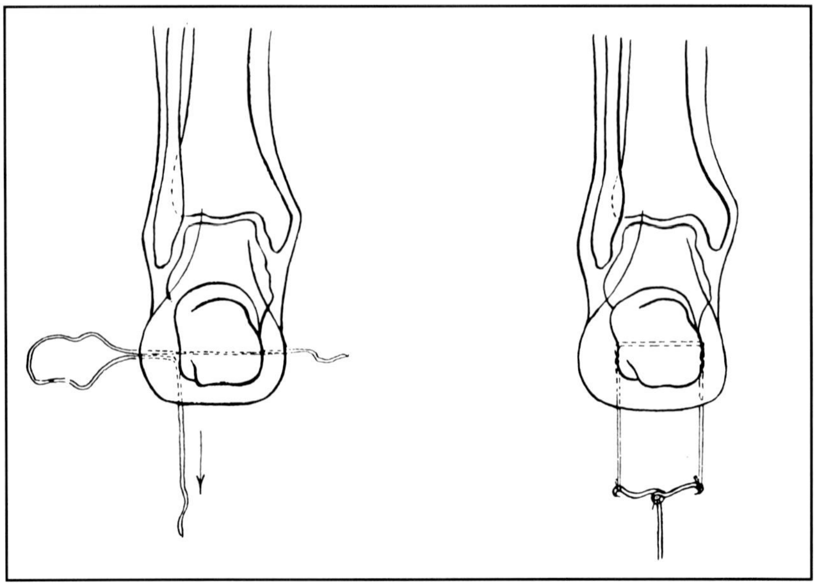

Figure 6.18 Klapp's method of applying traction to the *os calcis* using a wire. From Ottolenghi, *Tracción esqueletica* (Buenos Aires: Ateneo, 1946), 26.

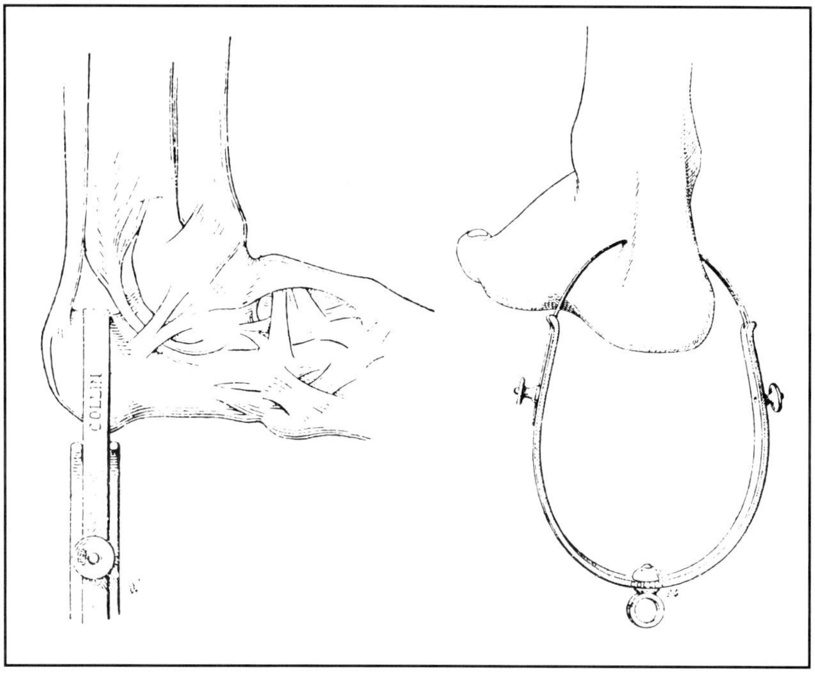

Figure 6.19 Finochietto's calcaneal stirrup. From R. Leriche, *Traitement des fractures* (Paris: Masson, 1917), 2:81.

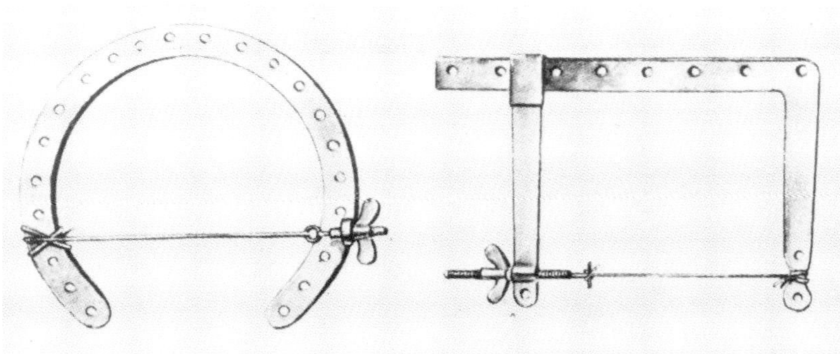

Figure 6.20 The first traction bails to make the wire rigid by applying tension. From Herzberg, "Zur Drahtextension am Ort der Wahl," *Zentralbl Chir* 47(1920): 1205.

In 1914 Rudolf Klapp of August Karl Gustav Bier's clinic in Berlin described a method of skeletal traction using an aluminum-bronze wire that was passed through the *os calcis* and brought out through the bottom of the heel[36] (figure 6.18). Klapp had developed this method while working in a military hospital in Belgrade during the Balkan War of 1912. He believed that this method was superior to the use of a pin because it reduced the chance of infection. However, the method was difficult to use because a hole had to be made in the bone with an awl and then the wire threaded through the hole. This problem was solved by means of a hollow awl through which the wire was passed. To avoid this problem, Enrique Finochietto designed a sharp pointed metal band that was passed through the soft

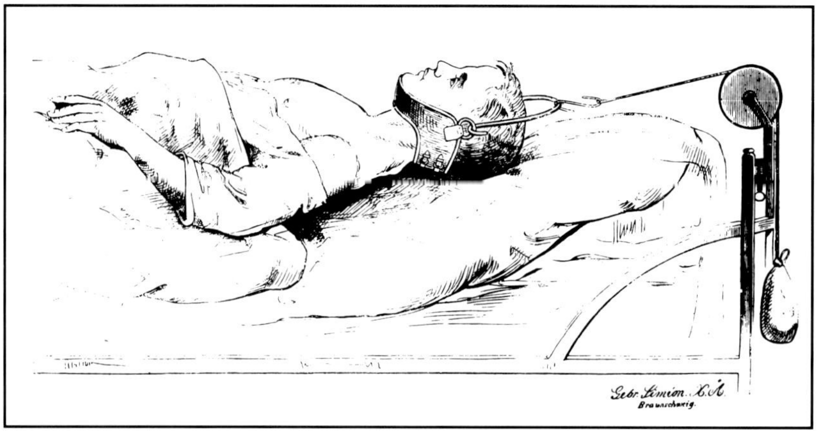

Figure 6.22 Cervical traction by means of a halter. From Richard Volkmann, "Die Krankheiten der Bewegungsorgane," in *Handbuch der allgemeinen und specillen Chirurgie*, ed. Pitha and Billroth (Erlangen: Enke, 1865), 2:752.

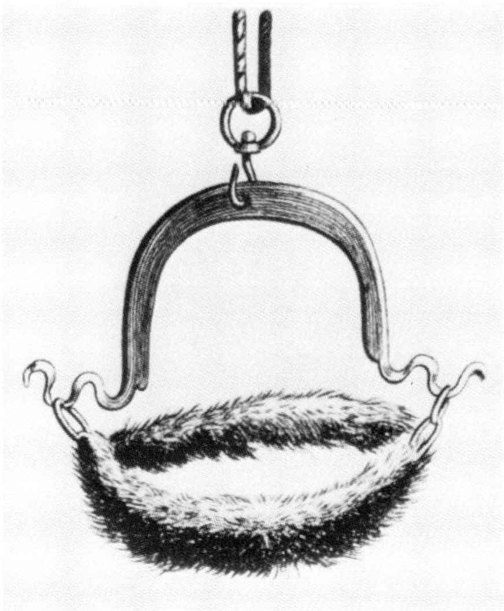

Figure 6.21 A sling for cervical traction. From Nuck, *Operationa et Experimenta Chirurgica* (Lyons: Batav, 1696), 86.

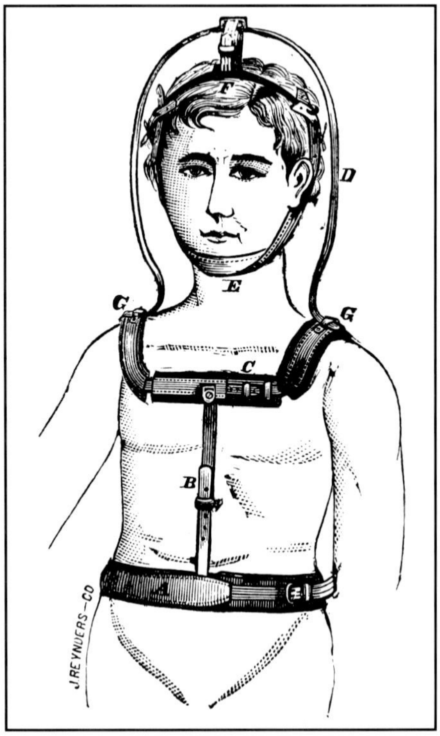

Figure 6.23 Cervical traction incorporated into a brace for the treatment of cervical spondylitis, probably tuberculosis. From L. A. Sayre, *Orthopedic Surgery and Diseases of the Joints* (New York: D. Appleton, 1876), 371.

tissues above the *os calcis* just anterior to the Achilles tendon[37] (figure 6.19). This band was then attached to a stirrup to which traction could be applied.

Wire traction was made more simple by the introduction of a traction bow by Erich Herzberg in 1918.[38] His second contribution was a traction bow to hold the wire stiff and rigid by applying tension[39] (figure 6.20). The final improvement made by Martin Kirschner was the perfection of a wire strong enough to be drilled through the bone with a drill guide.[40] The wire, the means of inserting it, and the tension bow to hold it rigid are all essential elements.

Although traction could be tolerated for short periods, continuous cervical traction by means of bandages and appliances applied to the head was limited by skin breakdown over the occiput and chin due to pressure necrosis. The sling described by Antonius Nuck in 1696 is characteristic of the most common method of cervical traction used[41] (figure 6.21). These traction methods were primarily for use in chronic diseases such as scoliosis, torticollis, and tuberculosis of the spine[42] (figures 6.22, 6.23).

The advantages of skeletal traction in the treatment of fractures of the extremities prodded surgeons to study the application of similar techniques to the skull for the treatment of injuries of the cervical spine.[43] In 1936 Thomas Hoen in Montreal passed wires through burr holes in the skull and used them to apply traction.[44] This method required an open operation with exposure of the dura. An interesting approach was described by Ben L. Neubeiser from St. Charles, Missouri.[45] It consisted of passing barbless fishhooks under the zygomatic arches just in front of the temporomandibular joints and using them to apply traction.[46] This method is still useful in an emergency when no other equipment is available. The technique was developed further by John Selmo, who substituted a flat hook for the fishhook[47] (figure 6.24).

William Edward Gallie applied skeletal traction to the skull by the simple expedient of ice tongs, set in place through tiny skin incisions over the most prominent part of the parietal bones. The points of the tongs were driven into the bone about one-eighth inch "by a sharp blow with a hammer"![48] W. Gayle Crutchfield first modified a set of tongs used for extremity traction and applied them to the skull.[49] Three years later, in 1936, he described the use of skull tongs of his own design.[50] Other types of skull tongs incorporating various modifications and improvements have been introduced[51] (figure 6.25).

The halo was introduced as a spinal skeletal traction fixation device in 1959 at Rancho Los Amigos Hospital in Downey, California.[52] Prototypes of the halo had been used by Leon Bloom in Houston and Neufeld in Los Angeles for the treatment of maxillofacial injuries, but the adaptation for use as a traction device for the cervical spine was the work of Jacqueline Perry, Roy Snelson, and Vernon Nickel.[53] The halo has become a popular method for the treatment of cervical spine fractures and dislocations because it can be applied easily, gives excellent control of the head, allows the application of strong traction, and can be incorporated into a rigid jacket or frame[54] (figure 6.26).

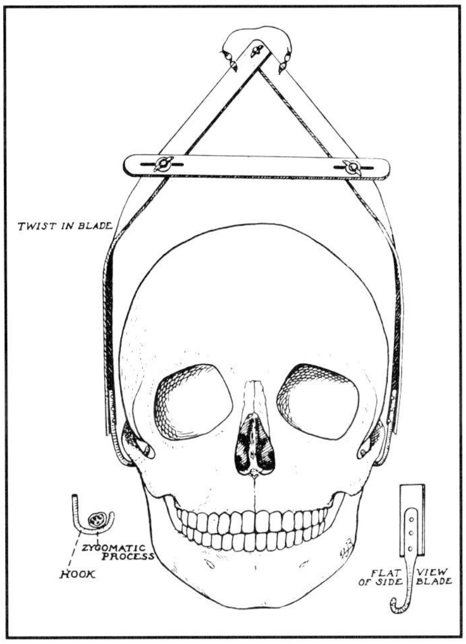

Figure 6.24 Skeletal traction on the skull by means of hooks under the zygoma. From Selmo, "Traction on the Zygomatic Process for Cervico-vertebral Injuries," *Am J Surg* 46(1939): 405.

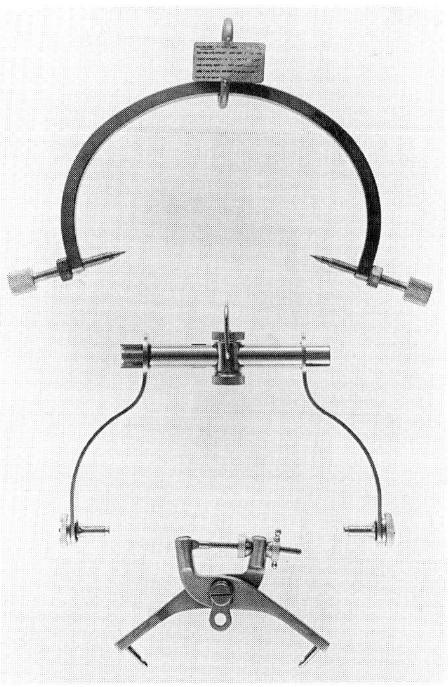

Figure 6.25 From top to bottom, the skull tongs of Gardner-Wells, Vinke, and Crutchfield.

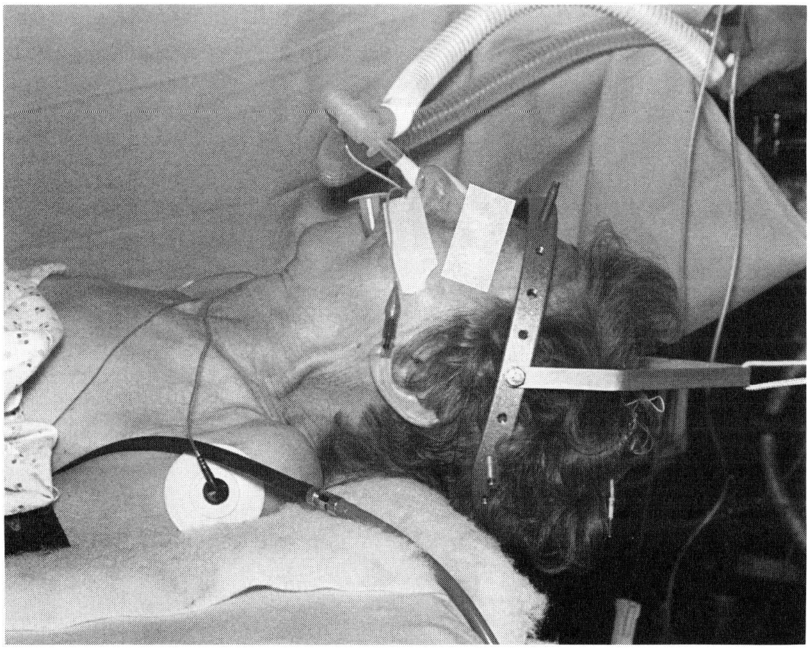

Figure 6.26 A halo being used to apply skeletal traction in a patient with an unstable cervical spine.

Notes

1. J.-F. Malgaigne, *Recherches historiques et pratiques sur les appareils employés dans le traitement des fractures en général depuis Hippocrate jusqu'à nos jours* (Paris: H. Cousin, 1841), 34.

2. W. C. Daniell, "Method of Treating Fractures of the Thigh Bone," *Am J Med Sci* 4(1829): 330–33; L. A. Dugas, "On the Best Plan of Treating Fractures in Country Practice," *South Med Surg J*, new ser., 10(1854): 69–78.

3. Gurdon Buck, "An Improved Method of Treating Fractures of the Thigh Illustrated by Cases and a Drawing," *Trans NY Acad Med* 2(1861): 232–50.

4. M. L. Mayor, *Mémoire sur l'hyponarthécie; ou, Sur le traitement des fractures par la planchette* (Geneva: n.p., 1827); J. N. Sauter, *Anweisung die Beinbruche der Gleidmassen* (Konstanz: n.p., 1812).

5. Emily A. Smith, *The Life and Letters of Nathan Smith, M.B., M.D.* (New Haven, Conn.: Yale University Press, 1914).

6. Nathan Smith, *Observations on Fractures of the Femur with an Account of a New Splint; Medical and Surgical Memoirs*, ed. with addenda by Nathan R. Smith, (Baltimore: W. A. Francis, 1831), 140.

7. N. Smith, *Observations*; Nathan Rhyno Smith, "A New Instrument for the Treatment of Fractures of the Lower Extremity," *Maryland and Virginia Med Surg J* 14(1860): 1–177.

8. J. T. Hodgen, "On the Treatment of Gunshot Fractures of the Femur and Tibia," *Am Med Times* 7(1863): 169–70.

9. Frank Hastings Hamilton, *A Treatise on Military Surgery and Hygiene* (New York: Bailliere Brothers, 1865), 411–12.

10. J. A. Bloxam, "Respecting the Treatment of Fractures of the Lower Extremities, in the Wards under the Care of Mr. Paget," *St. Bartholomew's Hosp Rep* 3(1867): 385–94.

11. F. G. Nifong, *The Hodgen Wire Cradle Extension Suspension Splint* (St. Louis: C. V. Mosby, 1918).

12. J. H. James, *The Retrospective Address in Surgery from July 1836 to July 1839* (Worcester: Henry Deighton, 1839).

13. Howard A. Kelly and Walter L. Burrage, "Swift, Joseph K.," *Dictionary of American Medical Biography*, 1st ed. (New York & London: D. Appleton & Co., 1928): 1183–84.

14. Samuel D. Gross, *The Anatomy, Physiology, and Diseases of the Bones and Joints* (Philadelphia: John Grigg, 1830), 50.

15. Josiah Crosby, "The Application of Extension in Fractures by Means of Adhesive Plaster," *NH J Med* 1(1850): 65; Crosby, "Substitute for the Gaiter, Report of the Standing Committee on Surgery, R. D. Mussey, Chairman," *Trans Am Med Assoc* 3(1850): 382–83; Crosby, "On the Application of Extension in Fractures by Means of Adhesive Plaster," *NY Med J*, 2d ser., 6(1851): 137–38.

16. Buck, "An Improved Method", 232–50.

17. E. F. Meyringh, *Ueber die Behandlung von Oberschenkel-Fracturen durch permanent Extension mit Gewichten* (Halle: Plotz'che, 1872).

18. Jules Tillie, *Traitement des fractures du fémur par l'extension continue* (Lille: Robbe, 1882).

19. Bloxam, "Respecting the Treatment of Fractures," 385–94.

20. Thomas Bryant, *The Practice of Surgery: A Manual* (London: J. & A. Churchill, 1872), 984.

21. J. D. Loeser, "History of Skeletel Traction in the Treatment of Spine Injuries," *J Neurosurg* 33(1970): 54–59.

22. Ernst Bardenheuer, *Leitfaden der Behandlung von Fracturen und Luxatonen der Extremitaten mittelst Feder-Resp. Gewichsextension* (Stuttgart: Enke, 1890).

23. R. H. Russell, "Theory and Method on Extension of the Thigh," *Brit Med J* 2(1921): 637–38; id., "Fractures of the Femur: A Clinical Study," *Brit Surg J* 11(1924): 491–502.

24. Malgaigne, *Traité des fractures et des luxations* (Paris: J. B. Baillière, 1847), 771–76, 795–99.

25. Carlos E. Ottolenghi, *Tracción esqueletica* (Buenos Aires: Ateneo, 1946), 9–10.

26. G. Vanghetti, *Amputazione, disarticulazione et protesi* (Florence, 1898).

27. Alessandro Codivilla, "Sulla correzione della deformità da frattura del femore," *Bull sci med Bologna*, ser. 8, 3(1903): 246–49; id., "On the Means of Lengthening in the Lower Limbs, the Muscles and Tissues Which Are Shortened through Deformity," *Am J Orthop Surg* 2(1905): 352–69.

28. F. Steinmann, "Eine neue Extensionmethode in der Fracturenbehandlung," *Zentralbl Chir* 34(1907): 938–42.

29. Ibid., 938–42.

30. Codivilla, "Ueber Nagelextension," *Zeit orthop Chir* 27(1910): 404–18; F. Steinmann, "Zur Geschichte der Nagelextension," *Zeit orthop Chir* 29(1911): 96–114; id., "Die Nagelextension," *Ergeb Chir Orthop* 9(1916): 520–60.

31. O. Hilgenfeldt, "Die Verwendung rostfreier Bildernagel in der Knochenbruchbehandlung," *Dtsch Zeit Chir* 244(1935): 433–44; Maurice Sinclair, *The Thomas Splint and Its Modifications* (London: Oxford University Press, 1927), 31–33.

32. E. Graser, "Die Kalkaneusezange nach v. Heineke, ein Vorlaufer der Nagel extension zur Behandlung von Knochenbruchen," *Münch med Wschr* 57(1910): 692.

33. Joseph Ransohoff, "Ice Tongs Extension for Simple Fractures of the Femur," *Trans Am Surg Assoc* 30(1912): 706–15.

34. M. G. Pearson and J. Drummond, *Fractured Femurs: Their Treatment by Caliper Extensions* (London: Oxford University Press, 1919).

35. R. H. Kennedy, "Traction-Suspension Treatment in Fractures," *J Bone Joint Surg* 15(1922): 320; id., "Treatment of Fractures of the Shaft of the Femur: An Analysis of 120 Cases," *Ann Surg* 107(1938): 419.

36. R. Klapp, "Besondere Formen der Extension," *Zentralbl Chir* 41(1914): 1209.

37. Enrique Finochietto, "Tracción supracalcaneana por medio de cintas," *La prensa médica* 2(1915): 61.

38. Erich Herzberg, "Fortschritte der Extensionbehandlung in der Kreigeschirurgie," *Zeit Chir* 144(1918): 120.

39. Herzberg, "Zur Drahtextension am Ort der Wahl," *Zentralbl Chir* 47(1920): 1205–7.

40. Martin Kirschner, "Verbesserung der Drahtextension," *Arch klin Chir* 148(1927): 651.

41. Antonius Nuck, *Operationes et Experimenta Chirurgica* (Lyons: Batav, 1696).

42. Bruno Valentine, *Geschichte der Orthopaedie* (Stuttgart: Georg Thieme, 1961), 24–61.

43. J. D. Loeser, "History of Skeletal Traction in the Treatment of Spine Injuries," *J Neurosurg* 33(1970): 54.

44. T. Hoen, "A Method of Skeletal Traction for the Treatment of Fracture Dislocation of the Cervical Vertebra," *Arch Neurol Psychiat* 36(1936): 158.

45. B. L. Neubeiser, "A Method of Skeletal Traction for Neck Extension," *J MO State Med Assoc* 30(1933): 495.

46. W. T. Peyton et al., "Hook Traction under the Zygomatic Arch in Cervical Spine Injuries," *SGO* 79(1944): 311.

47. John Selmo, "Traction on the Zygomatic Process in Cervico-vertebral Injuries," *Am J Surg* 46(1939): 405.

48. W. E. Gallie, "Skeletal Traction in the Treatment of Fractures and Dislocations of the Cervical Spine," *Ann Surg* 106(1937): 770.

49. W.G. Crutchfield, "Skeletal Traction for Dislocation of the Cervical Spine," *South Surg* 2(1933): 156.

50. W. G. Crutchfield, "Further Observations on the Treatment of Fracture Dislocations of the Cervical Spine with Skeletal Traction," *SGO* 63(1936): 513–17.

51. L. G. Barton, "The Reduction of Fracture-Dislocations of the Cervical Vertebrae by Skeletal Traction," *SGO* 67(1938): 94; W. J. Gardner, "Principles of Spring-loaded Points for Cervical Traction," *J Neurosurg* 39(1973): 543; T. H. Vinke, "A Skull Traction Apparatus," *J Bone Joint Surg* 30A(1948): 522.

52. J. Perry and V. L. Nickel, "Total Cervical-Spine Fusion for Neck Paralysis," *J Bone Joint Surg* 41A(1959): 37.

53. Nickel, letter to the author, 1981.

54. Nickel et al., "The Halo: A Spinal Skeletal Traction Fixation Device," *J Bone Joint Surg* 50A(1968): 1400.

CHAPTER SEVEN

External Skeletal Fixation for the Treatment of Fractures

SURGEONS TREATING fractures of the extremities complicated by associated injuries of the skin and soft tissues have always been caught on the horns of a dilemma: they would like to observe the condition of wounds, but at the same time they would like to maintain immobilization of fractures. Hippocrates resolved this dilemma for patients with injuries of the leg in the following manner (figure 7.1):

But one should sew two balls of Egyptian leather, such as are worn by persons confined for a length of time in large shackles, and the balls should have coats on each side, deeper toward the wound, but shorter toward the joints, and the balls should be well stuffed and soft, and fit well, the one above the ankle, and the other below the knee. Sideways it should have below two appendages, either of a single or double thong, and short, like loops, the one set being placed on either side of the ankles, and the other on the knee. And the upper ball should have others of the same kind in the same line. Then taking four rods, made of the cornel tree, of equal length, and of the thickness of a finger, and of such a length that when bent they will admit of being adjusted to the appendages, care should be taken that the extremities of the rods bear not upon the skin, but on the extremities of the balls. There should be three sets of rods, or more, one set a little longer than another, and another a little shorter and small, so that they may produce greater or less distension, if required. Either of these sets of rods should be placed on this side and that of the ankles. If these things be properly contrived, they should occasion a proper and equable extension in a straight line, without giving any pain to the wound; for the pressure, if there is any, should be thrown at foot and thigh. And the rods are commodiously arranged on either side of the ankles, so as not to interfere with the position of the limb; and the wound is easily examined and arranged. And, if thought

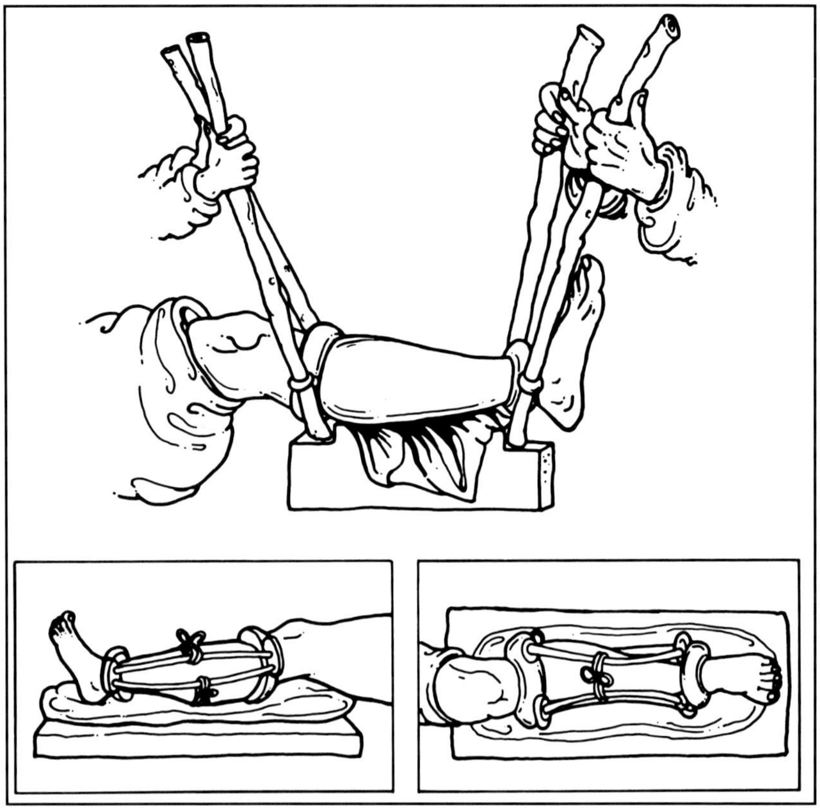

Figure 7.1 The method of Hippocrates for reducing a fracture of the tibia and fibula and retaining the reduction by an external fixation device. From *The Genuine Works of Hippocrates*, trans. Francis Adams (Baltimore: Williams and Wilkins, 1939), plate 8.

proper, there is nothing to prevent the two upper rods from being fastened to one another; and if any light covering be thrown over the limb, it will thus be kept off from the wound. If, then, the balls be well made, handsome, soft, and newly stitched, and if the extension by the rods be properly managed as has been already described, this is an excellent contrivance; but if any of them do not fit properly, it does more harm than good.[1]

A similar apparatus made of iron rings and rods was used by Paracelsus.[2] Another method described by Hippocrates, the fixation of fractures of the mandible by wiring or tying the adjacent teeth together, gave rise to the concept of fixing fractures by means of the insertion of pegs or pins into the fragments and holding the pins in an external device.

Malgaigne was the first to devise and to apply a practical method of external skeletal fixation.[3] This method was used in the treatment of displaced transverse fractures of the patella and consisted of two double hooks, which were inserted through the skin and engaged into the upper and lower borders of the patella. The hooks were then connected by a screw, which drew the fragments into apposition and maintained them in position during the healing period (figure 5.5).

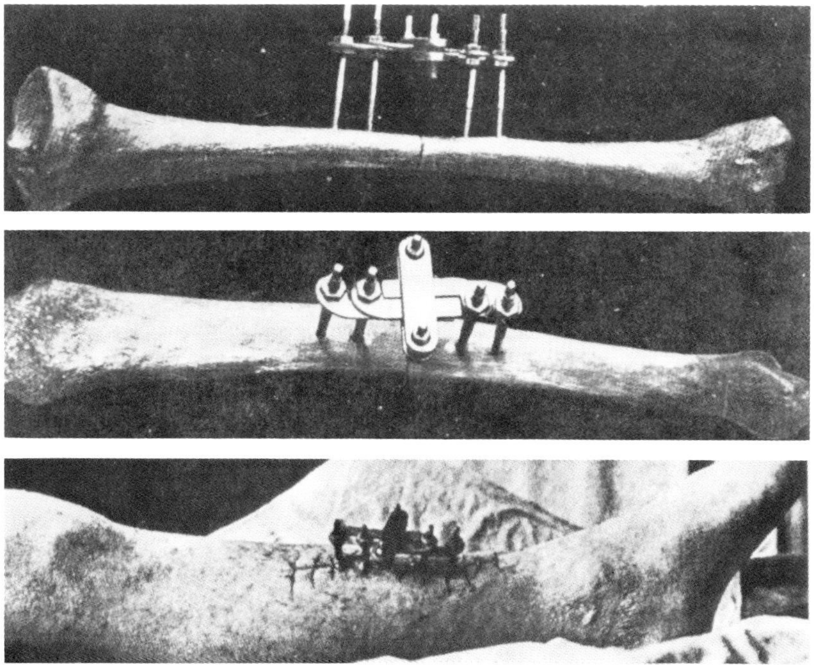

Figures 7.2a,b,c Views of the external skeletal fixation device of Parkhill. From Parkhill, "A New Apparatus for the Fixation of Bones after Resection and in Fractures with a Tendency to Displacement," *Trans Am Surg Assoc* 15(1897): 251–56.

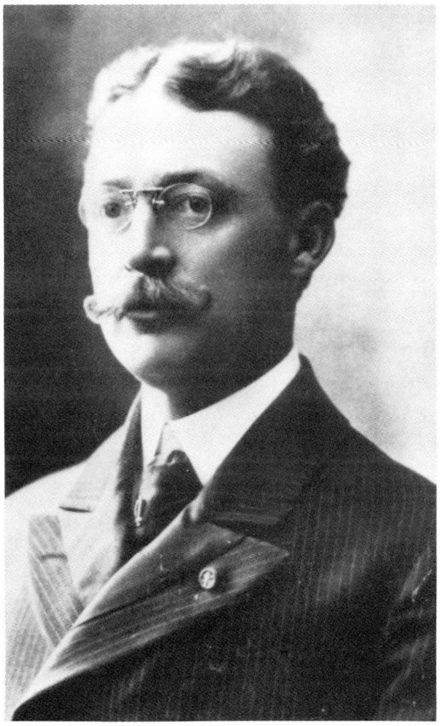

Figure 7.3 Clayton Parkhill (1860–1902), a pioneer in the development of external skeletal fixation.

The method was applicable to fractures of the patella because the bone was immediately beneath the skin and the risk of infection was small. A modification of Malgaigne's clamp was quickly applied to fractures of the olecranon by Philippe Rigaud.[4] Malgaigne also used a metal pin driven into the subcutaneous surface of the tibia to control angulation in tibial fractures[5] (figure 5.4). This method was revived by Carrell in 1931.[6]

In 1897 Clayton Parkhill of Denver (1860–1902) reported the results of the treatment of nine patients in whom he had used an external skeletal fixation device[7] (figures 7.2a,b,c). It consisted of four screws, two of which were inserted into each fragment. The external ends of the screws were fixed together by means of a series of small plates and bolts. In addition, the limbs were supported with a posterior splint made of plaster of paris. Eight of his patients had ununited fractures, and one patient had an unstable fracture of both bones of the leg. Union of the fractures occurred in eight of the nine patients. Surprisingly, when Parkhill presented his paper before the annual meeting of the American Surgical Association in May 1897, there was no discussion![8]

Clayton Parkhill (figure 7.3) was born in Pennsylvania and received his medical education at Jefferson Medical School in Philadelphia. After further training he began practice in Denver in 1885. There he was active as a teacher of anatomy and surgery in the Gross Medical School, later becoming professor of surgery and

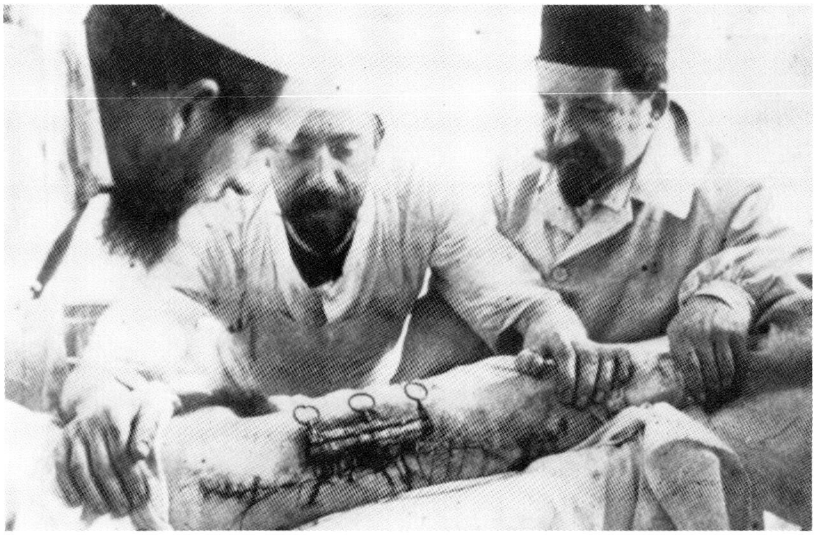

Figure 7.4 Albin Lambotte and his colleagues making the first application of his external skeletal fixation device. Photograph taken April 24, 1902 in the Stuyvenberg Hospital, Antwerp. From *Early Stages of Internal Fixation of Fractured Bones (Osteosynthesis) in Belgium* (Brussels: Imprimerie des Sciences, 1971), 57.

dean of the medical school of the University of Colorado. His promising career was interrupted when he was mobilized to serve as a medical officer during the war with Spain in 1898, and soon afterward was ended abruptly by an attack of appendicitis that proved fatal. As a result, he had no further opportunity to perfect his method of external skeletal fixation.

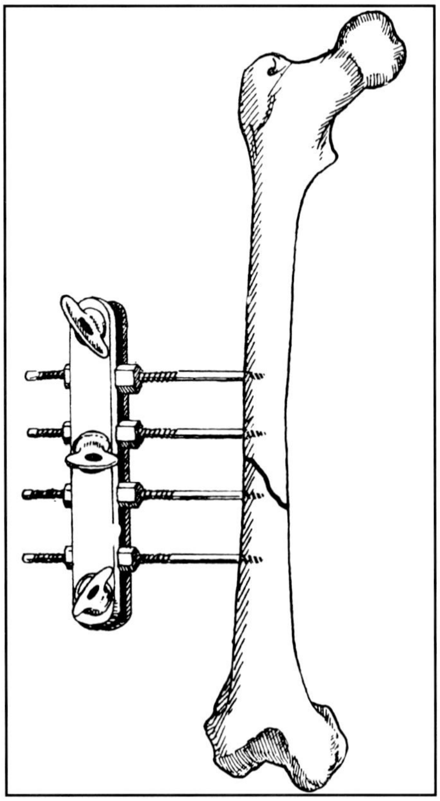

Figure 7.5 Lambotte's initial device. From Lambotte, *L'intervention opératoire dans les fractures récentes et anciennes* (Brussels: Henri Lamertin, 1907), 60.

In Belgium, Lambotte pursued development of his own methods of external skeletal fixation. He had heard of Parkhill's work but was unable to obtain a copy of his paper. His *fixateur de l'auteur*, first contemplated in 1900, was designed primarily for the treatment of fractures of the diaphysis[9] (figure 7.4). It had the advantage over Parkhill's apparatus in that no additional fixation other than that provided by the *fixateur* design was required (figure 7.5). Lambotte improved the design of the *fixateur* and enlarged the indications for its use in the treatment of fresh fractures, rapidly gaining extensive experience in its use.[10] He emphasized that the aftercare of the patient should include early active, assisted exercises to preserve and promote the functional rehabilitation of the injured extremity as a whole (figures 7.6a,b, 7.7, 7.8a,b). This development of an effective system of external skeletal fixation for the treatment of fresh fractures was one of the most original and important contributions made by Lambotte.

In Denver, Leonard Freeman continued Parkhill's work, treating fractures with his own method of external skeletal fixation[11] (figures 7.9, 7.10), while in New York, Howard Lilienthal described a method using pins or "gimlets" attached to rods by means of plaster of paris bandages[12] (figures 7.11a,b). This idea has since been revived, most recently by C. H. Wynn-Jones and A. R. Taylor, utilizing methylmethacrylate[13] (figure 7.12).

In 1913 Hey-Groves reported on the results of his experiments with transverse and comminuted tibial fractures in cats.[14] The fractures were fixed by means of external skeletal fixation. The apparatus was well tolerated and, in the absence of bone loss, the fractures healed well. He therefore applied his methods to patients, especially those with open or badly comminuted fractures[15] (figures 7.13a,b). On the basis of his experimental and clinical experience, Hey-Groves concluded:

> 1) *That the most rapid and perfect method of fracture repair follows "indirect fixation", namely fixation which does not directly interfere with the area of fracture.*
>
> 2) *That for such perfect results to be obtained by "indirect fixation", it is necessary for the method to ensure a) perfect anatomical restoration, b) fixation for the period required for union, and c) perfect freedom of all the soft parts and joints, so that the limb can be used directly when pain has ceased.*[16]

World War I stopped the growth of the use of external skeletal fixation because of the enormous numbers of severely injured combatants, the paucity of experienced and technically adept surgeons, and the stresses it put on the military and civilian medical services. In 1917, however, R. E. Humphrey did describe the use of external skeletal fixation in a patient with a gunshot fracture of the humerus[17] (figures 7.14a,b). During the immediate postwar period, external skeletal fixation was adapted for use in leg-lengthening procedures[18] (figure 7.15).

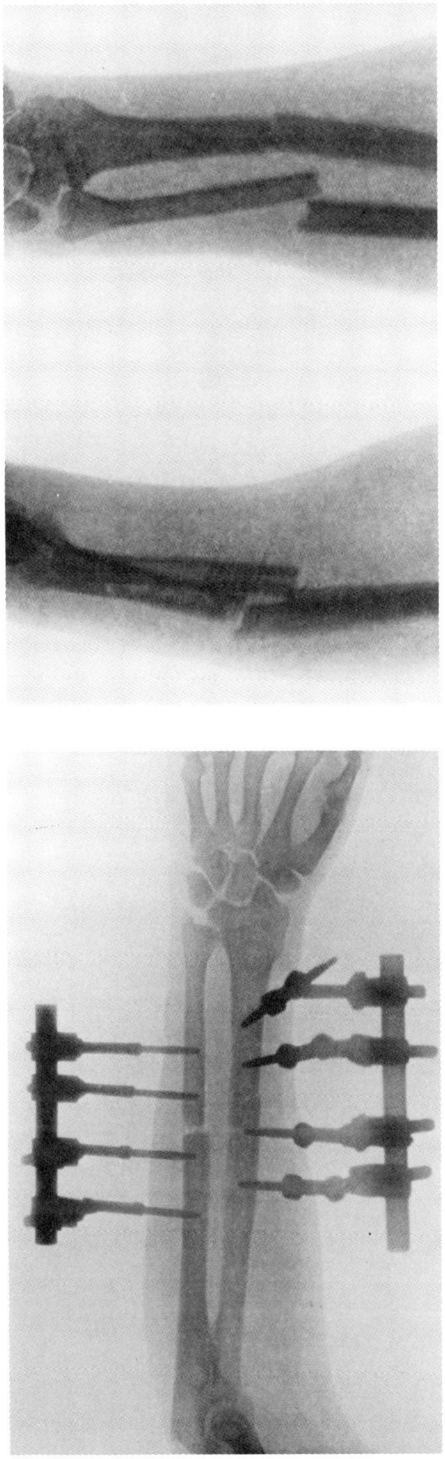

Figures 7.6a,b a) X rays of a fracture of both bones of the forearm treated by Lambotte in September, 1902, using external skeletal fixation. b) The fixation device in place. From Lambotte, *L'intervention opératoire*, figures 122 and 123.

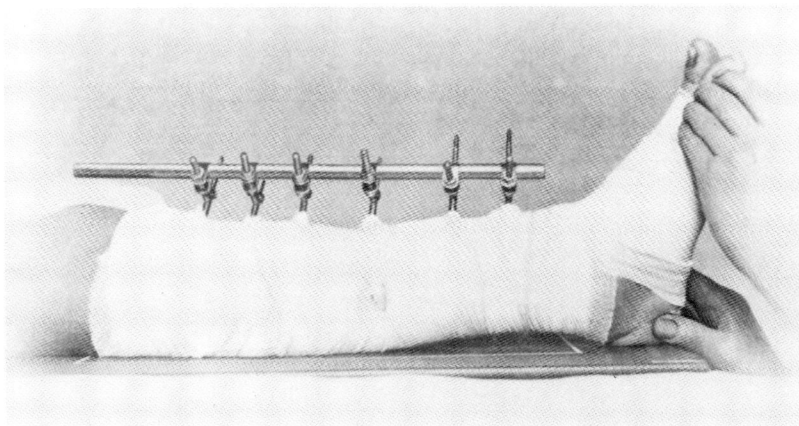

Figure 7.7 Lambotte's external skeletal fixation device applied to a fracture of the tibia. Note the absence of any additional external splinting. From Lambotte, *L'intervention opératoire*, figure 198.

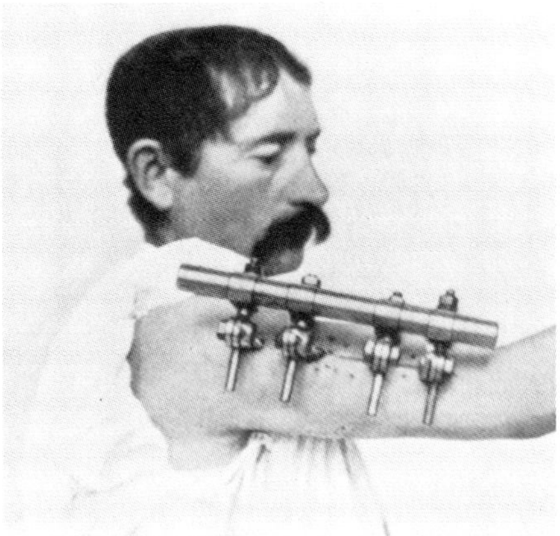

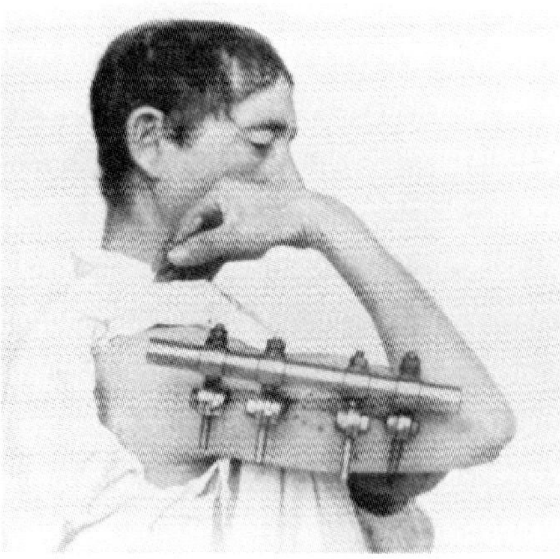

Figures 7.8a,b Lambotte's external skeletal fixation device applied to a fracture of the humerus, illustrating the range of motion in the elbow on the fifth postoperative day; a) extension, b) flexion. From Lambotte, *L'intervention opératoire*, figures 81 and 82.

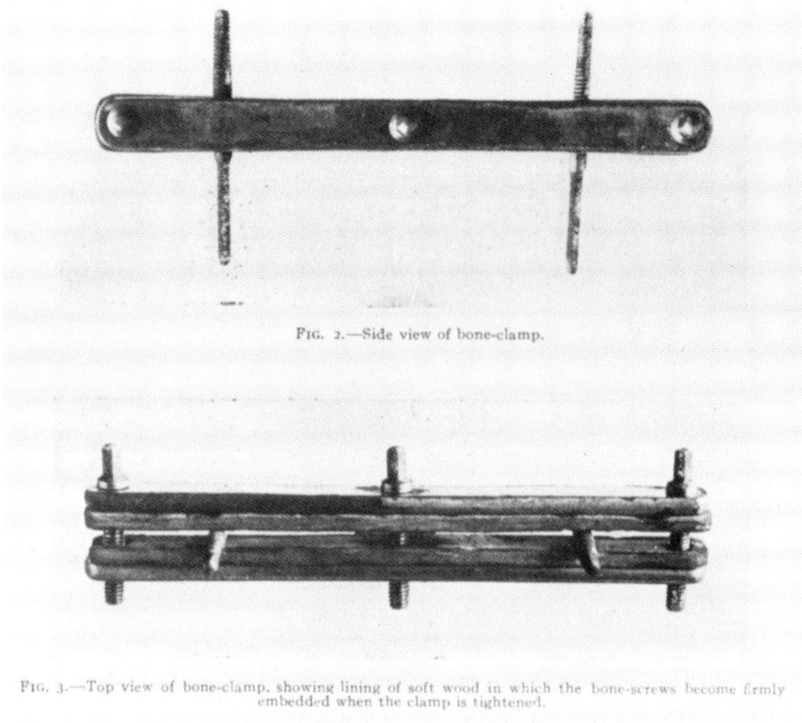

Figure 7.9 The bone clamp designed for external skeletal fixation by Freeman. From Freeman, "The Application of Extension to Overlapping Fractures, Especially of the Tibia, by Means of Bone Screws and a Turnbuckle, without Operation," *Ann Surg* 70(1919): 231–35.

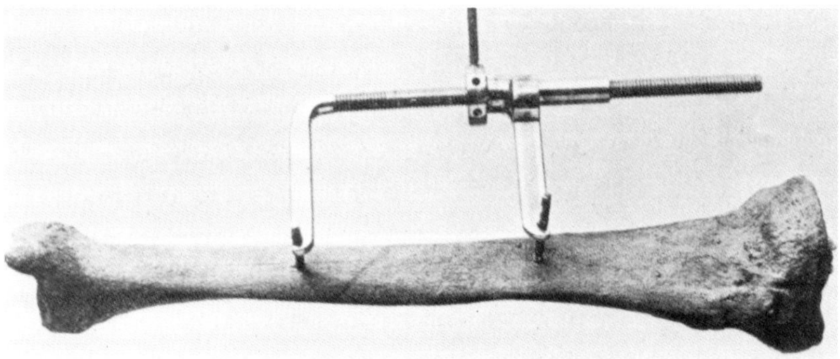

Figure 7.10 The method of "osteotaxis" used by Freeman. From Freeman, "Application of Extension," 231–35.

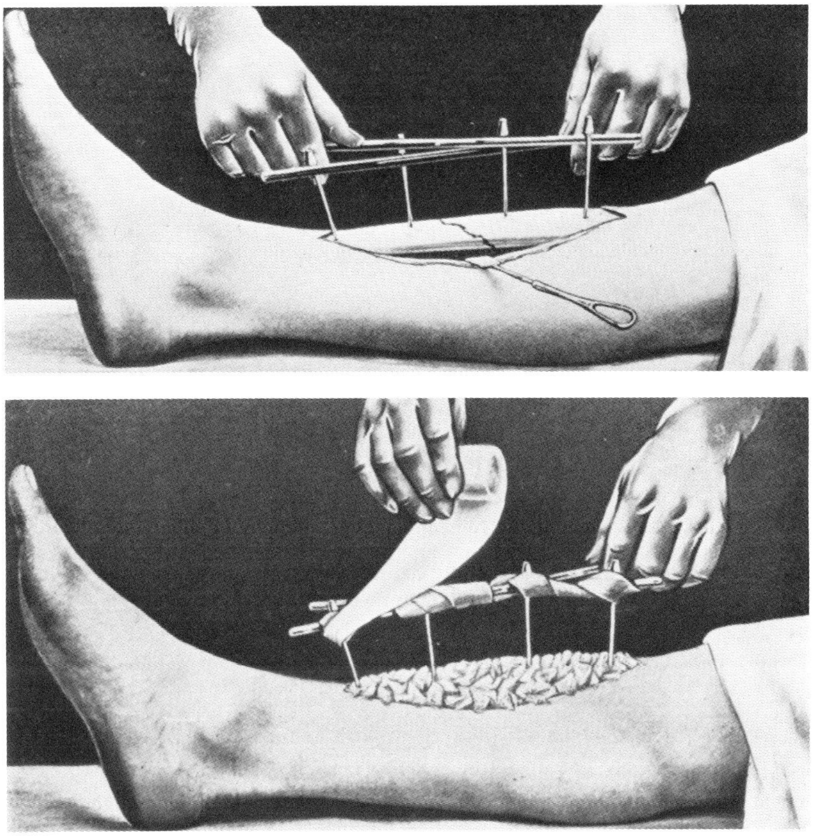

Figures 7.11a,b Lilienthal's method of external skeletal fixation using gimlets attached to rods by means of a plaster of paris bandage. From Lilienthal, "Safety in the Operative Fixation of Infected Fractures of Long Bones," *Trans Am Surg Assoc* 30(1912): 674–86.

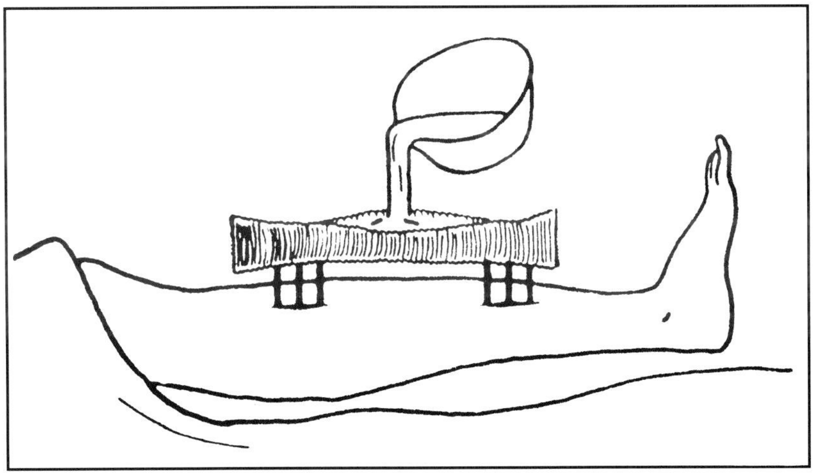

Figure 7.12 A recent modification of Lilienthal's method utilizing methylmethacrylate. From A. R. Taylor, "Wrinkle Corner: External Fixation of Fractures: A Simple Method," *Injury* 12(1980): 258–59.

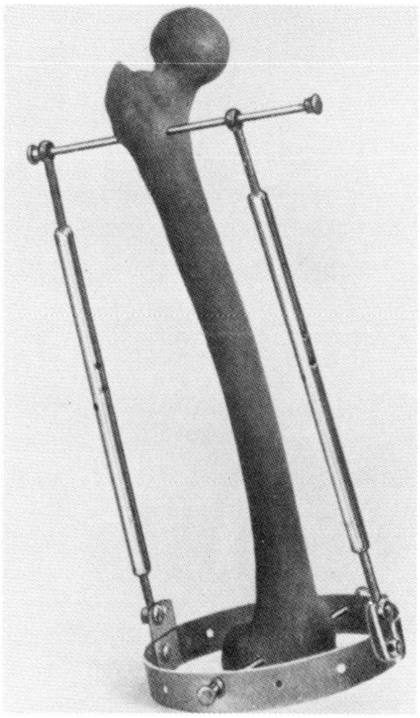
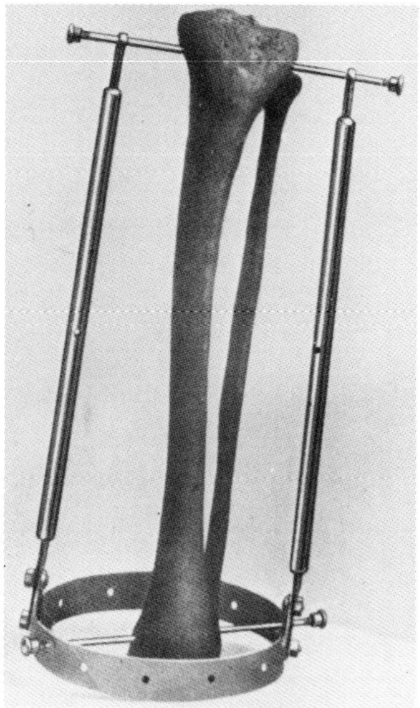

Figures 7.13a,b The external skeletal fixation devices of Hey-Groves. From Hey-Groves, *Modern Methods of the Treatment of Fractures* (Bristol: John Wright and Sons, 1916).

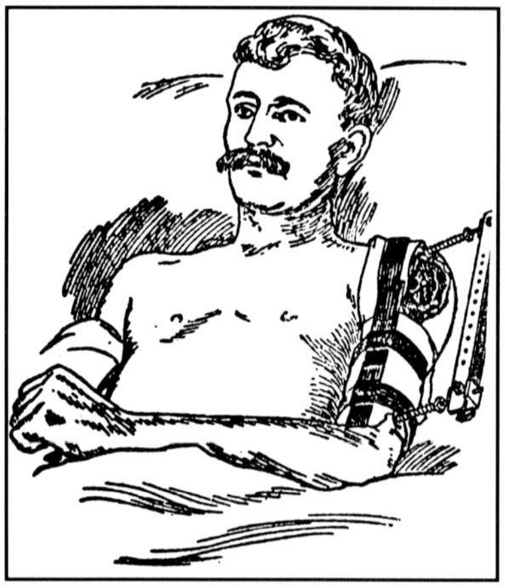
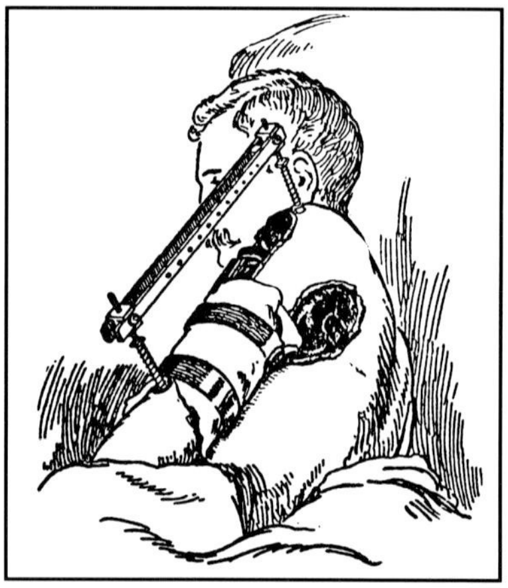

Figures 7.14a,b The treatment of a gunshot fracture of the humerus by an external skeletal fixation device. From Humphrey, "The Treatment of Septic Gunshot Fractures of the Long Bones by Means of a Steel Extension Appliance," *The Practitioner* 98(1917): 467–76.

In 1931 H. R. Conn described the successful use of external skeletal fixation in the treatment of a group of patients with fresh fractures.[19] He attributed previous failures with the method to poor design of the screws and to the use of metals that easily corroded. Conn used stainless steel screws with a narrow shoulder and a deeper thread (figures 7.16a,b). Similar improvements were being made in

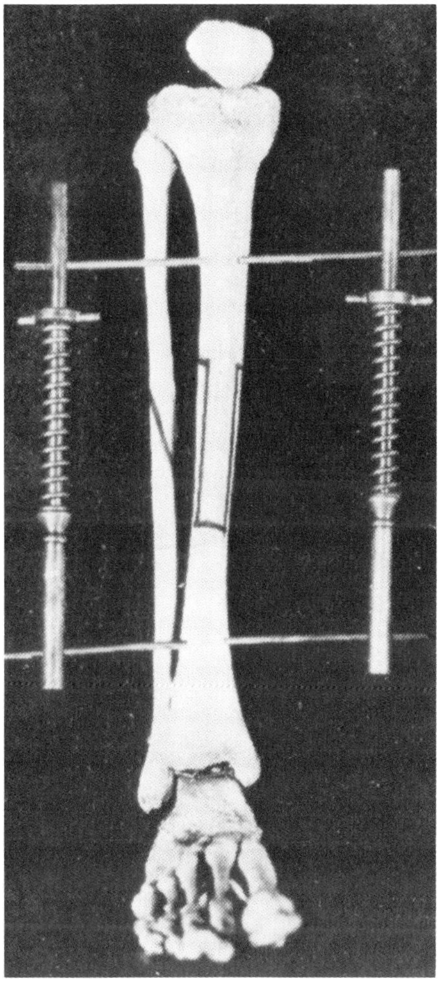

Figure 7.15 External skeletal fixation modified for use in leg-lengthening procedures. From Leroy Charles Abbott, "The Operative Lengthening of the Tibia and Fibula," *J Bone Joint Surg* 9(1927): 128–52.

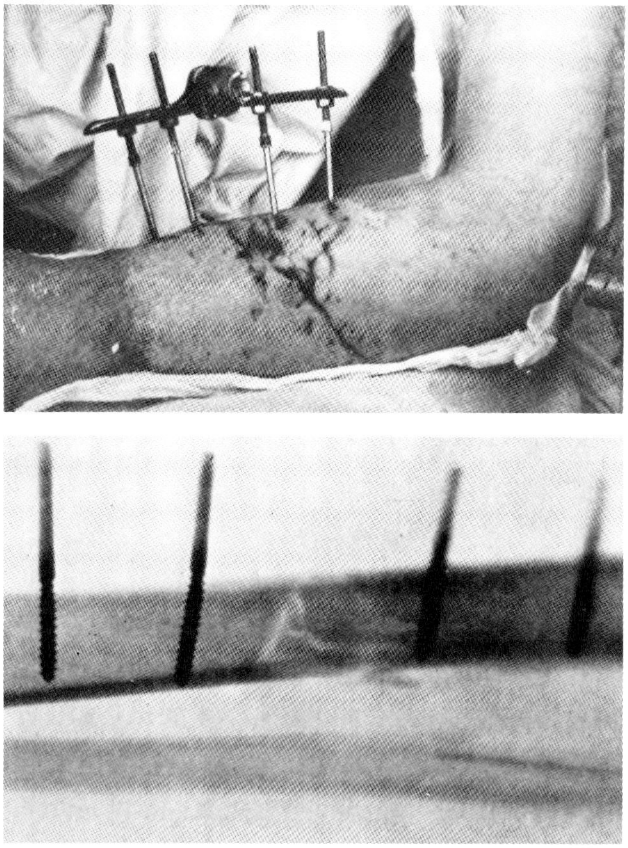

Figures 7.16a,b The external skeletal fixation device used by Conn in the treatment of open fractures. From Conn, "The Internal Fixation of Fractures," *J Bone Joint Surg* 9(1927), figures 3 and 4.

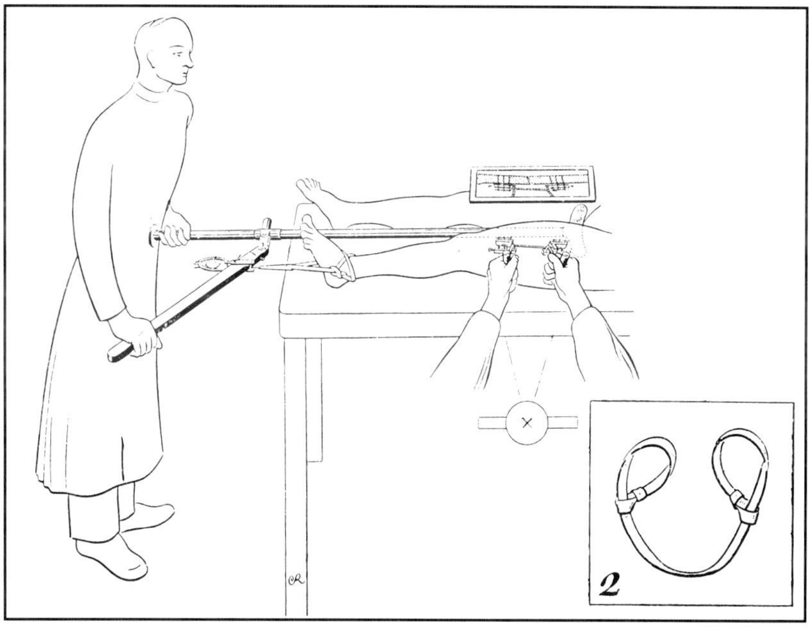

Figure 7.17 The application of *osteotaxis*, a term introduced by Hoffmann, using the "tracteur de Lambotte." From Hoffmann, "Osteotaxis: Ostéosynthèse externe par fisches et rotules," *Acta chir scand* 107(1954): 72–80.

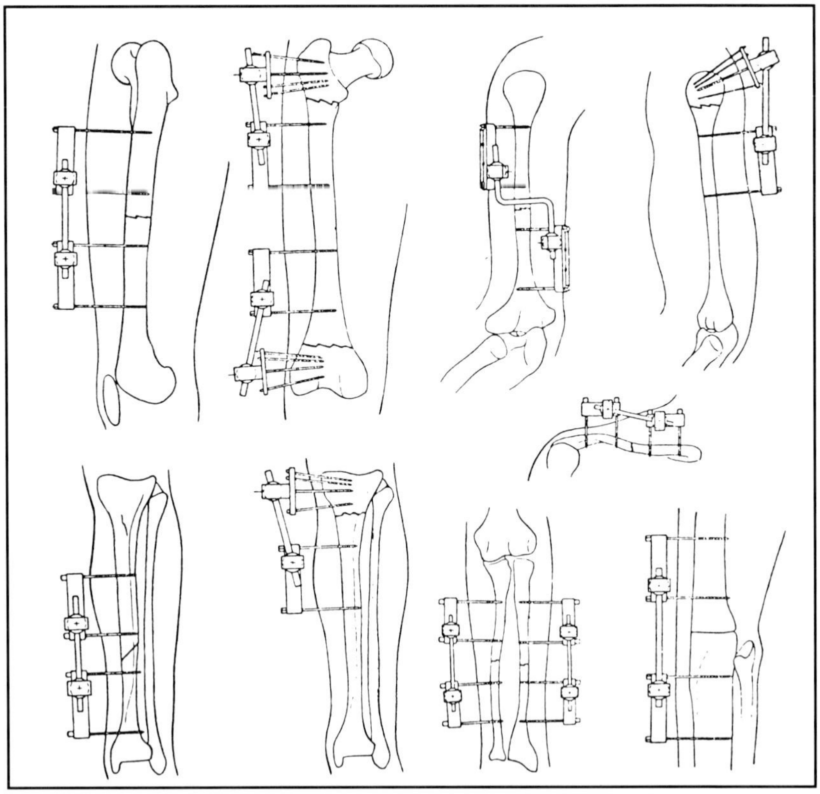

Figure 7.18 The schemes for external skeletal fixation advanced by Hoffmann in 1938. From R. Hoffmann, "'Rotules à os' pour la 'réduction dirigée,' non sanglante des fractures ('osteotaxis')," *Helv med acta*, 5(1938): 844.

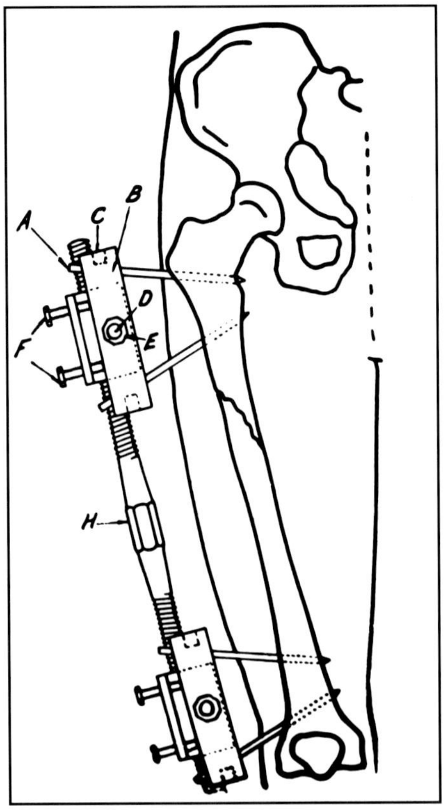

Figure 7.20 A diagram of Stader's apparatus originally developed for veterinary purposes in its application to femoral shaft fractures. From C. M. Shaar and F. P. Kreuz, Jr., "Treatment of Fractures and Bone and Joint Surgery with the Stader Reduction and Fixation Splint," *Surg Clin North Am* 22(1942): 1537–83.

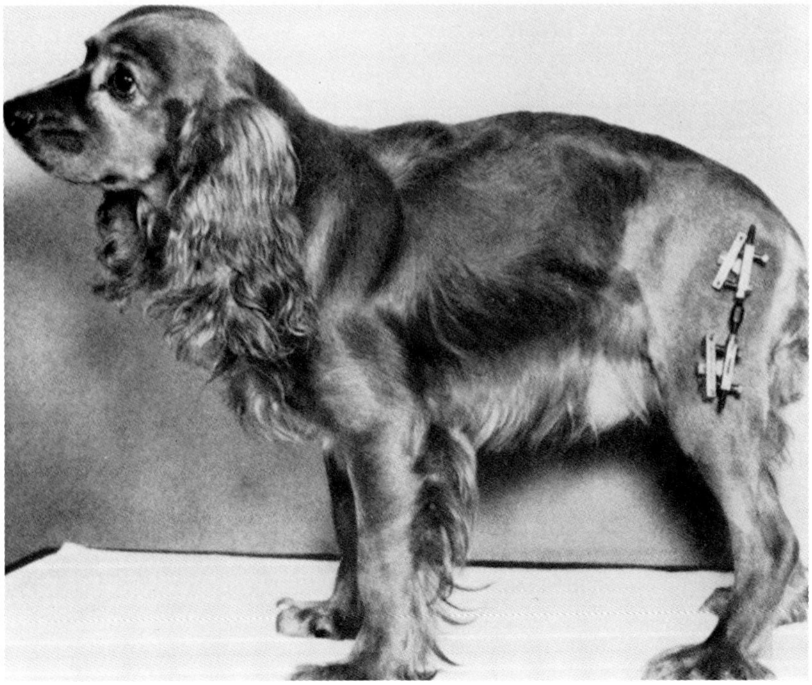

Figure 7.19 One of Otto Stader's patients being treated for a fracture of the femur. From K. M. Lewis et al., "The Stader Reduction Splints for Treating Fractures of the Long Bones," *Ann Surg* 116(1942): 623–36.

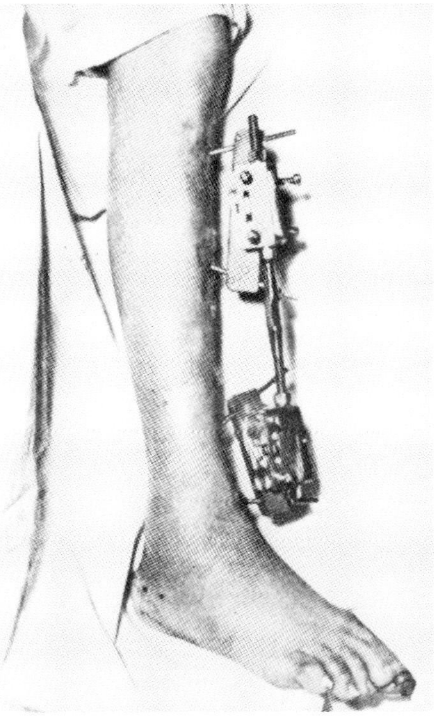

Figure 7.21 The application of the Stader splint to a fractured tibia. From Shaar and Kreuz, "Treatment of Fractures," 1537–83.

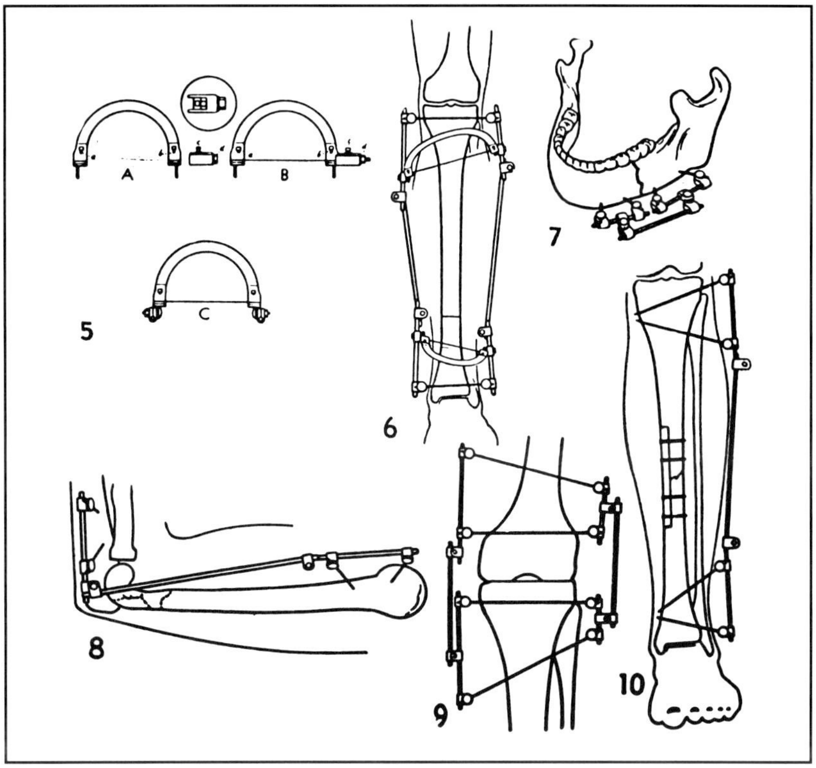

Figure 7.22 The system of Anderson. From Anderson, "Castless Ambulatory Method of Treating Fractures," *J Int Coll Surg* 5(1942): 458–62.

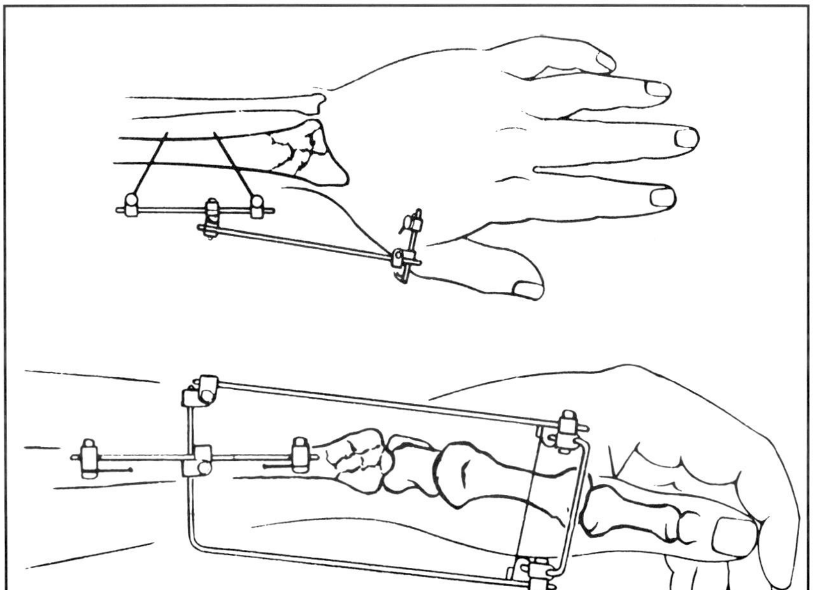

Figure 7.23 Anderson's method of treating comminuted fractures of the distal radius. From Anderson and O'Neill, "Comminuted Fractures of the Distal End of the Radius," *SGO* 78(1944): 434–40.

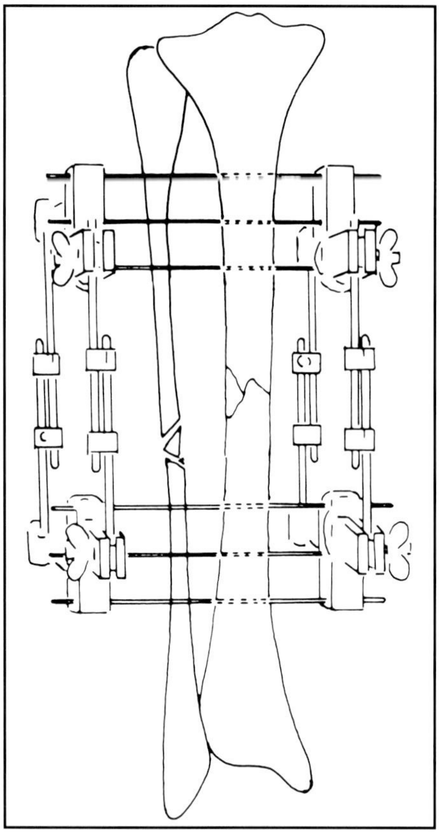

Figure 7.24 The double-frame method of Vidal-Adrey for the application of external skeletal fixation to the tibia. From G. Karlstrom and S. Olerud, "Stable External Fixation of Open Tibial Fractures," *Orth Rev* 6(1977): 25–39.

Belgium by S. Cuendet and Boever.[20] This work inaugurated a period of development. It was at this time that Raoul Hoffmann reported his work, coining the term *osteotaxis* for the method[21] (figures 7.17, 7.18).

In 1937 an American veterinarian, Otto Stader, developed a method of external skeletal fixation for the treatment of long-bone fractures in animals[22] (figure 7.19). One of Stader's "patients" was observed by surgeons from Bellevue Hospital, New York, and they persuaded him to adapt his apparatus for use in humans. During the next few years, Stader's splint was used extensively[23] (figures 7.20, 7.21). Another method was developed by H. H. Haynes and was used with good results.[24] As a natural evolution of his use of skeletal pins for the reduction of fractures in his "anatomic" or "self-aligning" splint for the treatment of fractures by pins in plaster of paris dressings, Roger Anderson replaced the plaster of paris with a system of rods and clamps.[25] Smaller versions of the equipment were designed for the treatment of fractures of the mandible and fractures of the distal end of the radius[26] (figures 7.22, 7.23).

The methods of Stader, Haynes, and Anderson were casualties of World War II, for although there were some favorable reports on their use at base hospitals, experience showed that the techniques were too specialized and time-consuming for use in an active theater of war.[27] As a result, external skeletal fixation was discredited as a method of treating fractures during the postwar period. The current revival of interest in its use is the result of continuing efforts of Raoul Hoffmann, Jacques Vidal, and others who have perfected the components of the apparatus and the technique of its application[28] (figure 7.24).

Notes

1. Hippocrates, *The Genuine Works of Hippocrates*, trans. Francis Adams (Baltimore: Williams and Wilkins Co., 1939), 193.

2. J.-F. Malgaigne, *Surgery and Ambroise Paré*, trans. and ed. Wallace B. Hamby (Norman, Okla.: University of Oklahoma Press, 1965), 224–25.

3. Malgaigne, *Traité des fractures et des luxations* (Paris: J. B. Baillière, 1847), 771–72.

4. P. Rigaud, "Nouvel appareil pour la fracture de l'olécrânone," *Revue méd-chir Paris* 7(1850): 50–51.

5. Malgaigne, *Traité des fractures*, 795–96.

6. W. B. Carrell, "End Results in 100 Fractures Treated by Internal Removable Fixation," *J Bone Joint Surg* 18(1936): 408–16; Carrell and P. M. Girard, "Removable Internal Fixation in Fractures," *JAMA* 96(1931): 670–73.

7. Clayton Parkhill, "A New Apparatus for the Fixation of Bones After Resection and in Fractures With a Tendency to Displacement," *Trans Am Surg Assoc* 15(1897): 251–56.

8. Parkhill, "Further Observations Regarding the Use of the Bone-Clamp in Ununited Fractures, Fractures with Malunion and Recent Fractures with a Tendency to Displacement," *Ann Surg* 27(1898): 553–70.

9. A. Lambotte, *L'intervention opératoire dans les fractures récentes et anciennes* (Brussels: Henri Lamertin, 1907), 59–67.

10. Lambotte, *Chirurgie opératoire des fractures* (Paris: Masson, 1913).

11. Leonard Freeman, "The Treatment of Oblique Fractures of the Tibia and Other Bones by Means of External Clamps Inserted Through Small Openings in the Skin," *Trans Am Surg Assoc* 28(1911): 70–93; id., "The Application of Extension to Overlapping Fractures, Especially of the Tibia, by Means of Bone Screws and a Turnbuckle, without Operation," *Ann Surg* 70(1919): 231–35.

12. Howard Lilienthal, "Safety in the Operative Fixation of Infected Fractures of Long Bones," *Trans Am Surg Soc* 30(1912): 674–86.

13. A. R. Taylor, "Wrinkle Corner: External Fixation of Fractures: A Simple Method," *Injury* 12(1980): 258–59; C. H. Wynn-Jones, "Wrinkle Corner: A Simple External Fixation Method Using Wire and Bone Cement," *Injury* 9(1978): 329–30.

14. E. W. Hey-Groves, "On the Treatment of Compound and Comminuted Fractures," *Brit Med J* 2(1913): 1079–80.

15. Hey-Groves, "On the Application of the Principle of Extension to Comminuted Fractures of the Long Bone, with Special Reference to Gunshot Injuries," *Brit J Surg* 2(1915): 429–43.

16. Hey-Groves, *On Modern Methods of Treating Fractures* (London: John Wright and Sons, 1916).

17. R. E. Humphrey, "The Treatment of Septic Gunshot Fractures of the Long Bones by Means of a Steel Extension Appliance," *The Practitioner* 98(1917): 467–76.

18. L. C. Abbott, "The Operative Lengthening of the Tibia," *J Bone Joint Surg* 9(1927): 128–52; Vittorio Putti, "The Operative Lengthening of the Femur," *JAMA* 77(1921): 934–35.

19. H. R. Conn, "The Internal Fixation of Fractures," *J Bone Joint Surg* 13(1931): 261–68.

20. S. Cuendet, "Procédé de réduction des fractures de la diaphyse des deux os de l'avant-bras, à l'aide de l'appareil à broches jumelées," in *Livre jubilaire offert au Docteur Albin Lambotte par ses amis et ses élèves* (Brussels: Vromant, 1936), 129–36; Boever, "Fixateur externe, nouveau modèle (Type Boever No.2)," *Le scalpel* 86(1938): 1175–76.

21. Raoul Hoffmann, "'Rotules à os' pour la 'réduction dirigée' non sanglante des fractures ('osteotaxis')," *Helv med acta* 5(1938): 844–80.

22. Otto Stader, "A Preliminary Announcement of a New Method of Treating Fractures," *N Am Vet* 18(1937): 37–38; id., "Treating Fractures of Long Bones with the Reduction Splint," *N Am Vet* 20(1939): 55–59.

23. K. M. Lewis et al. "The Stader Reduction Splint for Treating Fractures of Long Bones," *Ann Surg* 116(1942): 623–36; C. M. Shaar and F. P. Kreuz, Jr.: "Treatment of Fractures and Bone and Joint Surgery with the Stader Reduction and Fixation Splint," *Surg Clin North Am* 22(1942): 1537–83; Shaar et al.: "Fractures of the Tibia and Fibula: Treatment with the Stader Reduction and Fixation Splint," *Surg Clin North Am* 23(1943): 599–630; id., "End Results of Treatment of Fresh Fractures by the Use of the Stader Apparatus," *J Bone Joint Surg* 26(1944): 471–74.

24. H. H. Haynes, "Treating Fractures by Skeletal Fixation of the Individual Bone," *South Med J* 32(1939): 720–24; R. W. Johnson and John Lyford: "The Use of the Haynes Skeletal-Fixation Apparatus in Definitive Orthopaedic Surgery," *J Bone Joint Surg* 26(1944): 475–81.

25. Roger Anderson, "Castless Ambulatory Method of Treating Fractures," *J Inter Coll Surg* 5(1942): 458–62; id., "A Self-Aligning Method of Treating Fractures of the Long Bones," *J Inter Coll Surg* 7(1944): 1–8.

26. Anderson and Gordon O'Neill, "Comminuted Fractures of the Distal End of the Radius," *SGO* 78(1944): 434–40; J. M. Converse and F. W. Waknitz, "External Skeletal Fixation in Fractures of the Mandibular Angle," *J Bone Joint Surg* 24(1942): 154–59.

27. Oscar P. Hampton, ed., *Orthopedic Surgery in the Mediterranean Theater of Operations* (Washington, D. C.: Office of the Surgeon General, Department of the Army, 1957), 203–10; Charles Bradford and Phillip D.Wilson, "Mechanical Skeletal Fixation in War Surgery, with a Report of 61 Cases," *SGO* 75(1942): 468–76.

28. See, for example, Henry Connes, *Hoffman's Double Frame External Anchorage* (Paris: Gead, 1973); M. Fellander, "Treatment of Fractures and Pseudarthroses of the Long Bones by Hoffmann's Transfixation Method (Osteotaxis)," *Acta orthop scand* 33(1963): 132–150; Hoffmann, "Osteotaxis: Ostéosynthèse externe par fisches et rotules," *Acta chir scand* 107(1954): 72–80; Goran Karlstrom and Sven Olerud, "Stable External Fixation of Open Tibial Fractures," *Orthop Rev* 6(1977): 25–39; M. Lapeyrie et al.: "Notre expérience du fixateur externe d' Hoffmann en traumatologie récente," *J chir* 97(1969): 441–46; J. Vidal, "Notre expérience du fixateur externe d'Hoffmann," *Montpellier chir* 14(1968): 451–60.

CHAPTER EIGHT

The Treatment of Ununited Fractures

FRACTURE TREATMENT was not always successful; this, in spite of the fact that many fractures seem to heal satisfactorily with only limited treatment, or, indeed, none at all. In the middle of the nineteenth century, exhaustive reviews by Malgaigne and Ernst Julius Gurlt on this subject indicated that the incidence of nonunion was very small.[1] Joseph Amesbury was the only one of their contemporaries to admit to a substantial experience with the treatment of ununited fractures; he reported on a series of fifty-six such cases in 1828:

By the term nonunion or disunion, surgeons signify a fracture which has remained disunited a longer time than fractures in a similar situation, and at the same period of life, usually take in becoming united. In a more confined sense, however, these terms signify fractures which cannot be made to unite by the usual modes of treating fractures.

Experience has taught us, that the bones, as well as the softer textures, are endowed with vital powers, by the operation of which injuries inflicted upon them are repaired. If any breach of continuity is accidentally made in the osseous structure, that breach is soon closed; and the bone becomes again converted into one solid mass. But it should be remembered, that the bones, like the skin, nerves, blood-vessels, &c, require a period peculiar to themselves for the reparation of injuries. This period varies in different animals, and at different periods of life. The restorative process is, also, retarded or facilitated, according to the particular state of the constitution of the individual, the vital condition of the parts, the treatment adopted, &c. Thus we see that the process of union in bone is influenced by all those causes which effect the healing of soft parts. In man, if the constitution and the bone are healthy, and proper assistance be given by art, the process of re-union almost always goes on progressively to its completion; but, if this process has been disturbed by any cause, it often becomes slow and tedious; and in some cases, no osseous union has ever been produced.[2]

The factors resulting in a fracture's failure to heal were classified as constitutional and local.[3] Recognized among the systemic factors were *osteogenesis imperfecta* and congenital nonunion of the tibia.[4] Scurvy, pregnancy and lactation, and paralysis, cachexia, and senility were known to delay or completely inhibit the healing of fractures. The failure of pathological fractures associated with primary and metastatic tumors to heal was also well known.[5] Syphilis (and its treatment with mercury) was considered by all authorities to be a factor that inhibited healing. This relationship is difficult for us to understand today because the incidence of tertiary syphilis is small. However, even today, in a patient with *tabes dorsalis*, a minor, undisplaced, metaphyseal fracture can quickly show changes characteristic of a neuropathic joint with nonunion of the fracture.

Among the local factors identified as affecting fracture healing were wide separation of the fragments with interposition of soft tissues or foreign bodies— such as missles and sequestra. Loss of bony substance as a result of open fracture was known by Hippocrates to cause failure of healing, as evidenced by his Aphorism 19: "When a bone, cartilage, nerve, the slender part of the jaw, or prepuce, are cut out, the part is neither restored, nor does it unite."[6] Infection complicating open fractures, then as now, was considered a major cause of nonunion. Local ischemia as a result of initial damage to the nutrient arteries or to dressings compromised the circulation and was often an important consideration. Lastly, excessive motion at the fracture site due to inadequate fixation or too early resumption of function—factors usually under the control of the surgeon—were recognized to be failures of treatment.

The most frequent and most important fracture that commonly goes on to nonunion is the displaced intracapsular fracture of the neck of the femur, first described by Ambroise Paré in 1575. He attributed the difficulty in healing these fractures to lack of circulation: "More important than the fracture alone is that near the joints; the parts are bloodless and more difficult to treat and harder to cure. . . ."[7] Two hundred and fifty years later, Astley Cooper expressed a similar pessimistic point of view in his discussion of fractures of the thigh bone:

In all the examinations which I have made of transverse fractures of the cervix femoris entirely within the capsular ligament, I have never met with one, in which a bony union had taken place, or which did not admit of a motion of one bone upon the other. To deny its possibility, and to maintain that no exception to the general rule can take place, would be presumptuous, especially when we consider the varieties of direction in which a fracture may occur, and the degree of violence by which it may have been produced; as for example when the fracture is through the head of the bone, and there is no separation of the fractured ends; or when the bone is broken without the periosteum being torn; or if it be broken obliquely, partly within and partly externally to the capsular ligament; but all I wish to be understood to say is, that if it ever does happen, it is an extremely rare occurrence, and that I have not yet met with a single example of it.[8]

Cooper attributed the failure of healing to three factors: 1) failure to obtain and maintain an end-to-end reduction of the fracture; 2) lack of compressive forces across the fracture line; and 3) "the almost entire absence of ossific action in the head of the thigh-bone when separated from its cervix; its life being supported by the ligamentum teres, which has only a few minute vessels, ramifying from it to the head of the bone."[9] In contrast to these intracapsular fractures, extracapsular fractures of the upper end of the femur usually proceded to bony union if the patient survived. To support his clinical observations, Cooper carried out animal experiments, producing intra- and extracapsular fractures of the hip, demonstrating that while the former failed to heal, the latter always did. Dupuytren was not as pessimistic regarding the prognosis in patients with intracapsular fractures, recognizing that some of them would heal. He taught that the fractures were most frequent in elderly women, were associated with osteopenia, and required a long period of treatment before healing became solid.[10] By 1847, R. W. Smith could demonstrate many examples of healed intracapsular fractures, either undisplaced or impacted. In spite of these exceptions, the classification of fractures of the hip into intra- and extracapsular fractures remained important because of the difference in their prognosis for healing. There were many clinical similarities between the early and late presentations of these two types of fractures, so that the differential diagnosis between them was not always simple nor accurate.[11] While the anatomical landmarks described by Auguste Nélaton and Thomas Bryant were helpful in establishing the diagnosis of fracture of the hip (figures 8.1a,b), they were of little help in making this crucial differentiation.[12] As a young surgeon, William Stewart Halsted wrote a short paper describing a very complicated system of measurements addressing this problem.[13] The accurate delineation of the different types of hip fractures in living patients was not possible until well after the introduction of the X ray, and, in spite of years of investigation and trial, the results in the treatment of fractures of the neck of the femur remained so unsatisfactory that as late as 1935 it was characterized as the "unsolved fracture."[14]

In addition to intracapsular fractures of the hip, other intra-articular fractures commonly healed only by fibrous union. Displaced fractures of the patella and olecranon, like their counterparts in the hip, were not successfully treated by closed methods. In 1822,

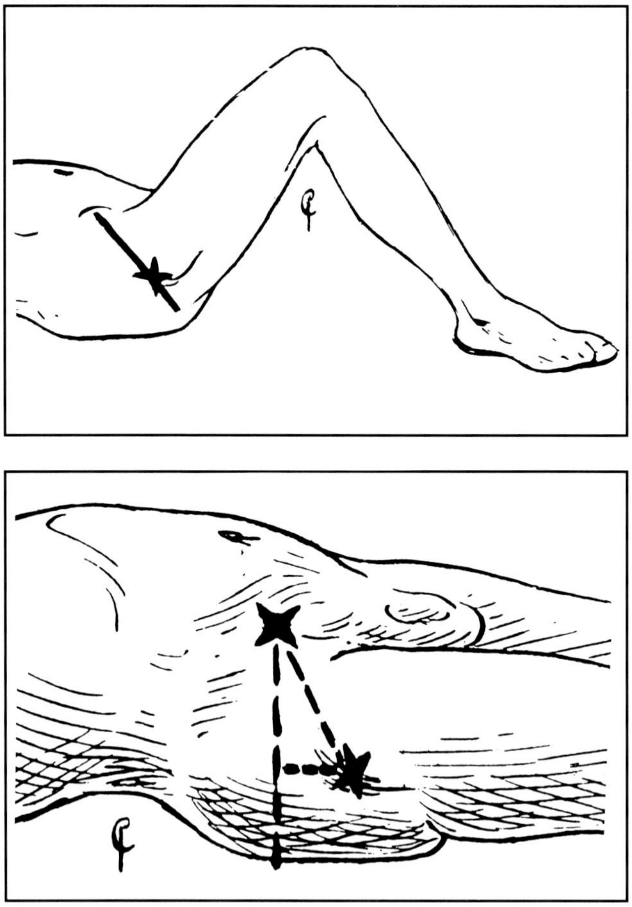

Figures 8.1a,b a) Nélaton's line: from the anterior spine of the ilium to the tuberosity of the ischium; and b) Bryant's triangle, the sides of which are lines from the anterior superior spine of the ilium to the greater trochanter and from the anterior superior spine perpendicular to the examining table. The greater trochanter is marked with a star in both drawings. Advancement of the tip of the trochanter proximal to Nélaton's line, or narrowing of the base of Bryant's triangle were evidence of femoral shortening and suggested a displaced fracture of the proximal femur. From Frederic J. Cotton, *Dislocations and Joint Fractures* (Philadelphia & London: W. B. Saunders & Co., 1910), 421, 423.

Cooper experimentally studied fractures of the patella in animals to determine if the presence of the synovial fluid between the fracture fragments prevented the fractures from healing. He compared the healing of vertical fractures and transverse fractures of the patella in rabbits. The vertical fractures did not become displaced and eventually healed. The transverse fractures became separated by the pull of the quadriceps apparatus and did not heal (figure 8.2). He concluded that displacement, rather than the presence of synovial fluid in the fracture line, was the cause of this failure.[15]

While solution of the problem of the displaced intra-articular fracture had to await the development of effective methods of open reduction and internal fixation, failure of healing of diaphyseal fractures—the classical cases of pseudarthrosis of long bones—was treated with a great variety of methods, some of which produced an occasional satisfactory result. Celsus believed that any treatment of an old fracture must reproduce the local conditions present in an acute fracture. "If the fracture is of long standing, the limb is stretched in order to reproduce the injury to some extent; the fractured ends must be separated by manipulation, so that when allowed to come into contact they rub one another; thus any fatty tissue is rubbed off, and the whole thing is like a fresh fracture."[16] This principle was applied in numerous ways.[17] Local circulation about the unhealed fracture was augmented by the application of blisters and irritating solutions to the skin, by percussion, damming and compression, by rubbing the bone ends together and using braces that permitted walking, and finally by the application of electricity. Invasive methods included the injection of various irritating solutions into the site of the pseudarthrosis or into associated sinus tracts, the insertion of setons and other foreign bodies into the fracture line or adjacent to it, and scraping, cauterization or resection of the bone ends with and without internal fixation. In 1873, George W. Norris, a Philadelphia surgeon, listed his options:

1st: To apply the method of cure by rest and compression. If the fracture has been regularly treated, and is not consolidated at the usual period, replace the limb in the apparatus, and insure to it a state of complete immovability; if the treatment of the injury has been altogether neglected, or has been inefficient, apply proper splints and moderate

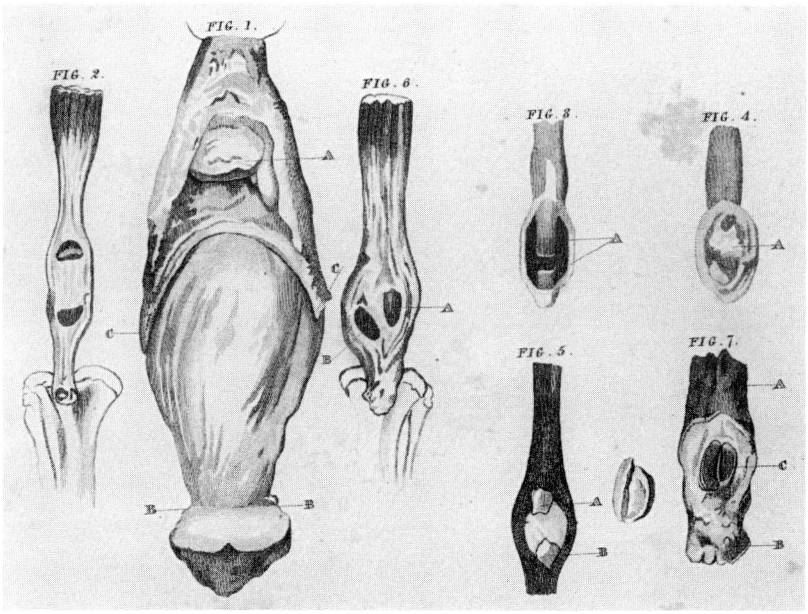

Figure 8.2 Astley Cooper's experiments on patellar fractures, showing the ununited transverse fractures and the healed verticle fractures. From Cooper, *A Treatise on Dislocations and on Fractures of the Joints* (London: Longman, Hurst, Rees, Orme and Brown, 1822), plate 10.

compression with a roller, and renew these as soon as they become in any degree lax.

2nd: If, from want of action in the seat of injury, rest and compression are in themselves insufficient to produce a cure, continue the state of immobility in which you have placed the limb, and apply blister, moxas, iodine, or some other stimulant to the seat of the fracture.

3rd: If both of these modes fail in producing a deposition of callus, apply frictions.

4th: If the methods mentioned fail to produce a change, or the patient has already been suffering from his injury for eight or ten months, and there is no contraindication to it, resort to the seton.

5th: If the case be one to which, from its long standing, or state of the injured parts, the seton is inapplicable, expose the fracture, and apply caustic potash to the fractured ends.

6th: If all of the above means have been carefully resorted to unsuccessfully, and not until then, resect the ends of the bone.

7th: Never resort to amputation of the member until fair trials have been made with all of these methods, and then only at the request of the sufferer, after he has found that the limb can be of no possible service to him.

In employing any of the above means, the obstacle to the occurrance of union which may exist, arising from the state of the constitution, should be carefully sought for and combatted by an appropriate treatment.[18]

Percussion and damming was Hugh Owen Thomas's favorite method of treating nonunion.[19] Percussion was applied by means of various hammers, sometimes with the patient under an anesthetic, but often not. The tissue about the fracture, and especially the subcutaneous periosteum, where possible, was bruised and became swollen and indurated. This congestion of the tissues about the fracture was encouraged by the application of tight bandages above and below the fracture, or damming. Thomas reported a series of thirty-nine cases treated by this method, generally with success:

J. T—, Fymon Craig, Devil's Bridge, South Wales, presented himself for treatment with an ununited fracture of the left humerus, caused by a "chaff cutter" driven by water power. The injury occurred nine months prior to his interview with me, January 6th, 1879. An examination of the injury made it doubtful whether the fractured points were in absolute contact. However, with this ill-omen, the operation of percussion was performed and repeated weekly for four weeks. The percussive force employed being only a moderate one, I also daily practiced "damming", for half-an-hour, the circulation around the fracture, so as to hinder subsidence of the tumefaction caused by the percussion. He was under my observation in hospital four weeks, during which period much progress was not observed. I applied no mechanical fixation beyond a sling around the wrist and neck which I requested him never to disturb until advised by me to do so. In this instance I did not administer an anesthetic during the several operations, as the force used was easily tolerated, and I thought it desirable to operate often rather than severely. On one of the occasions when I was performing the operation, a medical friend, who had often assisted me at like operations, chanced to enter the surgery, and at my request examined the patient's arm, after which he asked if I was going to continue the treatment. On my replying in the affirmative, my friend much amused left abruptly. However, as no harm could result by perservering in a thorough trial of this plan of treatment, I persisted. On leaving my hospital, he remained at home a month, and again presented himself, when, on examination, I found some slight improvement. I again made several moderate percussions, and the short periods of "damming" were continued. After a stay of one week he returned home, coming back again in four weeks, when I found much improvement. The treatment was again repeated, and after another stay of a week, he was sent home with instructions to "dam" the circulation, daily for half-an-hour, until his return. On his next visit May 6th, 1879, an examination of the fracture showed perfectly sound repair.[20]

Percussion and damming in the treatment of nonunion had advocates on the Continent as well as in the United States,[21] although August Bier, the great German enthusiast for hyperemia, did not recommend it for this indication.[22]

The use of braces for the functional support of paralyzed or diseased limbs was nothing new. In 1855, Henry H. Smith of Philadelphia described the application of braces to support the function of a limb disabled by an ununited fracture (figure 8.3). The title of his paper, "On the Treatment of Ununited Fracture by Means of Artificial Limbs which Combine the Principle of Pressure and Motion at the Seat of Fracture, and Lead to the Formation of Ensheathing Callus,"[23] describes the basic concepts still being applied to the treatment of ununited fractures treated in walking plasters and cast braces today.[24]

The application of electrical currents to ununited fractures also has a venerable history. In 1819, Alexander Stevens of New York made this comment:

The late Mr. Birch, one of the surgeons of St. Thomas' Hospital (whose assiduity in the instruction of his pupils it would be unjust not to mention with gratitude,) informed me that he had succeeded in procuring a firm osseous union, in several cases of ligamentous connexion of bones after fracture, by means of electricity. He stated, that, in his hands that remedy had never failed of success. One of his dressers, with whom

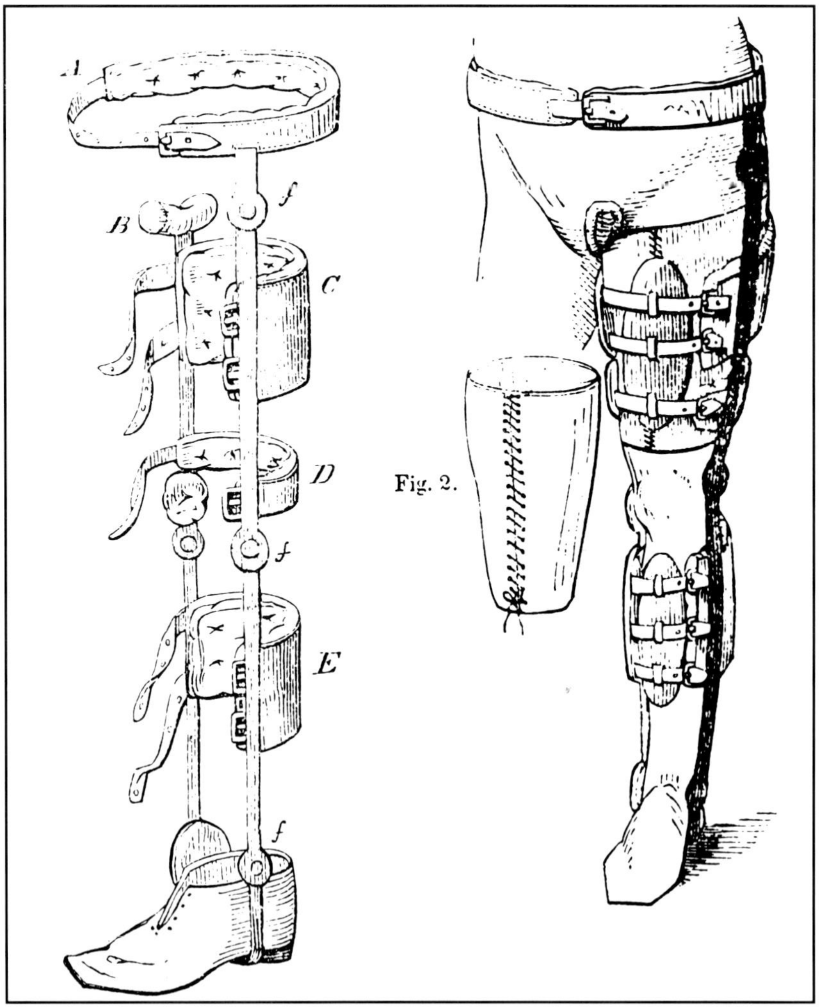

Figure 8.3 The brace used by Henry H. Smith for the treatment of nonunion of a fracture of the shaft of the femur. From Smith, "On the Treatment of Ununited Fracture by Means of Artificial Limbs which Combine the Principle of Pressure and Motion at the Seat of Fracture, and Lead to the Formation of Ensheathing Callus," *Am J Med Sci* 1(1855): 102–19.

I was intimately acquainted, saw two cases in which it produced the most happy effect.

One of these patients, whom I often visited during his illness, entered St. Thomas' Hospital in the month of January, 1812, with an unconsolidated fracture of the tibia, below the middle, of thirteen months standing. The leg below the fracture could be easily moved in any direction and without exciting much pain.

Shocks of electric fluid were daily passed through the space between the ends of the bones, both in the direction of the length of the limb and that of its thickness. The man, being somewhat weak, used bark and porter at the same time. After the limb was electrized, the ordinary apparatus for fractures of the leg was applied. At the expiration of two weeks, the limb had evidently become less flexible in the situation of the fracture; and after a continuance of the same treatment for six weeks, the man was able to walk and left the hospital cured.[25]

Valentine Mott reported no success with this method,[26] but in a series of continuing reports from the United States and other countries, other surgeons claimed success.[27] Guillaume Benjamin Duchenne de Boulogne, in his book on the medical applications of electricity published in 1855, did not include the treatment of fractures.[28] One hundred years later in Japan, Iwao Yasuda (1909–1983) described "piezoelectricity of bone" and the promotion of callus formation by electrical stimulation[29] (figure 8.4). The exploitation of these observations by C. Andrew L. Bassett and Robert O. Becker and by Zachary B. Friedenberg and Carl T. Brighton has led to the development of the techniques currently employed in the treatment of ununited fractures by electricity.[30]

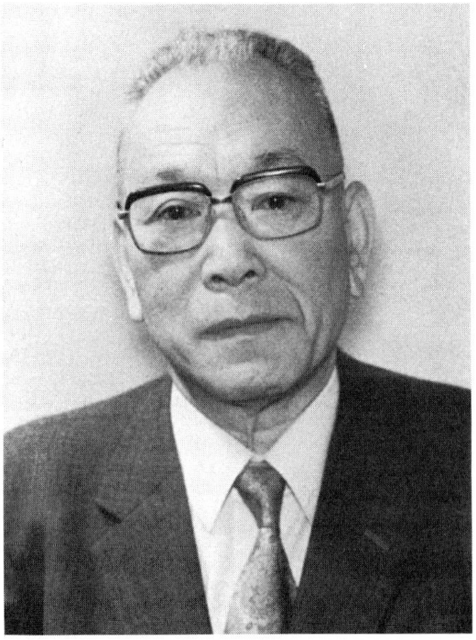

Figure 8.4 Iwao Yasuda (1909–1983), whose work established the use of electrical stimulation of fracture healing on a scientific basis.

A seton is a method of producing counterirritation or local inflammation by means of the passage of a bundle of sutures or horsehairs, an umbilical tape, or some other foreign material through the skin and subcutaneous tissue using a large needle. Although part of the armamentarium of surgeons for centuries, the seton was not applied to the treatment of ununited fractures until 1802. At that time, Philip Syng Physick, considered by many to be the Father of American Surgery, first applied the method to the treatment of an ununited fracture of the humerus.[31] The patient, Isaac Patterson, was described in a paper entitled "A Case of Fracture of the Os Humerus, in which the Broken Ends of the Bone Not Uniting in the Usual Manner, a Cure Was Effected by Means of a Seton." Patterson was a twenty-eight-year-old sailor who had suffered a fracture of the shaft of the humerus twenty months previously during a storm at sea. The fracture was two and one-half inches above the elbow and was freely movable in all directions. Physick proposed to use a seton consisting of a skein of silk to excite inflammation and suppuration, which would in turn lead to the formation of granulation tissue promoting ossification:

The operation being agreed to, it was performed on the 18th of December, 1802, twenty months after the accident happened. Before passing the needle, I desired the assistants to make some extension of the arm, in order that the seton might be introduced as much as possible between the ends of the bone. Some lint and a pledget were applied to the orifices made by the seton-needle, and secured by a roller. The patient suffered very little pain from the operation. After a few days the inflammation (which was not greater than what is commonly excited by a similar operation through the flesh, in any other part) was succeeded by a moderate suppuration. The arm was now again extended, and splints applied. The dressings were renewed daily for twelve weeks, during which time no amendment was perceived; but soon afterwards the bending of the arm at the fracture was observed to be not so easy as it had been, and the patient complained of much more pain than usual whenever an attempt was made to bend it at that place. From this time the formation of the new bony union went on rapidly, and on the fourth of May, 1803, was so perfectly completed, that the patient could move his arm, in all directions, as well as before the accident happened. The seton was now removed, and the small sores occasioned by it healed up entirely in a few days. On the 28th May, 1803, he was discharged from the hospital, perfectly well, and he has since repeatedly told me that his arm is as strong as it ever was.[32]

This case was widely reported in medical literature around the world and was the first method of fracture treatment by a surgeon in the United States to receive international attention. Reports of successful treatment of ununited fractures by use of a seton were quickly reported by Mott and John Baxter in New York.[33]

In Germany, Johann Friedrich Dieffenbach reported the use of ivory pegs placed in holes bored adjacent to the fracture in the treatment of ununited fractures, the ivory foreign body performing the same function as a seton.[34] A similar case was reported from Bernhard von Langenbeck's clinic.[35] Richard Volkmann carried this technique a step further when he used the ivory pegs not just to incite inflammation but also for internal fixation of the ununited fracture after realignment.[36]

Other, more aggressive surgical approaches to the treatment of ununited fractures were also tried. Charles White of Manchester reported in 1770 "An Account of an Operation successfully performed upon a broken Leg, in which the fractured Tibia was not united, though thirty-six Weeks had elapsed after the Accident."[37] In this case, the fracture was exposed through an incision four inches long. The fracture fragments themselves were then exposed and the periosteum scraped. The wound was left open and the bone ends were dressed with butter of antimony during the next few weeks. The resulting reaction led to the healing of the fracture. Other surgeons, including John Rhea Barton of Philadelphia, succeeded in promoting the union of fractures by applying various caustic substances to the bone ends.[38] The pseudarthrosis itself, or the surgical treatment by scraping, cauterization or excision, often resulted in the creation of defects in the substance of the bone. To bring the ends together at the operation was not difficult. To maintain them in apposition was more than the external splints could be relied upon to accomplish. Faced with such a problem, J. Kearny Rodgers of New York resorted to tying the ends together with silver wire. The wire was brought out through the wound and later was pulled away as the fracture healed, with two inches of shortening. An account of this case was published in 1827.[39] Louis-Henri Laloy reported upon this method in 1839,[40] and Eben K. Sanborn described such a case in New England in 1860.[41]

The introduction of antiseptic and aseptic surgical techniques during the latter part of the nineteenth century made these older surgical methods of treating ununited fractures obsolete and permitted the development of the surgical methods used today.

The use of materials such as ivory, deer antler, and other animal bones in the treatment of fractures had been primarily for fixation and the promotion of an inflammatory reaction. The study of bone grafts to replace defects in bone and to promote healing of fractures began with the work of Ollier, Barth, George Axhausen and Sir William Macewen; this work has been ably summarized by Hey-Groves.[42] The literature on this subject accumulated rapidly and was often confusing and contradictory. Samuel W. Chase and Charles H. Herndon were able to cite 855 references on the subject by 1955.[43] J. Spencer Speed opened a discussion of the use of bone grafts in the treatment of ununited fractures in this way:

> *In no other field of surgery has experimental work given us so little that is practical or dependable as in the work done in connection with bone grafts. The literature is full of very carefully planned research on various phases of this subject, yet when it has all been read and the results of the numerous investigators have been tabulated, there is so much conflicting evidence that few positive conclusions can be drawn.*[44]

Good clinical papers stressing the natural history and pathology of ununited fractures, such as that by Marshall R. Urist, Robert Mazet, Jr., and Franklin C. McLean, were scarce.[45]

The first serious study of heterografts was made by Svante Orell, who processed animal bone by boiling and defatting to produce "os purum."[46] When this had been implanted and had provoked an inflammatory ingrowth of capillaries, the implant was called "os novum." The material was made available commercially and was quite widely used immediately before World War II.[47] After World War II, experiments with processed heterografts were continued by Bassett and his associates in New York (with Boplant) and by Richard Maatz, an associate of Gerhard Kuntscher's in Kiel (Kiel bone).[48]

At the same time methods for processing heterografts were being investigated, similar consideration was being given to the processing of homografts. Bone banks came into use after World War II and have enjoyed variable success.[49] The most sophisticated and successful of these was the program developed for the Naval Hospital in Bethesda by George W. Hyatt.[50]

One thing that all surgeons could agree upon was that fresh, autogenous bone was the best material to use in the treatment of ununited fractures by bone grafting. Homografts and heterografts were second choices and were employed when bone of sufficient quantity or quality could not be obtained from the patient. The techniques for bone grafting became well established.[51] The observation that the application of compression across the fracture site alone was sufficient to promote the healing of some ununited fractures simplified the care of some patients.[52] The indications for treatment were further clarified by the observations of Swiss surgeons that there were two types of diaphyseal pseudarthroses.[53] The first was characterized by a proliferative healing reaction—the "elephant's foot"—and could be treated by immobilization alone with rigid fixation. The second showed atrophy and absorption of bone without an established healing reaction and required autogenous bone grafting and rigid fixation for successful union.

Notes

1. Joseph-François Malgaigne, *Traité des fractures et luxations*, vol. 1(Paris: J. B. Baillière, 1847); Ernst Julius Gurlt, *Handbuch der Lehre von den Knochenbruchen*, vol. 1 (Hamm: Grote, 1862).

2. Joseph Amesbury, *Observations on the Nature and Treatment of Fractures of the Upper Third of the Thigh-Bone, and of Fractures of Long Standing* (London: Underwood, 1828), 193–95.

3. George W. Norris, "On the Occurence of Non-Union after Fractures," in *Contributions to Practical Surgery* (Philadelphia: Lindsay & Blakiston, 1873), 9–111.

4. O. J. Ekman, *Dissertatio Medica Descriptionem et Casus Aliquot Osteomalaciae Sistens* (Uppsala: J. Edman, 1788), 130–35; J. Paget, *Studies of Old Case-Books* (London: Longmans, Green, 1891), 130–35.

5. Guilliame Dupuytren, *On the Injuries and Diseases of the Bones*, trans. and ed. F. LeGros Clark (London: Sydenham Society, 1846), 32–33.

6. Hippocrates, *The Genuine Works of Hippocrates*, trans. Francis Adams (Baltimore: Williams & Wilkins, 1939), 318.

7. Ambroise Paré, *The Case Reports and Autopsy Records of Ambroise Paré*, comp. and ed. Wallace B. Hamby (Springfield, Ill.: Charles C. Thomas, 1960), 80–82.

8. Astley P. Cooper, *A Treatise on Dislocations and Fractures of the Joints* (London: Hurst, Reese, Orme and Brown, 1822), 127–28.

9. Ibid., 131.

10. Dupuytren, *Injuries and Diseases of the Bones*, 187–88.

11. Robert William Smith, *A Treatise on Fractures in the Vicinity of Joints, and on Certain Forms of Accidental and Congenital Dislocations* (Dublin: Hodges and Smith, 1847), 30–33.

12. Auguste Nélaton, *Eléments de pathologie chirurgicale* (Paris: Germer Baillière, 1847–48), 2:441; Thomas Bryant, "Clinical Lecture on the Diagnostic Value of the Ilio-femoral Triangle in Cases of Injury of the Hip-joint," *Lancet* 1(1876): 119–20.

13. William Stewart Halsted, "The Effects of Adduction and Abduction on the Length of the Limb in Fractures of the Neck of the Femur," *NY Med J* 39(1884): 317–18.

14. Kellogg Speed, "The Unsolved Fracture," *SGO* 60(1935): 341–52.

15. Cooper, *Treatise on Dislocations*, 213–15.

16. Celsus, *De medicina*, with an English translation by W. G. Spencer (Cambridge, Mass.: Harvard University Press, 1953), 3:555.

17. R. R. Crawford, "A History of the Treatment of Non-Union of Fractures in the 19th Century, in the United States," *J Bone Joint Surg* 55A(1973): 1685–97.

18. Norris, "On the Occurence of Non-Union," 102–3.

19. Hugh Owen Thomas, *The Principles of the Treatment of Fractures and Dislocations*, Part VI (London: H. K. Lewis, 1886),40–41.

20. Ibid.

21. J. B. Roberts, "Continuous Passive Hyperemia in Delayed Union of Fractures and in Hastening the Consolidation of Fractures," *SGO* 5(1907): 16–18.

22. August Bier, *Hyperamie als Heilmittel*, 2d edition (Leipzig: F. C. W. Vogel, 1905).

23. Henry H. Smith, "On the Treatment of Ununited Fracture by Means of Artificial Limbs which Combine the Principle of Pressure and Motion at the Seat of Fracture, and Lead to the Formation of Ensheathing Callus, " *Am J Med Sci* 29(1855): 102–19.

24. Augusto Sarmiento and L. L. Latta, *Closed Functional Treatment of Fractures* (Berlin: Springer Verlag, 1981), v–vi.

25. Abel Boyer, *A Treatise on Surgical Diseases and the Operations Suited to Them*, trans. Alexander H. Stevens (New York: T. & J. Swords, 1816), 2:387.

26. Valentine Mott, "Two Cases of Ununited Fractures Successfully Treated by Seton," *Med Surg Reg* 1, pt.2 (1820): 375–79.

27. For example, J. Burman, "Case of Ununited Fracture Treated by Galvanism," *Prov Med Surg J* (1847): 654–55; A. C. Garratt, *Electro-Physiology and Electro-Therapeutics* (Boston: Ticknor and Fields, 1861), 657–59; L. LeFort, "Pseudarthrose du fémur et de l'humérus; traitment par l'électrolyse," *Gaz hôp civ milit* 61(1888): 35; and F. D. Lente, "Cases of Ununited Fractures Treated by Electricity," *NY Med J* 5(1850): 317.

28. Guillaume Benjamin Duchenne de Boulogne, *De l'électrisation localisée et son application à la physiologie, à la pathologie et à la thérapeutique* (Paris: J. B. Baillière, 1855).

29. Iwao Yasuda, "Fundamental Aspects of Fracture Treatment," *J Kyoto Med Soc* 4(1953): 395–406.

30. C. Andrew L. Bassett and Robert O. Becker, "Generation of Electric Potentials by Bone in Response to Mechanical Stress," *Science* 137(1962): 1063-64; Zachary B. Friedenberg and Carl T. Brighton, "Bioelectric Potentials in Bone," *J Bone Joint Surg* 48A(1966): 915–23.

31. G. F. Sheldon and R. G. Sheldon, "Philip Syng Physick, M. D., 1768–1837, The Father of American Surgery," *Bull Am Coll Surg* (May 1979): 17–27.

32. Phillip Syng Physick, "A Case of Fracture of the Os Humerus, in Which the Broken Ends of the Bone Not Uniting in the Usual Manner, A Cure Was Effected by Means of a Seton," *Med Repository* 1(1804): 122–24.

33. John Baxter, "Case of the Efficacy of the Seton in Artificial Joint after a Fracture of the Fore-Arm," *Med Record* 7(1824): 30–31; Mott, "Two Cases of Ununited Fractures," 375–79.

34. J. S. Bushman, "New and Successful Operation for Pseudarthrosis," *Am J Med Sci*, new ser., 14(1847): 477–78; Johann Friedrich Dieffenbach, "Neue sichere Heilmethode des falschen Gelenkes oder der Pseudarthrose," *Wschr ges Heilk Berlin* 46(1846): 729–34; 47(1846): 745–52; and 48(1846): 761–65.

35. H. Friedberg, "Pseudarthrose der Tibia in Folge einer Fractur mit Dislocation der Fragemente. Anwendung von Elfenbeinzapfen. Heilung.," *Dtsch Klin-Berl* (1852): 207.

36. H. R. Ranke, "Pseudarthrose des Unterschenkels; treppenformige Resection mit Aneinandernnietung der Fragmente durch Elfenbeinstifte. Heilung," *Berl klin Wschr* 12(1875): 221–22.

37. Charles White, *Cases in Surgery with Remarks*, part 1 (London: W. Johnston, 1770), 79–93.

38. John Rhea Barton, "Observations on the Cure of Ununited Fractures by the Application of Caustics," *Am Med Rec* 9(1826): 275–78.

39. J. Kearny Rodgers, "Case of Ununited Fracture of the Os Brachii, Successfully Treated," *NY Med Phys J* 6(1827): 521–23.

40. Louis-Henri Laloy, *De la suture des os appliquée aux résections et aux fractures avec plaie* (Paris: Rignoux, 1839).

41. Eben K. Sanborn, "The Silver Wire in Ununited Fracture, with a Case," *Am J Med Sci* 39(1860): 339–42.

42. E. W. Hey-Groves, "Methods and Results of Transplantation of Bone in the Repair of Defects Caused by Injury or Disease," *Brit J Surg* 5(1917–18): 185–242.

43. Samuel W. Chase and Charles H. Herndon, "The Fate of Autogenous and Homogenous Bone Grafts," *J Bone Joint Surg* 37A(1955): 809–41.

44. J. Spencer Speed, "Bone Grafts in Ununited Fractures," *South Surg* 23(1930): 179–88.

45. Marshall R. Urist et al., "The Pathogenesis and Treatment of Delayed Union and Non-Union," *J Bone Joint Surg* 36A(1954): 931–67.

46. Svante Orell, "Studien über Knochenimplantation und Knochenneubildung, Implantation von 'Os Purum' sowie Transplantation von 'Os Novum'," *Acta chir scand* 74, suppl.(1934): 31; id., "Surgical Bone Grafting with 'Os Purum,' 'Os Novum,' and Boiled Bone," *J Bone Joint Surg* 19(1937): 873–85.

47. C. W. Goff, "The Os Purum Implant," *J Bone Joint Surg* 26(1944): 758–67.

48. Bassett and D. R. Creighton, Jr., "A Comparison of Host Response to Cortical Autographs and Processed Calf Heterographs," *J Bone Joint Surg* 44A(1962): 842–54; R. Maatz and A. Bauermeister, "A Method of Bone Maceration," *J Bone Joint Surg* 39A(1957): 153–66.

49. L. F. Bush, "The Use of Homogenous Bone Grafts," *J Bone Joint Surg* 29(1947): 620–28.

50. George W. Hyatt, "The Founding of the U.S. Navy Tissue Bank," *Transplant Proc* 8(1976): 17–20.

51. D. B. Phemister, "Splint Grafts in the Treatment of Delayed and Non-Union of Fractures," *SGO* 52(1931): 376–81; J. S. Speed, "Bone Grafts," *South Surg* 23(1930): 179–88.

52. R. Judet et al., "Traitement des pseudarthroses par la compression osseuse simple," *Mém Acad Chir* 82(1956): 402–7.

53. E. Müller et al., *Operative Frakturenbehandlung* (Berlin: Springer Verlag, 1963), 123.

CHAPTER NINE

The Healing of Fractures

CONTROVERSY REGARDING the process of fracture healing has existed since antiquity. Malgaigne (figure 9.1), a thorough student of Greek and Roman medical literature, contrasted the idea of Hippocrates that callus formation depends on factors produced by the bone marrow with the view of Galen, who believed that the essential factors were brought to the site by the blood vessels.[1] These two theories of fracture healing competed for centuries. The experimental study of fracture healing began in 1684, when Antonius de Heyde, a Dutch physician, studied callus formation in frogs and concluded that it arose from the coagulation of the blood in the fracture hematoma.[2] Two developments provided the impetus for research on the healing of fractures. The first was the appreciation of bone as a living structure, stemming from the work of Clopton Havers (?–1702). In his book *Osteologia Nova; or Some New Observations of the Bones and the Parts Belonging to Them* (figures 9.2a,b), published in London in 1691, Havers described the architecture of bone and the canals containing the blood vessels, which became known as the Haversian canals.[3]

The second development was the application of a vital staining method to the study of bone growth. The plant known as madder or *Rubia tinctorum* has been used as a dye for cloth and leather since biblical times. The first mention of madder's ability to stain the bone in living animals appeared in a Dutch treatise published in 1564.[4] It was John Belchier (1706–1785), a favorite student of Cheselden, who first called the attention of the scientific community to this phenomenon. In a paper entitled "An Account of the Bones of Animals Being Changed to a Red Colour by Aliment Only," published in the *Philosophical Transactions* of the Royal Society of London in 1735, he described how the bones of bran-fed hogs that

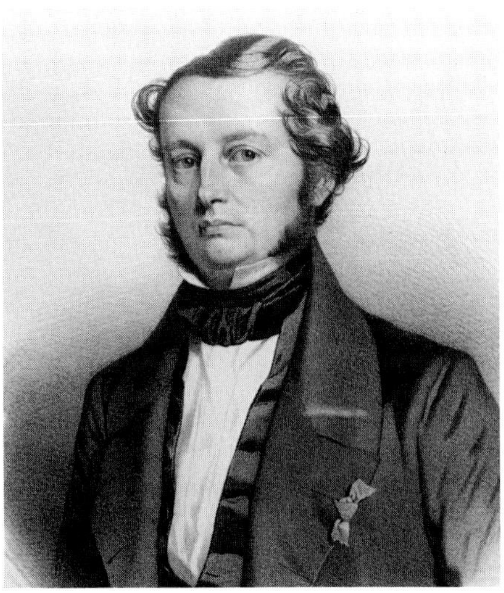

Figure 9.1 Joseph-François Malgaigne (1806–1865)

had been boiled in a caldron with cloth to rid the cloth of an excess of the dye madder were found to have been stained by the dye. The dye did not affect the cartilage or the soft tissue, only the calcified bone.[5] This observation was quickly put to use by students of fracture healing.

The first of these students was Henri Louis DuHamel du Monceau (1700–1781), a French naturalist (figure 9.3). DuHamel was not a physician. He took an active part in the management of his estates and became an expert in botany and agriculture. However, he had an avid interest in all natural phenomena, as was characteristic of the savants of his generation. Hearing of Belchier's observations, he immediately repeated the experiments on chickens, pigeons, turkeys and lambs on his farm, reporting the results to the Royal Academy of Sciences in France in a series of papers.[6] It was from these observations on bone growth that he derived his ideas on the healing of fractures. He summarized these observations in a letter to his friend Charles Bonnet (1720–1793), the Swiss naturalist who first clarified the mechanism of parthenogenesis:

> 1) *The structure of the wood is unlike its bark. The structure of the bone is dissimilar to periosteum.*
>
> 2) *The wood grows in size by the addition of thin layers which form between the wood and the bark. The bone grows in size*

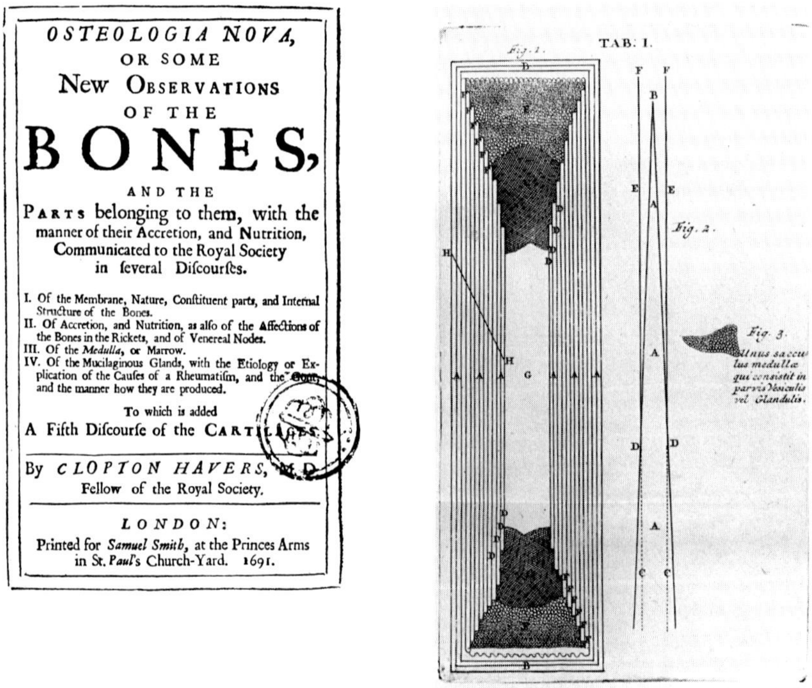

OSTEOLOGIA NOVA,
OR SOME
New OBSERVATIONS
OF THE
BONES,
AND THE
PARTS belonging to them, with the manner of their Accretion, and Nutrition, Communicated to the Royal Society in ſeveral Diſcourſes.

I. Of the Membrane, Nature, Conſtituent parts, and Internal Structure of the Bones.
II. Of Accretion, and Nutrition, as alſo of the Affections of the Bones in the Rickets, and of Venereal Nodes.
III. Of the *Medulla*, or Marrow.
IV. Of the Mucilaginous Glands, with the Etiology or Explication of the Cauſes of a Rheumatiſm, and the Gout, and the manner how they are produced.

To which is added
A Fifth Diſcourſe of the CARTILAGES.

By CLOPTON HAVERS, M.D.
Fellow of the Royal Society.

LONDON:
Printed for *Samuel Smith*, at the Princes Arms in St. *Paul's* Church-Yard. 1691.

Figure 9.2a,b a) First edition of the work in which Clopton Havers first described the Haversian canals (1691). b) Haversian canals, as illustrated in the Latin translation of Havers's *Osteologia Nova* (Leiden: Georg Wishoff, 1734). The title was later changed to *Novae quaedam observationes de ossibus.*

by the addition of thin layers forming between the periosteum and the bone.

3) *The cortical layers of bone form, just as in the wood, between the wood and the bark. I will not assert that the new products of the periosteum, which differs from the remainder, are formed between the periosteum and the bone. I have no proof of this.*

4) *I cannot help but believe, as some have thought, that the layers of wood have their origin in a gelatinous secretion collecting between the bark and the wood, not in an organized form, and that this humor, the cambium, becomes organized, little by little, becoming solid and turning into wood.*

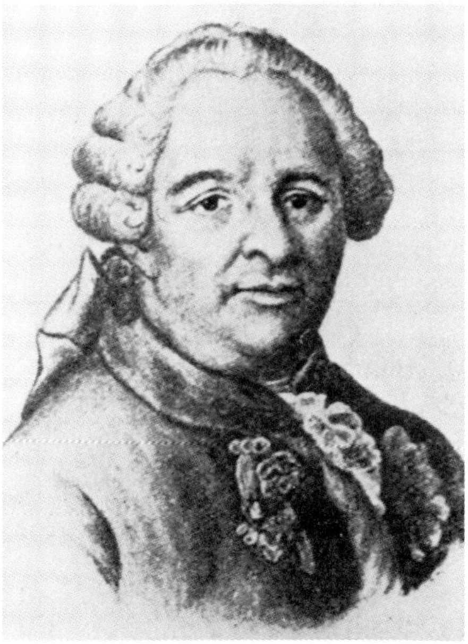

Figure 9.3 Henri Louis DuHamel du Monceau (1700–1781). From R. Osgood, *The Evolution of Orthopaedic Surgery* (St. Louis: C. V. Mosby, 1925), 20.

5) *The bark is truly the organ which produces the layers of wood, and I have seen it form under strips of bark partially detached from the wood. In looking at fractures of the bone and at the formation of layers of new bone, it appears to me that the periosteum can be regarded as the organ which forms the osseous layers.*

6) *The diseased exterior of a tree which is split cannot be healed by its bark since it is separated from the interior wood. Certain healthy bones, which overlie a dead bone or a part of a bone which is dead, can be regarded similarly, and can heal by material secreted by the periosteum.*

7) *In a young tree, wood stripped of its bark and protected from the sun and wind can produce a new layer under which new wood can form. The bare bone of a young animal, protected from contact with air, can also produce a tissue under which it forms new layers of bone.*

8) *If one leaves the wood, bare of its bark and exposed to air, the wound will not heal in from the edges of the bark. Similarly, exposing the bone to air by causing a defect in the periosteum or by a slough caused by an absorbent or spiritous medication results in exfoliation and a sore; and when the compact bone is dense, the defect will not heal in from the edges of the wound.*

9) *In grafts and in broken branches, one observes the bark producing material of the same type which forms the layers of wood, spreading out between the torn woody fibers; this substance becomes hard, and a woody layer forms over the fracture, making a cover which hides the process. In the long bones and in firm callus in adult animals with fractures, I have drilled the area to expose the structure. I have found*

traces of a substance close to the developing bone, which I believe was produced by the periosteum, extending between the cavities and the bony layers and covering all of the fracture.

10) *In healed broken branches, one always sees a local thickening in the area of the break. Fractures of the bones of adults are always associated with such a thickening which is called callus.*[7]

By drawing analogies between the processes he had observed in trees and in animals, DuHamel concluded that the periosteum was the important element in the healing of fractures. One wonders whether Nicholas Andry (1658–1742), who was familiar with DuHamel and his work, was influenced by such analogies when he used a young tree to illustrate his idea of how to straighten a crooked limb.

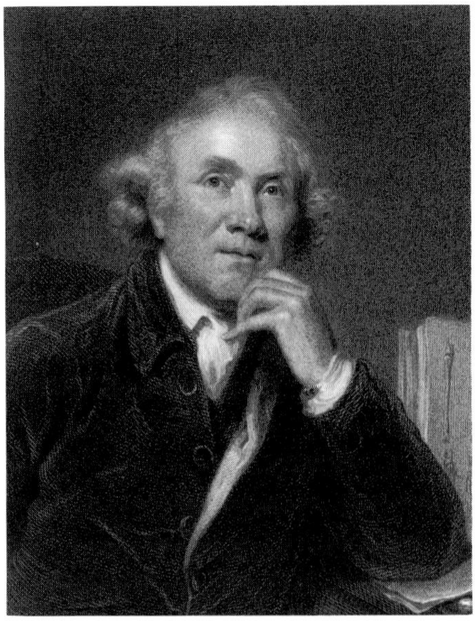

Figure 9.4 John Hunter (1728–1793)

The importance of the role of the periosteum in fracture healing was immediately challenged by Albrecht von Haller (1708–1777), the distinguished Swiss scholar and surgeon, who, on the basis of similar experiments using madder, concluded that bone was not formed by the periosteum, but was a product of the arteries, which could lay down bone anywhere within cartilage or beneath the periosteum.[8] John Hunter (1728–1793) was influenced by Haller's work and carried out extensive experiments on growing animals using madder (figure 9.4). He emphasized that new bone was not only laid down during growth, but was also absorbed, thus explaining the phenomenon of remodeling. He also clearly demonstrated that the bones grew in length as a result of growth at the epiphyses, an observation that had been made initially by Stephen Hales (1677–1761) in 1717.[9] Hunter concluded: "The space between the broken surfaces of the bone and other parts are first filled with extravasated blood from the ruptured vessels. This blood coagulates, and in time becomes vascular, as in the same mode of union of the soft parts, forming a callus."[10] A good summary of the controversy between DuHamel and his followers and those of Haller and Hunter was published by Fougeroux de Bondarey (1732–1789).[11] In 1799, Antonio Scarpa (1747–1832) observed that bone formation at the site of the healing fracture was similar to that occurring during the normal growth and development of the skeleton.[12] The next important contribution to the problem was based on human material.

It was from observations and experiments on patients at the Hôtel Dieu in Paris that Guilliaume Dupuytren derived his ideas of fracture healing—for example, bending fractures of the forearm in children.[13] On the basis of his broad clinical experience and his intensive work in the dissection room, Dupuytren summarized his ideas on the healing of fractures as follows:

Convinced by my experiments that Nature never accomplishes the immediate union of a fracture, save by the formation of two successive deposits of callus, I have been induced to name one provisional and the other permanent. The former of these is usually perfected in about thirty or forty days, and which comprises the ossification due to the vessels of the periosteum, the filamentous tissue, sometimes even of the muscles and of the medullary tissue, has not always strength enough (especially in oblique fractures), when the splints and other supports are removed, to resist the power of the muscles or such passive force as may be applied, even to a moderate extent, to the seat of injury; and the brittleness of this provisional callus is such that the bone more readily yields at the point where it is deposited than at any other part. The second (permanent) callus, formed by the reunion of the surfaces of the fracture, possesses a solidity superior even to that of the bone itself, so that the latter would sooner break at any other point than where the former is deposited. The production and organization of the permanent callus is never completed under eight, ten, or twelve months, a period which is further marked by the disappearance of the provisional callus, and the renewed continuity of the medullary canal.

The following are the principal phenomena which may be observed during the time that elapses between the occurrence of the fracture and the complete and exact reunion of the broken bone; their succession is so constant and unvarying, that they may be referred to five different periods. The first extends over the eight or ten days which immediately succeed the accident, and presents the following characters: at the moment that the fracture occurs, the periosteum and medullary membrane, the filamentous tissue, and sometimes even the muscles are torn; blood escapes from the ruptured vessels, and surrounds the fragments, is poured into the medullary canal, and distends the neighbouring filamentous tissue. After a time the vessels retract, and their mouths are closed, the blood ceases to escape, and a mild inflammation is set up in all these parts. The filamentous tissue, reddened by a multitude of small vessels, becomes distended, condensed, and thickened, losing its elasticity, and acquiring a remarkable consistence; irregular prolongations are sent from it into the interstices of the muscles, by which their organization is altered, and they are made to participate altogether or in part in the changes which are going on; their texture is transformed into one closely allied to the condensed filamentous tissue, and they are united and confounded with the periosteum, which, in turn, is also thickened by a network of delicate red vessels distributed over its surface. The medulla being broken through and mingled with blood, at first swells out and hardens, and subsequently becomes of a greyish colour. The medullary canal is contracted in its diameter by the encroachment of the thickened lining membrane, which assumes a reddish, fleshy, or pulpy appearance, resulting from a sort of gelatinous infiltration. The coagulum which results from the primary extravasation is absorbed and disappears. A stringy and viscid matter, sometimes presenting a gelatinous appearance, is poured out between the ends of the bone; occasionally likewise a reddish substance is developed in the same posi-

tion, springing from the inequalities which present themselves; they grow and extend towards each other in the form of rosy points, and ultimately meet and interlace with each other. This production, the nature of which is but little understood, never acquires any great amount of thickness or density; it becomes continuous internally with the medullary membrane, and externally is identified with the congested soft parts; it is not always met with, and then the viscid and gelatinous matter of which mention has been made is alone present. Both of these structures, whether found separately or together, appear to play an important part in the production of the callus, but of the permanent callus only. The fragments of the bone are, in short, surrounded by the gorged soft parts, which are converted into a homogeneous tissue of a lardaceous consistence, and red colour, but varying in intensity.

The second period then commences, and comprises the interval between the tenth or twelfth day and the twentieth or twenty-fifth. The gorged condition of the surrounding soft parts diminishes, the muscular tissue resumes its distinctive characteristics, but the filamentous tissue continues condensed. The tumefaction is more concentrated immediately about the fracture, and gradually assumes a more circumscribed character until it forms a distinct tumour isolated from all surrounding structures, not even excepting the tendons, which play in grooves channeled for them along its surface, or in perfect canals traversing its structure; such is the callus. This tumour is thicker on a level with the fracture than at any other point, and insensibly diminishes in density on either of the fragments. Its tissue is homogeneous, its colour white or whitish, its consistence firm, and its resistance analogous to that of the fibrocartilages, giving out a similar sound when cut with a sharp knife. The deepest part of this structure, that which is formed by and continuous with the periosteum, is found to contract more close adhesions to the bones the nearer it approaches to the fracture, at which point it is difficult to separate them. If, however, this separation is effected with the aid of the handle of a scalpel, it is perceived that they are formed of longitudinal fibres parallel to those of the bones, and analogous to the fibre of tendons; or they may exist in the form of cartilaginous or osseous striae, according to the more or less advanced condition of the provisional callus. Towards the extremities of the tumour formed by the callus, the periosteum becomes more distinct and easy to detach from the bone. The medullary membrane, swollen, tumid, and identified with the matter by which it is infiltrated, sometimes obliterates the canal, not only on a level with the fracture, but for some distance on either side of it; thus filling up the space usually occupied by the medulla, which is proportionately diminished in quantity; the cylinder which it forms passes rapidly into a cartilaginous state, and still more quickly into bone, becoming identified at the seat of fracture with the whitish, rosy red, or violet-coloured, viscid, or gelatinous substance, as the case may be, which is interposed between the fragments; on the other hand, it is lost in the callus externally. Whilst in this condition it is still possible for the callus to yield opposite the fracture, but crepitus is rarely reproduced.

The third period extends from the twentieth or twenty-fifth day to the thirtieth, fortieth, or sixtieth, according to the rapidity of the work of reproduction, and the age, constitution, and health of the patient. The conversion into cartilage commences at the centre of the tumour, and proceeds towards its circumference, and ossification speedily succeeds; thus little by little, the whole mass of callus becomes converted into bone. The periosteum, which is abnormally thick, then ceases to present any trace of the solution of continuity to which it had been subjected; and the muscles and tendons become free, though their natural mobility is not quite restored, on account of the induration of the filamentous tissue. If at this epoch, a section of the callus is made, the fractured ends of the bone are still found movable on each other, the condition of the intermediate substance not being as yet sensibly changed; and the tissue of the callus presents all the characteristics of the spongy texture of bone.

The fourth period includes the interval between the fiftieth or sixtieth day and the fifth or sixth month. The substance of the provisional callus becomes condensed, and passes from the condition of a spongy to that of a compact tissue, and the medullary canal is obliterated by osseous matter of greater or less density. The substance intervening between the fragments is reduced to a mere line of a different colour from the bone itself; it gradually assumes more consistence, loses it colour, and ultimately, towards the end of this period, becomes ossified: the definitive or permanent callus is then formed.

The fifth and last period embraces all the time which elapses between the fourth or sixth, and the eighth, tenth, or twelfth months. The temporary callus gradually diminishes in thickness, and at last disappears; the periosteum recovers its natural texture and density, and the muscles and tendons are restored to perfect liberty; the internal deposit of bone disappears, and the canal is insensibly re-established; the medullary membrane is repaired, and the medulla is reproduced. The process of consolidation is then completed.[14]

Dupuytren used this scheme of fracture healing in a very practical way to determine at what point a healing fracture could still be realigned by further manipulation and at what stage external splinting could be removed. His information was gained in the dissecting room, where subjects with fractures who died in the hospital were examined and the pathological anatomy of the fractures thoroughly studied. It was only a short step from the study of the pathological anatomy of fractures to the study of the biomechanics of fractures. Dupuytren became the first to study the mechanisms of common fractures by subjecting fresh cadavers to controlled manipulations that produced fractures and then dissecting them to determine their pathological anatomy. Such investigations formed the basis of his important work on ankle fractures.[15] His student Jules Gilles Thomas Maisonneuve continued this work and, on the basis of anatomical dissections and cadaver experiments, contributed more data on the biomechanics of ankle fractures.[16]

Auguste Nélaton used fresh cadavers to study fractures of the distal radius. The forearms were disarticulated at the elbows and the olecranon removed. With the hand fixed in a position of flexion or extension and the forearm vertical, its upper end was struck by a mallet. The resulting fracture of the radius was then carefully dissected and the type correlated with the mechanism of injury.[17] Amédée Bonnet, in Lyons, carried out extensive experiments on fresh cadavers of all ages to study the mechanism of meniscal injuries. In older patients, his manipulations resulted in fractures; in young adults, ligament avulsions; and in children, epiphyseal separations.[18] Johann Honigschmied carried out similar experiments in Germany.[19] Our knowledge of epiphyseal separations was advanced by a macabre series of experiments on the fresh cadavers of children of various ages.[20]

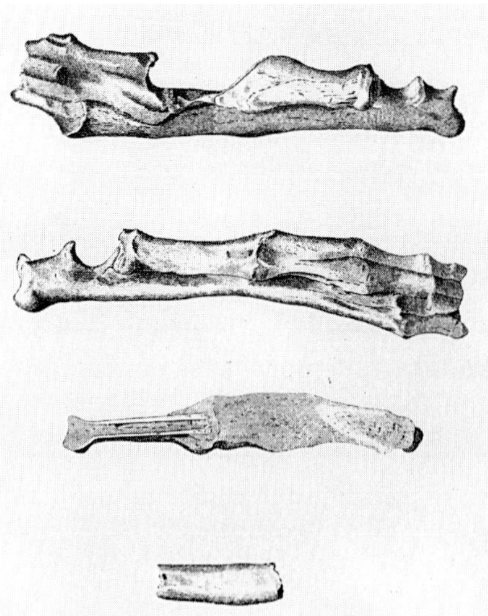

Figure 9.5 Some of the results of Syme's experiments on the regeneration of bone in the dog's radius. From Syme, "On the Power of the Periosteum to Form New Bone," *Proc Roy Soc Edinb* 14(1840): 158–62.

Paul Jules Tillaux and Léon Gosselin continued to study ankle fractures by such methods fifty years after Dupuytren.[21] In 1905, Lilienfeld of Leipzig carried out the first cadaver experiments in which X rays were taken of the injuries.[22] A classification of tibial plateau fractures was prepared by Frank Ellsworth Blaisdell on the basis of cadaver experiments in 1922,[23] and similar work was done in 1963 and 1965 by J. C. Kennedy.[24] It is hard for us now to imagine the abundance of fresh, unembalmed, human cadavers that were available for dissection in the major European centers during the nineteenth and the early part of the twentieth centuries. Although such dissections and experiments are sometimes carried out today, the conclusions to be drawn from such investigations are colored by the fact that the tissues are not optimal because they are from embalmed cadavers or amputation specimens and from subjects that are, almost without exception, from the oldest age group.

The work of DuHamel remained fresh in the minds of investigators. James Syme, in Edinburgh, carried out experiments on dogs, experiments that have been repeated literally a hundred times, demonstrating the ability of the periosteum to generate bone (figure 9.5). In addition, he noted the importance of the periosteum in the formation of the involucrum in cases of osteomyelitis.[25] Marie Jean Pierre Flourens repeated the experiments of DuHamel, using alizarin as well as madder, and came to the same general conclusions regarding the important role of the periosteum. In addition, he noted that as the bone grew with the accretion of periosteal new bone formation, there was an accompanying resorption of the medullary layers.[26]

The emergence of cellular pathology in the middle of the nineteenth century led to a further understanding of the processes of bone growth. In 1845, John G. Goodsir (1814–1867), an anatomist in Edinburgh, first established the fact that bone formation was the function of specific cells, which he named *osteoblasts.*[27] Interestingly, the source of these cells in the process of fracture healing is still in dispute.[28] The work of John Tomes and Campbell DeMorgan in 1853 demonstrated that techniques required for the study of the histology of bone were well developed. Using them, they were the first to demonstrate bone remodeling on a microscopic basis.

In newly-formed bone situated near ossifying cartilage, the Haversian spaces are exceedingly numerous and large, frequently affording room for the development of two or more systems, while in older bone they are far less numerous, and generally less in size. . . . This is a very important fact, as it demonstrates that the old tissue is removed in masses, and a new one develops in its place. It has long been taught that the older particles of an internal tissue are removed by absorption and new ones substituted, and this throughout the life of the individual. But the authors believe that they have demonstrated it for the first time.[29]

The year 1853 also saw the publication by Rudolph Virchow (1821–1902) of the first description of the uncalcified matrix of bone or osteoid.[30] Carl Gegenbaur in 1864 demonstrated that osteoblasts were present in both the periosteal layer and in the endosteum.[31] By 1873, the specific cell responsible for bone resorption, the osteoclast, had been identified and named by Rudolph A. Kolliker (1817–1905).[32]

These histological techniques were not immediately applied to the study of fracture healing. Louis Xavier Ollier (1825–1901) carried out extensive studies on bone growth, bone grafting, and fracture healing that have been summarized by Hey-Groves.[33] Although Ollier's work was published in 1867, it contains nothing but gross observations, which were interpreted generally to support DuHamel's ideas on the importance of the periosteum.[34] The role of the periosteum was finally put in perspective by the work of William Macewen (1848–1924) of Glasgow in his book *The Growth of Bone: Observations on Osteogenesis.*[35] His work unfortunately contains no histological material for interpretation, but it marked the first time that aseptic surgical procedures were used for animal experiments. These experiments emphasized the role of the periosteum as a limiting membrane and its inability to promote bone formation by itself. We see this function of the periosteum well illustrated in cases of scurvy with healing, of osteomyelitis with involucrum formation, and of osteogenic sarcoma at Codman's triangle. Macewen was a surgeon of astounding scope, recognized as one of the pioneers of neurosurgery, as well as for having carried out the first successful pneumonectomy.[36]

The discovery of X rays by Wilhelm Conrad Roentgen in 1895 was quickly followed by the appearance of articles describing the blood supply to healing fractures using arteriography. In 1906, Gustav Delkeskamp described changes in the normal vessel patterns in fractures in dogs, using mercury as a contrast material.[37] Robert Dax studied the importance of the circulation for healing fractures, with emphasis on the nutrient artery.[38] Anatole Kolodny's experiments on dogs with fractures pointed out the importance of the periosteal blood supply for the healing of fractures.[39] Robert W. Johnson, Jr., used specimens injected with India ink to delineate the role of the nutrient artery, the metaphyseal arteries, and the periosteal arteries.[40] K. Houang, a student of Robert Danis in Brussels, studied the role of the nutrient artery in fracture healing and noted that ligation of this artery could provoke calcification of the medullary canal.[41] In Turin, Stefano Teneff demonstrated that a few days after fracture there was a rapid proliferation of vessels into the fracture hematoma, coming both from the periosteal and endosteal vessels, and a wide system of anastomoses of these vessels developed.[42] J. Ladanyi and F. Hidvegi studied the blood supply in the callus of fractures following various types of fixation.[43] Perhaps the most important studies of the blood supply of bones and their role in the healing of fractures are those of José Trueta and F.C. Rhinelander, which arrived at opposite conclusions. Trueta emphasized the importance of the periosteal vessels, while Rhinelander emphasized the endosteal vessels.[44]

Most investigations of the healing of fractures have dealt with only one facet of a complex phenomenon. In a way, the literature resembles the tales of blind men describing an elephant, each accurate to a degree, but as a whole incomplete. One of the first major works to synthesize this work and to place fracture healing within the framework of our knowledge of bone as a tissue was the monograph by René Leriche and A. Policard.[45] Leriche (1879–1955) was educated in Lyons, traveled widely in Europe and the United States, and was the chief of the Surgical Clinic of the University of Strasbourg from 1924 to 1939. His experience in World War I aroused his interest in sympathetic dystrophies, which he treated with sympathetic blocks and periarterial sympathectomy. Vascular surgeons are all acquainted with Leriche's syndrome: impotence, absent femoral pulses, and claudication. He was a thoughtful surgeon and philosopher whose book, *La chirurgie à l'ordre de la vie*, received critical acclaim and wide circulation.[46] His colleague, A. Policard (1881–1972), was the professor of histology at the University of Lyons. The preface to their book expresses their enthusiasm for the scientific method as it was applied to this problem:

This book is the fruit of ten years of collaboration. For ten years we have unceasingly observed the numerous aspects of the normal and pathological evolution of bone, have reflected on the problems to which they give rise, and have sought the various solutions in every direction, through histology, radiography, experiment, and direct observation of man, each of us using for that purpose his particular field and pouring into a common fund the result of his own observations.

Thus, little by little, we have been forced to a new understanding of everything concerned with the development, life, evolution, diseases, and regeneration of bone.

It seemed to us that the time had arrived for an exposition of the synthesis of those things which we had observed and deduced.

Certain individuals will perhaps think that it would have been preferable to have been more analytic and more documentary, to have confined ourselves to explaining facts without making a constructive effort, thus permitting others to draw their conclusions in such a complex matter. It is the old quarrel of objective and subjective literature.

We are frankly prejudiced.

Having ourselves tried to penetrate the meaning of things, we shall show how one may understand today the intimate construction of bone. Claudel has said somewhere: "Do not trust thine eye alone, but without reserve, all that is thyself." [N'appliquez point à la vérité de l'oeil seul, mais tout cela sans réserve qui est toi-même.]

This we have done, persuaded that it is legitimate to choose one's opinion even though it is no longer in harmony with contemporary views.

Medical works of our time too frequently have the appearance of manuals of history or anthology. They should be a critical and systematic exposition of actual science.

Like Louis XI kissing the figures on his hat each time he uncovered himself, we have thought ourselves obliged to salute our predecessors, each time we have uncovered ourselves, without daring to make the choice of separating the good grain from the tares.

Then, this done, without reaching the bottom of things, we have placed in juxtaposition in parallel lines the facts and theories, without condensation, without reaching a conclusion, without showing frankly the extent of our ignorance.

It would be well to end the poor method of popularization which retards progress.

Without doubt, in criticizing the past one exposes oneself to criticism. It matters little. All loyal pursuit of truth brings one nearer to it even if one does not attain it.

Certainly facts are facts, and we should not forget the past, on the edifice of which we have elevated ourselves in order to advance in our own time; but, in this past we should make a choice instead of continually musing on outworn dogmas. When a thing is indeed dead, let us say so, and do not allow a doubt to linger on with the possibility of its revival.

In the question of osteogenesis, masses of observations and experiments have been accumulating for a long time. Every day the problem instead of becoming simpler becomes more complex. After having indicated what has been accomplished, there is perhaps some utility in stating clearly the problems, the solutions of which should be sought.

This book was conceived in this spirit. For ten years we have read everything that we could procure on the subject of osteogenesis. We have retained that which seemed good to us, comparing it with our own observations. That which has been revealed to us by this work is set forth here, the whole having a unity, so to speak, which gives rise to a theory.

This theory is of a general character. It applies to all the modalities of osteogenesis. It allows an understanding of its diverse peculiarities. It explains disconnected and obscure pathological facts.

It always takes into consideration the individual tissues themselves, and not their relationship to the whole individual. The phenomena of the life of tissues are automatic. They mutually reveal themselves, as in a stream. One runs a great risk of a mistake in interpreting them otherwise.

One need not be surprised to find, in the course of these pages, sentences like the following: "This question is absolutely unknown," "The problem is entirely unsolved," etc. We would consider that we have fulfilled one of the prime objects we have in view if this book can place someone on the road to fruitful researches.

The problem of osteogenesis has passed through many phases. It has been histological, and surgical, and at the present time it is, above all, chemical. It is useless now for the histologists to repeat what has been done so many times, and for the surgeons to experiment on the periosteum, on grafts, and on the osteogenesis of repair. It is now the turn of the chemists and physicists. They alone can open up new horizons by giving us some of the certainties we lack. When they have solved certain pending questions, it will be possible to resume with profit the studies of the past. We can then progress, and, perhaps, have bone formed at will, accelerate the union of fractures, and prevent the pathological and physiological rarefactions of bone. But for this to occur, it is necessary for us to ask them some definite questions.

We shall see in the course of these pages how much the division into water-tight compartments, which always prevails in the biological sciences, has impeded the progress toward knowledge.

We have tried to establish connections and to indicate clearly the problems that it is necessary to solve before progress can be made.

This book is dedicated to Ollier.

We did not know Ollier. We were not his pupils. We have often been called on to contradict him. After having proved the exactness of the facts that he observed, we have finally overthrown his theories.

Nevertheless, it seems to us that, were he still living, he would understand us. In any case, we have tried to follow his spirit and to guide ourselves by his method, considering him above all as one of the originators of contemporary scientific surgery.[47]

A quarter of a century later, Franklin C. McLean (1888–1968) and Marshall R. Urist (b. 1914) published a similar monograph, in which they attempted to unify our knowledge of bone and fracture healing.[48] It is interesting to note that one of the most significant observations on fracture healing made in the first half of this century was made by Danis, who noted that fractures that were rigidly and internally fixed could heal without any callus at all— *soudure autogène.*[49]

Notes

1. Joseph-François Malgaigne, *Traité des fractures et luxations* (Paris: J. B. Baillière, 1847), 113.

2. Ibid.

3. Clopton Havers, *Osteologia Nova; or, Some New Observations of the Bones and the Parts Belonging to Them* (London: S. Smith, 1691).

4. G. R. Cameron, "The History of Madder (*Rubia tinctorum*)," *Ann Med Hist* 4(1932): 466–73.

5. John Belchier, "An Account of the Bones of Animals Being Changed to a Red Colour by Aliment Only," *Phil Trans Roy Soc London* 30(1735): 287–300.

6. Henri Louis DuHamel, "Observations sur la réunion des fractures animaux," *Mém Acad Roy Sci* (1741); "Sur le développement et la crue des os des animaux," *Mém Acad Roy Sci* (1742); "Sur les os," *Mém Acad Roy Sci* (1743).

7. DuHamel, "Lettre: Sur la formation des os dans les animaux et du bois dans les arbres," *J méd*, septembre (1757), 165–67.

8. Albrecht von Haller, *Deux mémoires sur la formation des os, fondées sur les expériences* (Lausanne: M. M. Bousquet, 1758).

9. Stephen Hales, *Vegetable Statistics* (London: Innys & Woodward, 1717).

10. John Hunter, *The Works of John Hunter, F.R.S., with Notes*, ed. James F. Palmer (London: Longman, Rees, Orme, Brown, Green and Longman, 1835), 1:501.

11. Fougeroux de Bondarey, *Auguste Denis; Mémoires sur les os, pour servir de réponse aux objections proposées contre le sentiment de M. DuHamel du Monceau; Rapportée dans les volumes de l'Académie Royale des Sciences; avec les mémoires de M. M. Haller et Bordenave, qui ont donné lieu à ce travail* (Paris: H. L. Guerin & L. F. Delatour, 1760).

12. Antonio Scarpa, *De Penitiori Ossium Structura Commentarius* (Leipzig: J. F. Hartnoch, 1799).

13. Hannah K. Barsky, *Guillaume Dupuytren: A Surgeon in His Place and Time* (New York: Vantage, 1984), 111–24; Guillaume Dupuytren, "Sur quelques cas particuliers de fractures ou de courbures des os survenus à des enfants," *Bull Faculté Méd Paris* 2(1811): 152–60.

14. Dupuytren, *On the Injuries and Diseases of Bones*, trans. and ed. F. Le Gros Clark (London: Sydenham Society, 1847), 41–45.

15. Dupuytren, "Sur la fracture de l'extrémité inférieure du péroné, les luxations et les accidents qui en sont la suite," *Annuaire méd-chir hôp Paris* (1819), 1–227.

16. Jules Gilles Thomas Maisonneuve, "Recherches sur la fracture du péroné," *Arch gén méd*, 3ème sér., 7(1840): 165–87.

17. Auguste Nélaton, *Eléménts de pathologie chirurgicale* (Paris: Germer Baillière, 1844), 1:740.

18. Amédée Bonnet, *Traité des maladies des articulations* (Paris: J. B. Baillière & Germer Baillière, 1845), 2:178–94.

19. Johann Honigschmied, "Leichenexperimente über die Zerreissungen der Bander im Sprunggelenk mit Rucksicht auf die Entstehung der indirecten Knochelfracturen," *Dtsch Zeit Chir* 8(1977): 239–60.

20. J. T. E. Foucher, "De la divulsion des épiphyses," *Congrès méd France* 1(1867): 63–72.

21. Léon Gosselin, "Rapports," *Bull Acad Méd*, 1872, 817–25.

22. Lilienfeld, "Die Luxation ossis lunati volaris eine Luxatio ossis capitati dorsalis," *Arch klin Chir* 76(1905): 641–60.

23. Frank Ellsworth Blaisdell, "Fracture of the Tibial Spine," *AMA Arch Surg* 5(1922): 561–77.

24. See J. C. Kennedy, "Complete Dislocation of the Knee," *J Bone Joint Surg* 45A(1963): 889–904; id., "Experimental Tibial Plateau Fractures," *J Bone Joint Surg* 50(1968): 1552–34.

25. James Syme, "On the Power of the Periosteum to Form New Bone," *Proc Roy Soc Edinb* 14(1840): 158–62.

26. Marie Jean Pierre Flourens, "Recherches sur le développement des os et des dents," *Archs Mus Hist nat*, 1842, 315–460.

27. John G. Goodsir, *Anatomical and Pathological Observations* (Edinburgh: Black, 1845).

28. B. McKibbin, "The Biology of Fracture Healing in the Long Bones," *J Bone Joint Surg* 60B(1978): 150–62.

29. John Tomes and Campbell DeMorgan, "Observations on the Structure and Development of Bone," *Phil Trans Roy Soc London* 143(1853): 109–39.

30. Rudolph Virchow, "Das normale Knochenwachsthum und die rachitische Storung desselben," *Virchows Arch path Anat Physiol* 5(1853): 409–505.

31. Carl Gegenbaur, "Ueber die Bildung des Knochengewebes," *Jena Zeit Naturw* 1(1864): 343–69.

32. Rudolph A. Kolliker, *Die normale Resorption des Knochengewebes* (Leipzig: Vogel, 1873).

33. E. W. Hey-Groves, "Methods and Results of Transplantation of Bone in the Repair of Defects Caused by Injury or Disease," *Brit J Surg* 5(1917–18): 185–242.

34. Louis X. E. L. Ollier, *Traité expérimental et clinique de la régénération des os* (Paris: Masson, 1867).

35. William Macewen, *The Growth of Bone: Observations on Osteogenesis; An Experimental Inquiry into the Development and Reproduction of Diaphyseal Bone* (Glasgow: James Maclehose, 1912).

36. A. K. Bowman, *The Life and Teaching of Sir William Macewen* (London: William Hodge, 1942), 340–45.

37. Gustav Delkeskamp, "Das Verhalten der Knochenarterien bei Knochenerkrankungen und Frakturen," *Fortschr Geb Röntgenstr* 10(1906): 219–24.

38. Robert Dax, "Ueber die Beziehungen der Zirkulationsstorungen zur Heilung von Frakturen der langen Rohrenknochen mit besonderer Berucksichtigung der Arteria nutritia," *Bruns Beitr klin Chir* 104(1916): 313–42.

39. Anatole Kolodny, "The Periosteal Blood Supply and Healing of Fractures," *J Bone Joint Surg* 5(1923): 698–711.

40. Robert W. Johnson, Jr., "A Physiological Study of the Blood Supply of the Diaphysis," *J Bone Joint Surg* 9(1927): 153.

41. K. Houang, "Le rôle des artères nourricières des os longs dans la formation du cal et la calification de la cavité médullaire," *Presse méd* 42(1934): 2074–76.

42. Stefano Teneff, "Experimental Studies in Vascularization of Bony Callus," *J Int Coll Surg* 13(1950): 186–191.

43. J. Ladanyi and F. Hidvegi, "Blood Supply of Experimental Callus Formation," *Acta morphol Acad Sci Hung* 4(1954): 35–44.

44. A. X. Cavadias and José Trueta, "An Experimental Study of the Vascular Contributions to the Callus of Fractures," *SGO* 120(1965): 731–47; F. C. Rhinelander and R. A. Baragry, "Microangiography in Bone Healing," *J Bone Joint Surg* 44 A(1962): 1273–98; Trueta, *Studies of the Development and Decay of the Human Frame* (Philadelphia: W. B. Saunders, 1968), 9–11.

45. René Leriche and A. Policard, *Les problèmes de la physiologie normale et pathologique de l'os* (Paris: Masson, 1926).

46. Leriche, *La chirurgie à l'ordre de la vie* (Paris: La Presse Française et Etrangère, 1944).

47. Leriche and Policard, *The Normal and Pathological Physiology of Bone*, trans. Sherwood Moore and J. Albert Key (London: Henry Kimptom, 1928), 7–10.

48. Franklin C. McLean and Marshall R. Urist, *Bone: An Introduction to the Physiology of Skeletal Tissue* (Chicago: University of Chicago Press, 1955).

49. Robert Danis, *Théorie et pratique de l'ostéosynthèse* (Paris: Masson, 1949).

CHAPTER TEN

The Impact of Roentgen's Discovery on the Treatment of Fractures

PERHAPS NO EXAMPLE better illustrates the dependence of medical progress on the progress made in the basic sciences than the effect of the discovery of X rays on the treatment of fractures. Professor Wilhelm Conrad Roentgen, director of the Physical Institute of the University of Wurzburg, on a Friday evening, November 8, 1895, was repeating the experiments of Heinrich Rudolf Hertz and Phillipp Lenard on cathode rays. In the darkened room, he suddenly observed a bright fluorescence of some crystals lying on the table some distance away from the tube. Stimulated by this observation, he carried out an intensive investigation, the results of which were embodied in a brief paper, "On a New Kind of Rays," submitted for publication on December 28, 1895. This report, which mentioned the first photograph of the bones of a living hand, was published in the annals of the Physical Medical Society of Wurzburg during the first week of 1896.[1] Its appearance set off a chain of events that has affected all mankind. Public reaction to the discovery was instantaneous, and its practical applications in medicine were recognized immediately by doctors and laymen alike. The *Frankfurter Zeitung* for Tuesday, January 7, 1896, carried the following note:

At the present time, we wish only to call attention to the importance this discovery would have in the diagnosis of disease and injuries of the bones, if the process can be developed technically so that not only the human hand can be photographed, but the details of other bones may be shown without the flesh. The surgeon then could determine the extent of a complicated bone fracture without the manual examination which is so painful to the patient; he could find the position of a foreign body, such as a bullet or piece of shell, much more easily than has been possible heretofore and without any painful examinations with a probe. Such photographs also would be extremely valuable in diagnosing bone dis-

eases which do not originate from an injury and would help to guide the way in therapy.[2]

The dissemination of information about the new rays proceeded with such speed that when a translation of Roentgen's article appeared in the February 14, 1896 issue of *Science*, it was accompanied by notes and reproductions of X-ray photographs made by M. I. Pupin of Columbia College, Edwin B. Frost of Dartmouth College, and Arthur W. Goodspeed of the University of Pennsylvania.[3] In 1896 alone, 995 scientific books and articles dealing with X rays were published in the world's scientific literature, as well as countless newspaper and magazine articles directed at the public.[4] How did this come about?

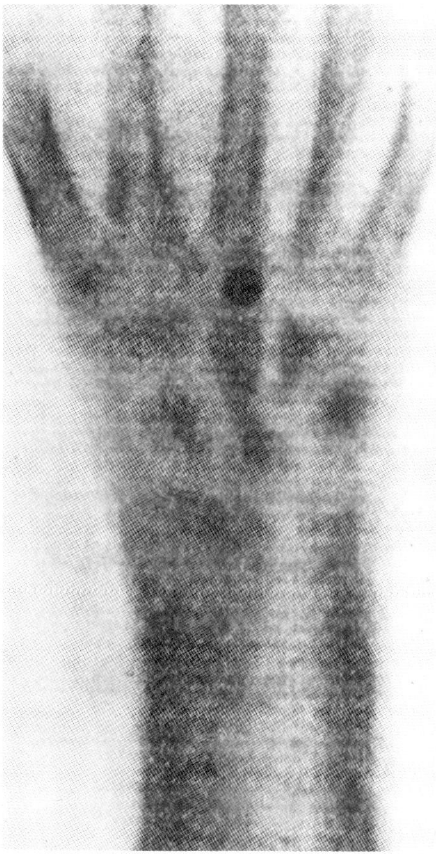

Figure 10.1 An X ray of the wrist of a twelve-year-old boy showing a bullet. This is the earliest clinical X ray published, only months after Roentgen's discovery of X rays. From R. Jones and O. Lodge, "The Discovery of a Bullet Lost in the Wrist by Means of the Roentgen Rays," *Lancet* 1(February 22, 1896): 476–77.

Roentgen's original publication was a model of scientific exposition. It contained a complete description of the equipment and methods employed. It was rapidly translated into many languages and was published in scientific journals throughout the world. The equipment needed to reproduce his experiments was available in every physical laboratory. As a result, any investigator could demonstrate the action of X rays simply by following Roentgen's directions. However, Roentgen took no part in the ensuing race to develop practical applications for his discovery, although he used his apparatus to take an occasional photograph for his medical colleagues.[5]

The first newspaper account of Roentgen's discovery to appear in Britain was published in the London *Standard* on Tuesday, January 7, 1896. Robert Jones may have learned about the new rays even sooner through the good offices of Mrs. Wimpfheimer, a volunteer worker in his Sunday charity clinic, who called his attention to the earlier report in the *Frankfurter Zeitung*.[6] In any event, Jones and a colleague, Oliver Lodge, a professor of physics, University College, Liverpool, soon built a working X-ray apparatus. In the *Lancet* for February 22, 1896, less than two months after Roentgen's announcement, Jones and Lodge published a brief note, "The Discovery of a Bullet Lost in the Wrist by Means of the Roentgen Ray."[7] The patient was a twelve-year-old boy who had been shot in the wrist. The bullet was located by X ray, but it was a time-consuming process: "rather more than two hours exposure was given" (figure 10.1)! This paper fulfills all of the criteria for the first published case in which X rays were used in the diagnosis of a medical problem.[8]

Robert Jones (1857–1933) (figure 10.2) was born in Wales. After finishing his medical education in Edinburgh he began a surgical practice in Liverpool, where he was closely associated with his uncle, Hugh Owen Thomas. Very early in his career, he developed a special interest in orthopedic problems and in the treatment of fractures. His administrative abilities were tested in his position as the surgeon to the workers who constructed the Manchester Ship Canal. This experience later helped him through the difficult days of World War I, when he was in charge of the orthopedic service for the British

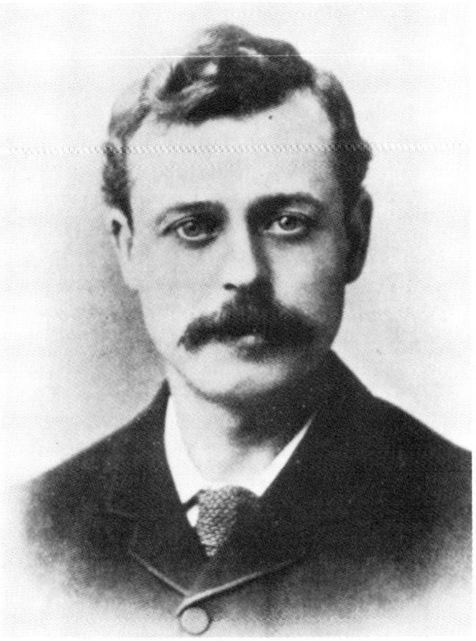

Figure 10.2 Robert Jones (1857–1933) as a young man. From F. Watson, *The Life of Sir Robert Jones* (London: Hodder & Stoughton, 1934).

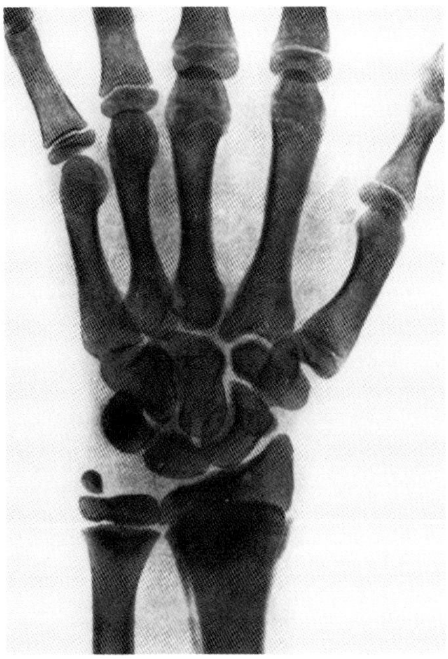

Figure 10.3 A skiagram taken in the fourth week after separation and displacement backwards of the lower epiphysis of the radius, with fracture of the styloid process of the ulna. From John Poland, *The Epiphyses: With a Skiagraphic Atlas Showing the Development of the Bones of the Wrist and Hand; with 19 Skiagrams* (London: Smith, Elder & Co. 1898).

army. His association with orthopedists from the United States before, during, and after the war made him an influential figure. "As a teacher he was preeminent, not in the role of didactic pedagogue, but in the role of a leader able to enthuse men, and through them he advanced the art and science of his specialty."[9] Jones continued to be an advocate of the use of X rays all his life, and was one of the founders of the specialty of radiology in Britain.[10] Of particular interest is his description of the fracture of the base of the fifth metatarsal, which has become known as Jones's fracture.[11] It occurred in his own foot and was the first eponymic fracture to be defined by X ray.[12] Shortly before his death, Jones had this to say about the value of the X ray in medical practice:

> *Radiography here, as in all branches of medicine, is an essential aid to diagnosis. No matter how experienced we may be, we cannot afford to dispense with it, even in the apparently simple and obvious case. Not only should we insist upon procuring a film, but it is equally important that we should welcome the radiologist's reading of it. Some surgeons resent this and say, "Give me the film so that I can read it for myself," but this is an arrogant and stupid attitude, and not to the patient's advantage.*[13]

Other early exponents of the use of X rays for diagnostic purposes were John Poland, whose monumental work on epiphyseal injuries was accompanied by an atlas of X rays showing the bones of the wrist and hand (figure 10.3), and Sidney Rowland, who suggested that X rays of the wrist in children might be used to establish their age.[14] In France, Gabriel Maunoury wrote about the use of X rays in the diagnosis and treatment of fractures.[15]

The first serious investigation of the possible value of X rays in diagnosis was carried out by the Prussian War Ministry. On February 4, 1896, it was announced that a systematic study of the anatomical and pathological preparations in the pathological museum was being carried out to determine if fractures and metallic foreign bodies could be discovered by this method.[16] The results were published later in the year.[17]

In April 1896, the British Army Medical Department, having concluded that the value of X rays was undisputed, took steps to supply an expedition into the Egyptian Sudan with X-ray equipment for use in the field.[18] Two complete sets of apparatus were sent up the Nile, where they were used to localize foreign bodies and to diagnose fractures. A report on the value of X rays in localizing bullets appeared in May 1896 from an Italian military hospital in Naples engaged in treating soldiers wounded in Ethiopia.[19] The Greco-Turkish War of 1897 provided another convenient testing ground. The soldiers on both sides were treated by Red Cross medical units supplied with X-ray apparatus. In their reports, both the British unit with the Greek Army and the German unit with the Turkish Army emphasized the value of X rays in the diagnosis of fractures and gunshot wounds.[20] It was felt that X-ray facilities should be available in the first medical units at which wounds could be examined and treated properly. Arthur Kuttner's conclusion was that "we possess a new aid in the x-ray which is so valuable that the wounded have a right to have it employed in their care."[21]

The medical department of the U.S. Army was not slow in adopting the use of X rays. During the war with Spain in 1898, seventeen X-ray units were in use in general hospitals and on hospital ships. A complete report of the accumulated experience was published in 1900.[22] It was profusely illustrated and showed the value of X rays in diagnosing fractures, demonstrating their form, the amount of comminution, foreign bodies, and other information that could not have been demonstrated easily by previously available techniques. The army had its martyrs to this new science. Elizabeth Fleischmann Ascheim was a pioneer in the use of X rays at the Presidio Division Hospital in San Francisco, now Letterman General Hospital. Working without protection she fell victim to cancer, as did Lt. Col. Eugene Garland Northington.[23]

The use of X rays in the study of fractures and gunshot wounds led to an abrupt change in the methods of treating these injuries. The technique of localizing metallic foreign bodies was rapidly perfected. The number, size, and distribution of metal fragments and comminuted pieces of bone could be determined with ease and accuracy. The probe, the tool of the military surgeon for centuries, was abandoned. It was soon recognized that all metallic foreign bodies could not be removed without the added trauma of an extensive exploration of the wound, and that it was not always necessary to remove all of these fragments to obtain healing. A large amount of meddlesome surgery could be avoided.

The discovery of X rays stirred wide public interest. The appeal of the new technique was not limited to physicians. Photographers, charlatans, and "electricians" seized upon it and proceeded to exploit it, each to his own ends. Public interest was expressed in cartoons, humorous verse, and advertisements for such products as X-ray proof garments to preserve feminine modesty. Shoe stores featured X-ray photographs of feet cramped in poorly fitted shoes and X-ray machines for fitting shoes were soon put on the market. Thomas A. Edison gave a public demonstration of X rays in New York City during March 1896. Visitors were allowed to view their hands and arms under a flouroscope, and the exhibit proved to be a great attraction. Such extensive publicity resulted in a demand for X-ray services on the part of patients. Physicians were subjected to inexorable pressures by their patients to purchase the necessary equipment, and as a result they began, willy-nilly, using X-ray photographs as a regular part of their armamentarium.

Patients with fractures old and new sought to have their injuries photographed by the new process. Because the taking of X-ray photographs was not limited to physicians, independent studios advertised and catered to the curious and disgruntled. The inevitable result was a rash of suits for malpractice against physicians. The situation was aggravated not only by faulty technique, which frequently distorted the photographs, but also by errors of interpretation due to inexperience. In April 1896, the Court of the Queen's Bench in Montreal was the first court to admit X-ray evidence of injury.[24] Courts in England and France quickly followed suit.[25] In the United States, an eastern judge refused to accept X-ray photographs as evidence, ruling that, "there is no proof that such a thing is possible. It is like offering the photograph of a ghost."[26] A Denver judge took a different tack. In a suit filed against a surgeon on April 14, 1896, Judge Owen LeFevre handed down the following opinion regarding four X-ray photographs entered as exhibits:

> *The defendant's counsel objected to the admission of evidence of exhibits, the same being photographs produced by means of the x-ray process, on the ground that, being photographs of an object unseen by the human eye, there is no evidence that the photograph accurately portrays and represents the object so photographed. This rule of law is well settled by a long line of authorities and we do not dissent therefrom as applied to photographs which may be seen by the human eye. The reason for this salutory rule is so apparent to the profession that as a rule of evidence we will not discuss it. We, however, have been presented with a photograph taken by means of a new scientific discovery, the same being acknowledged in the arts and in science. It knocks for admission at the temple of learning; what shall we do or say? Close fast the doors or open wide the portals?*
>
> *These photographs are offered in evidence to show the present condition of the head and neck of the femur bone, which is entirely hidden from the eye of the surgeon. Nature has surrounded it with tissues for its protection and there it is hidden; it cannot, by any possibility, be removed nor exposed that it may be compared with its shadow as developed by means of this new scientific process. In addition to these exhibits in evidence, we have nothing to do or say as to what they purport to represent; that will, without doubt, be explained by eminent surgeons. These exhibits are only pictures or maps to be used in explanation of a present condition, and therefore, are secondary evidence, and not primary. They may be shown to the jury as illustrating or making clear the testimony of experts.*[27]

Since that time, juries have been impressed upon countless occasions by X-ray photographs of fractures, seeing with their own eyes if the bones were crooked or straight. The threat of legal action for malpractice based on such evidence furnished, perhaps, the most potent stimulus for the rapid adoption of the routine use of X-rays in the treatment of fractures.

As is the case with all innovations in medical practice, the exploitation of Roentgen's discovery was enthusiastically espoused by some physicians, observed skeptically or ignored by many, and actively opposed by a few. One of the most enthusiastic supporters was Henry W. Cattell of the University of Pennsylvania, who as early as March 6, 1896, wrote:

> *The manifold uses to which Röntgen's discovery may be applied in medicine are so obvious that it is even now questionable whether a surgeon would be morally justified in performing a certain class of operation without having first seen pictured by these rays, the field of his work, a map, as it were, of the unknown country he is to explore.*[28]

A Boston physician later in the same year expressed the opinion that no well-equipped hospital in the land could do justice to its patients unless it possessed a complete X-ray apparatus.[29] Similar opinions were echoed from Baltimore and St. Louis and seemed to represent an attitude that developed spontaneously throughout the country.[30]

The voice of skepticism was raised in a leading editorial in the *Medical News*, February 22, 1896:

> *As far as our present knowledge goes, the positive advantages to medicine seem to be limited to three conditions; fractures, dislocations and tumors of bones, encysted bullets, needles or pieces of glass in the tissues, and earthy calculi. In the first class of conditions, its advantages would appear to be slight unless great advances upon present powers and methods can be made. The Tactus eruditus is certainly a delicate and reliable sense in investigating fractures and dislocations, and it is questionable how much help can be obtained by such blurred shadow pictures as can at present be obtained. In recent cases of fracture or dislocation, the delay and discomfort to the patient necessarily involved in the application of the method would be practically an insuperable objection to its use for purposes of diagnosis. . . .*[31]

This opinion as to the practical value of X rays resulted from high expectations and the failures and disappointments that necessarily attended the development of the new technique. An example was the long exposure times required to produce adequate contrast; in 1907, exposure times were five to ten seconds for the upper extremity, fifteen to twenty seconds for the lower, and twenty to thirty seconds for the shoulder and chest.[32] A. L. McCosh gave a resume in July 1896 of the recent progress in the treatment of fractures that omitted all mention of the use of X rays.[33] The following year, 1897, David W. Cheever in his Shattuck Lecture entitled "The New Surgery" hailed the advent of a great new epoch as a result of the development of anesthesia and antiseptic surgery, with no mention of Roentgen's discovery.[34] Bigelow's famous book, *The Mechanism of Dislocations and Fracture of the Hip*, was reprinted in 1900 without the addition of a single X-ray photograph of these conditions, an addition that would have been of inestimable value.[35] The following note from a review of the third edition of Stimson's *A Practical Treatise on Fractures and Dislocations* (1901) illustrates the inertia characteristic of many authorities: "The plates added include a number of very interesting skiagrams, although the author rarely receives information of practical importance from the x-ray in fractures which could not be obtained by other means."[36]

This attitude was reflected in the report of the Committee of the American Surgical Association on the medico-legal relations of the X rays in 1900. This most interesting document consists largely of complaints by members who have been sued for malpractice on the basis of X-ray evidence. It concludes: "The routine employment of the x-ray in cases of fractures is not at present of sufficient advantage to justify the teaching that it should be used in every case."[37] The position of the association was not reversed officially for thirteen years, when its committee on fractures recommended the routine use of X rays in all cases of fractures and dislocations.[38]

The first ten years following the discovery of X rays were a time of trial and error. But the incidence of burns, epilation, misinterpretation, and technical failure could not obscure the real value of the method. The use of X rays stimulated the improvement of equipment and a greater understanding of both the normal and anomalous anatomy as seen on the X-ray photograph. John Poland's book on the epiphyses, published in 1898, was accompanied by an atlas of skiagrams showing the development of the bones of the wrist and the hand, prepared by his friend William Webster.[39] The work of Robert Kienbock, Etienne Destot, and Thomas Dwight helped to define the differences between the normal, the anomalous, and the pathological anatomy as seen on the X ray.[40] The value of X rays in the treatment of fractures at the end of this period was summarized in this way by David Walsh:

> *To sum up: in dealing with bone injuries successful radiography, compared with previous methods, offers the following advantages. It substitutes speed, accuracy, and finality for delay and doubt; it affords exact evidence that may confirm or modify the diagnosis of the surgeon; it may furnish both grounds for prognosis and hints for treatment; it may save the patient the pain of useless and perhaps dangerous manipulations, as well as the risk of anesthetics; it provides a permanent record of the precise nature of the injury; it may prove a safeguard for the patient and for his medical attendant, both in the present and the future, and lastly has a special value for teaching purposes.*[41]

Walsh's last comment was particularly perceptive, for the introduction of the use of X rays in the diagnosis and treatment of fractures wrought a fundamental change in the method of teaching students how to care for these injuries. Previously, the student was fortunate

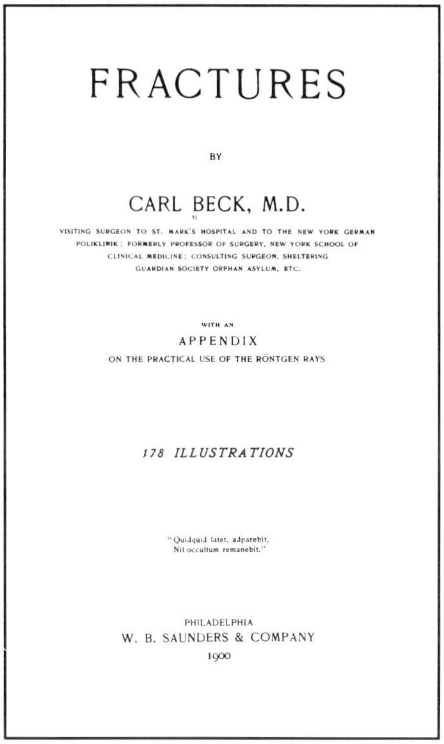

FRACTURES

BY

CARL BECK, M.D.

VISITING SURGEON TO ST. MARK'S HOSPITAL AND TO THE NEW YORK GERMAN POLIKLINIK; FORMERLY PROFESSOR OF SURGERY, NEW YORK SCHOOL OF CLINICAL MEDICINE; CONSULTING SURGEON, SHELTERING GUARDIAN SOCIETY ORPHAN ASYLUM, ETC.

WITH AN

APPENDIX

ON THE PRACTICAL USE OF THE RÖNTGEN RAYS

178 ILLUSTRATIONS

"Quidquid latet, adparebit,
Nil occultum remanebit."

PHILADELPHIA
W. B. SAUNDERS & COMPANY
1900

Figure 10.4 Beck's book on fractures was dedicated to Wilhelm Conrad Roentgen.

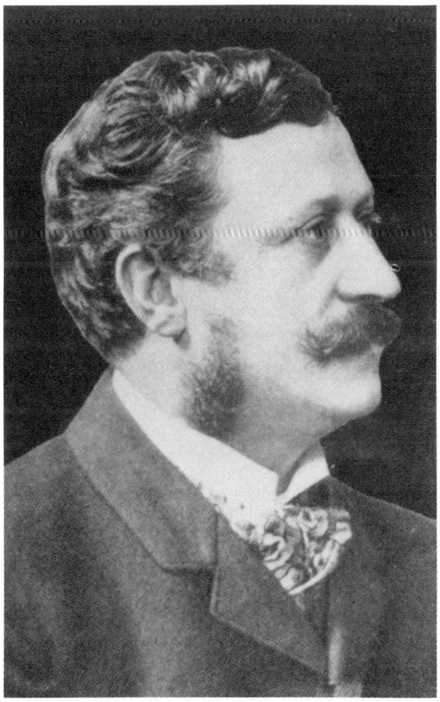

Figure 10.5 Carl Beck (1856-1911)

if he could follow a few patients with fractures from the time of the accident until healing occurred. He was forced to rely on the description of the clinical examination at various stages to provide a picture of the course of events during this period. X-ray photographs provided a permanent record of the patient's condition. They could be shown to students at any stage of treatment. Didactic diagrams of typical fractures could be discarded in favor of X-ray photographs of real fractures. This development greatly improved the clinical atmosphere of the lecture room. The opportunity of observing the rarer varieties of fractures and dislocations became available to all, since the X-ray photographs of these cases were preserved. The clinical X-ray conference became a most important feature of any program for teaching the treatment of fractures.

The need for new textbooks incorporating information about fractures gained by the use of X rays was expressed as early as 1897:

> *We were certainly justified in supposing that our knowledge of fractures had nearly reached its limit; but the Roentgen rays have opened up new fields for investigation, and we find that there is still much to learn. . . . A complete new set of data must now be accumulated and reviewed.*[42]

Eugene R. Corson remarked, "There will have to be a new treatise on fractures and dislocations, based upon the x-ray. There are many surprises in store, many surgical bugaboos will go, and many revelations will simplify much which is still obscure."[43]

In 1900, Carl Beck published his book *Fractures; With an Appendix on the Practical Use of the Röntgen Rays.* It was dedicated to "Wilhelm Conrad Röntgen, without whose discovery much of this book could not have been written."[44] This was the first book on the diagnosis and treatment of fractures based upon the routine use of X rays and is the prototype of all of our standard textbooks on fractures (figure 10.4).

Carl Beck (1856–1911) (figure 10.5) was born in Germany and educated at the University of Heidelberg. He emigrated to the United States in 1882 and became one of the best known of the German-American surgeons in New York City. He had a special interest in X rays, spent some time with Roentgen learning about them, and among other accomplishments, was the first to visualize gall stones on an X ray. An important part of his book is an appendix entitled "The Practical Use of the Röntgen Rays," which describes the technical details of taking and developing the plates. The work also discusses at length all of the problems of arriving at an accurate diagnosis, particularly emphasizing anomalous bones that can be mistaken for fracture fragments. The quality of the pictures that he obtained was surprisingly good (figure 10.6).

Technical factors are all important in the successful use of X rays for the diagnosis and treatment of fractures. At first, only one view was taken, usually in the anterior-posterior projection. It was quickly recognized that this was not sufficient. Ernest Amory Codman, a pioneer in radiology in the United States, emphasized that two or more views must be taken.[45] Special views were introduced for the visualization of particular anatomical areas. It is well accepted now that "one view is no view and two may not be enough."[46] Stephen Bronson Dewing has described the evolution of the X ray from glass plates to cellulose nitrate films and later to cellulose acetate "safety" films. The change to safety film was accelerated by the fire in the X-ray section of the Cleveland Clinic in 1929, which resulted in the deaths of 125 people.[47] Dewing also discussed the introduction of intensifying screens, grids, and high vacuum tubes with reliable high-voltage energy sources that have gradually increased the capability of X rays to penetrate the thicker portions of the body with continually shorter exposures.

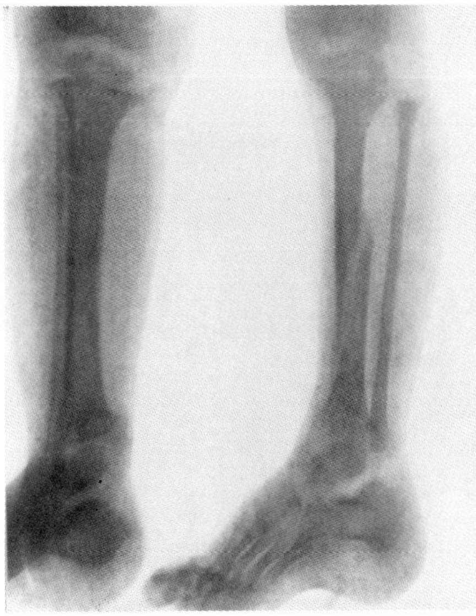

Figure 10.6 An example of the quality of the X rays obtained by Beck. From Beck, *Fractures: With an Appendix on the Practical Use of the Roentgen Rays* (Philadelphia: W. B. Saunders, 1900).

It was not long after the introduction of X rays into medical practice that a new species of physician-specialist arose, the radiologists, and they began to contribute their observations to medical literature. One of these was Edward W. H. Shenton (1872-1955). After fourteen years of experience with X rays at Guy's Hospital, Shenton published a book in 1911, *Disease in Bone and Its Detection by the X-rays*, in which he described what has come to be known as "Shenton's line" (figure 10.7).

> *This line in all positions of the joint, i.e. abduction, adduction, etc., of the femur, is the same, an unbroken arch formed by the top of the obturator foramen, and the inner side of the femoral neck. Immagination must connect these two lines before a perfect arch is formed, but a glance at Figure 28 will show that this line is a reality and not solely immaginative. There are many lesions of the hip joint which will disturb this line. Congenital dislocation is a good example.*[48]

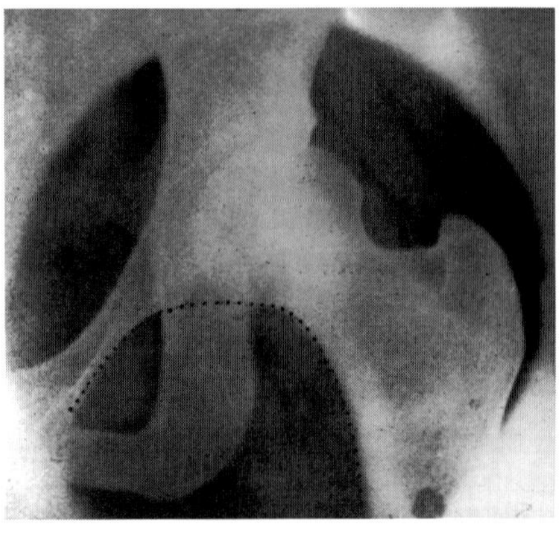

Figure 10.7 Shenton's line. From E. W. H. Shenton, *Disease in Bone and Its Detection by X-rays* (London: Macmillan, 1911), 42.

This is just one of many examples of the early contributions of radiologists to the diagnosis of fractures.

The fluoroscope, so named by Thomas A. Edison, has remained virtually unchanged since Roentgen first detected the "new rays" on such a screen. Its ubiquity, low cost, and ease of operation encouraged physicians and surgeons to use it extensively in the diagnosis and treatment of fractures. Before the introduction of the X ray, the surgeon examined the fracture "through a glass darkly," and the diagnosis often remained obscure, the reduction incomplete, and the entire procedure undocumented. Easy access to the fluoroscope led to its abuse with excessive doses of radiation being absorbed by patients, and especially by the operators, often with tragic results. The use of fluoroscopy in the operating room could be very cumbersome (figure 10.8). Great efforts were made to improve the quality of the images seen on the fluoroscope. As early as 1942, W. Edward Chamberlain, on the basis of his observation of the techniques of electron microscopy and television, predicted their use in enhancing

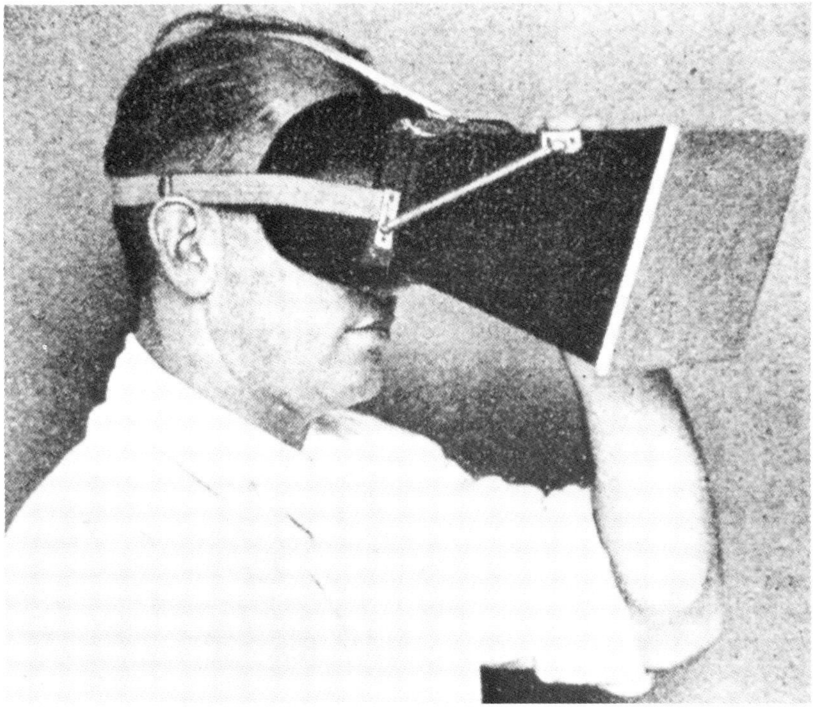

Figure 10.8 A head-mounted flouroscopic screen for intraoperative viewing. From Lorenz Böhler, *Technik der Knochenbruchbehandlung im Frieden und im Kriege*, (Vienna: W. Maudrich, 1943), 3:1669.

fluoroscopic images.[49] The developments of the next two decades, including image intensification tubes, wide-angle optical image amplifiers, and television applications, improved the quality of X-ray images immensely while reducing the levels of radiation exposure required; these advances also eliminated the use of fluoroscopy in most operating rooms, but the use of the fluorscope in the treatment of fractures persists in many parts of the world. The development of computerized tomography by Sir Godfrey Newbold Hounsfield and A. M. Cormack has added yet another dimension to our diagnostic capabilities and has proven very useful in the diagnosis and understanding of obscure fractures and bony injuries.[50]

The impact of Roentgen's discovery on the treatment of fractures has thus been enormous. Continuing technical innovations are enabling surgeons to gather increasing amounts of information about the injuries they are called upon to treat. It is doubtful, however, if ever again we will see such an explosion of public and professional interest compressed into such a short period as that which immediately followed the introduction of the use of X rays in the treatment of fractures.

Notes

1. Wilhelm C. Roentgen, "Ueber eine neue Art von Strahlen," *Sber phys-med Ges Würz*, 1895, 132–41.

2. Otto Glasser, *Wilhelm Conrad Roentgen and the Early History of the Roentgen Rays* (Springfield, Ill.: Charles C Thomas, 1934).

3. Roentgen, "On a New Kind of Rays," *Science* 3(1896): 227–37.

4. Glasser, *Wilhelm Conrad Röntgen und die Geschichte der Röntgenstrahlen* (Berlin: Julius Springer, 1931), 298–337.

5. Fessler, "Radiousfraktur, nach Prof. Roentgen photographiert," *Münch med Wschr* 43(1896): 201–2.

6. David Walsh, *The Roentgen Rays in Medical Work*, 4th edition, New York: William Wood, 1907).

7. Robert Jones and Oliver Lodge, "The Discovery of a Bullet Lost in the Wrist by Means of the Roentgen Rays," *Lancet* 1(February 22, 1896): 476–77.

8. Charles G. Roland, "Priority of Clinical X-Ray Reports: A Classic Dethroned," *Can J Surg* 5(1962): 247–51.

9. M. S. Henderson, "Sir Robert Jones," obituary, *SGO* 57(1933): 120.

10. C. T. Holland, "Sir Robert Jones," obituary, *Brit J Radiol* 6(1933): 116.

11. Jones, "Fracture of the Fifth Metatarsal Bone, " *Liverpool Med-Chir J* 22(1902): 103–7; id., "Fracture of the Base of the Fifth Metatarsal Bone by Indirect Violence," *Ann Surg* 35(1902): 697–700.

12. Leonard F. Peltier, "Eponymic Fractures: Robert Jones and Jones's Fracture," *Surgery* 71(1972): 522–26.

13. Jones, "Manipulation as a Therapeutic Measure," *Proc Roy Soc Med* 25(1931–32): 1405.

14. John Poland, *The Epiphyses: With a Skiagraphic Atlas Showing the Development of the Bones of the Wrist and Hand, with 19 Skiagrams* (London: Smith, Elder, 1898); Sidney Rowland, *A Series of Collotype Illustrations with Descriptive Text, Illustrating Applications of the New Photography to Medicine and Surgery* (London: Rebman, 1896).

15. Gabriel Maunoury, "De la radiographie dans l'étude des fractures," in Congrès International de Médicine XIII, *Comptes rendues, Section de chirurgie générale* ([Paris]: 1900), 329–47.

16. "News Brief," *Münch med Wschr* 43(1896): 114.

17. "Versuche zur Festellung der Verwertbarkeit Roentgen'scher Strahlen für medicinische-chirurgische Zwecke," *Veröff Geb Milit-Sanitwes* 10(1896): 1–45.

18. "The Value of the New Photography in Military Surgery," *Brit Med J* 1(1896): 1059.

19. "News Brief," *Münch med Wschr* 43(1896): 114.

20. F. C. Abbott, "Surgery in the Graeco-Turkish War (1897)," *Lancet* 1(1899): 80, 152–56.

21. Arthur Kuttner, "Ueber die Bedeutung der Roentgenstrahlung für die Kriegs-chirurgie," *Bruns Beitr klin Chir* 20(1898): 167–230.

22. W. C. Borden, *The Use of the Roentgen Ray by the Medical Department of the U.S. Army in the War with Spain (1898)* (Washington, D.C.: Government Printing Office, 1900).

23. Holland, "Roentgenology," *Science* 97(1943): 2518.

24. "Roentgen Rays in Court," *Med Record (NY)* 49(April 4, 1896): 491.

25. "The New Photography in Court," *Literary Digest* 12(April 11, 1896): 707; "The Roentgen Rays in the Witness Box," *JAMA* 27(1896): 168.

26. Sanford Withers, "The Story of the First Roentgen Evidence," *Radiology* 17(1931): 99-101.

27. Ibid.

28. H. W. Cattell, "Application of the X-Rays to Surgery," *Science* 3(1896): 344–46.

29. Eugene R. Corson, "Some Observations on Colles' Fracture by the Aid of the X-Ray," *Med Record (NY)* 51(1897): 649–53.

30. A. V. L. Brokaw, "An Exhibition of Radiographs with Remarks," *Trans South Surg Assoc* 10(1898): 80; H. Helferich, *Atlas and Epitome of Traumatic Fractures and Dislocations*, 5th edition, ed. Joseph Bloodgood (Philadelphia: W. B. Saunders, 1902), 5–6.

31. Editorial, "Possibilities of the X-rays in Surgery," *Literary Digest* 12(1896): 554.

32. Walsh, *Roentgen Rays in Medical Work.*

33. A. L. McCosh, "Resume of Recent Progress in Surgery: The Treatment of Fractures," *Medical News* 69(1896): 46–48.

34. D. W. Cheever, "The New Surgery," *Med Comms Mass Med Soc* 17(1897): 373–87.

35. H. J. Bigelow, *The Mechanism of Dislocations and Fracture of the Hip* (Boston: Little Brown, 1900).

36. Book Review, "A Practical Treatise on Fractures and Dislocations by Lewis A. Stimson, 3d edition," *Ann Surg* 34(1901): 719.

37. "Report of the Committee of the American Surgical Association on the Medico-Legal Relations of the X-Rays," *Trans Am Surg Assoc* 18(1900): 429–61.

38. *Reports of the Committee of the American Surgical Association on the Treatment of Fractures for 1913, 1914, 1915, 1916, 1917, 1918, and 1921* (American Surgical Association).

39. Poland, *The Epiphyses.*

40. Robert Kienbock, "Über traumatische Malazie des Mondbeins und ihre Folgezustande: Entartungsformen und Kompressionfrakturen," *Fortschr Geb Röntgenstr* 16(1910): 78–103; Etienne Destot, *Le poignet et les accidents du travail: Etude radiographique et clinique* (Paris: Vitot, 1905); id., *Traumatismes du pied et rayons X* (Paris: Masson, 1911); Thomas Dwight, *Variations of the Bones of the Hands and Feet* (Philadelphia: J. B. Lippincott, 1907).

41. Walsh, *Roentgen Rays in Medical Work.*

42. Leonard Freeman, "Some Fractures of the Lower End of the Radius as Seen by the Roentgen Ray," *Ann Surg* 25(1897): 470–74.

43. Corson, "Some Observations on Colles' Fracture," 649–53.

44. Carl Beck, *Fractures: With an Appendix on the Practical Use of the Roentgen Rays* (Philadelphia: W. B. Saunders, 1900).

45. Ernest Amory Codman, "The Roentgen Ray and Its Relation to Fractures," in Charles Locke Scudder, *The Treatment of Fractures* (Philadelphia: W. B. Saunders, 1900).

46. K. F. Lee, letter to the author, 30 August, 1985.

47. Stephen Bronson Dewing, *Modern Radiography in Historical Perspective* (Springfield, Ill.: Charles C Thomas, 1962), 75–76.

48. Edward W. H. Shenton, *Disease in Bone and Its Detection by the X-Rays* (London: Macmillan, 1911), 42.

49. W. Edward Chamberlain, "Fluoroscopes and Fluoroscopy," *Radiology* 38(1942): 383–413.

50. Sir Godfrey Newbold Hounsfield, "A Method of an Apparatus for Examination of the Body by Radiation such as X- or Gamma-Radiation," United Kingdom Patent No. 1283915 (1972).

APPENDIX A

Anesthesia for the Treatment of Fractures and Dislocations

THE CHIEF OBSTACLE to the reduction of fractures and dislocations is the reaction of the surrounding muscles, which contract vigorously and exhibit a persisting protective spasm. Although Suśruta is said to have used henbane (*Hyoscyamus niger*) and Indian hemp (*Cannabis sativa indica*), and Theodoric a soporofic sponge to promote analgesia and muscle relaxation, ethanol was probably the most readily available agent, with intoxication being present at the time of injury or speedily induced in anticipation of the ordeal.[1] Cooper and Physick induced fainting by copious phlebotomy, often with the patient in an upright position, immersing the patient in a warm bath, and the administration of an emetic.[2] Rendered weak by this onslaught, the patient could hardly resist the manipulations of his surgeon. With the introduction of subcutaneous tenotomy and myotomy, the resisting muscles and/or their tendons were divided to aid in the reduction of fractures and dislocations, especially if treatment had been delayed.[3]

The induction of a general anesthesia using ether or chloroform carried with it a substantial risk, because a useful degree of muscular relaxation required a deep level of anesthesia. For this reason, techniques utilizing local and hematoma blocks were welcomed. In 1885, John R. Conway of Bellevue Hospital in New York described the use of hematoma blocks of a 4 percent cocaine solution for the reduction of fractures of the distal radius and a dislocated elbow.[4] The use of hematoma blocks, usually with 1 percent solutions of cocaine became widespread.[5] Cocaine was replaced by procaine in 1926.[6]

In 1908, August Bier (1861–1949), who had administered the first spinal anesthetic to a human ten years before, introduced his method of intravenous regional anesthesia using cocaine.[7] Joseph Ransohoff described an intra-arterial method of regional anesthesia two years later.[8] Because cocaine and later procaine were not suitable for this type of block, the method was neglected. In 1963, it was revived by C. McK. Holmes, who used lidocaine, a more effective agent.[9] As a result, "Bier blocks" for regional anesthesia for the treatment of fractures, particularly in the upper extremity, are widely used.

Notes

1. Ralph H. Major, *A History of Medicine* (Springfield, Ill.: Charles C. Thomas, 1954), 1:72; Theodoric, *The Surgery of Theodoric*, trans. Eldridge Campbell and James Colton (New York: Appleton-Century-Crofts, 1960), 1:212–13.

2. Astley Cooper, "On Dislocations," in Astley Cooper and Benjamin Travers, *Surgical Essays*, 3d edition (London: Cox and Son, 1818), 1:22; J. S. Dorsey, *Elements of Surgery*, 3d edition (Philadelphia: E. Parker, 1823), 1:226.

3. Amédée Bonnet, *Traité des sections tendineuses et musculaires* (Paris: J. B. Baillière, 1841), 618–22; Johann Friedrich Dieffenbach, *Die Operative Chirurgie* (Leipzig: Brockhaus, 1845), 1:794–802; John B. Roberts, *Notes on the Modern Treatment of Fractures* (New York: D. Appleton, 1899), 20–22; Charles Locke Scudder, *The Treatment of Fractures*, 4th edition (Philadelphia: W. B. Saunders, 1904), 383.

4. John R. Conway, "Cocaine as an Anesthetic in Fractures and Dislocations," *NY Med J* 42(1885): 632–33.

5. Guido Lerda, "Die praktische Anwendung der Localanasthesie bei Frakturen," *Zentralbl Chir* 34(1907): 1417–20.

6. Ira Cohen, "Local Anesthesia in the Reduction of Fractures," *JAMA* 86(1926): 1896–97.

7. August Bier, "Ueber einen neuen Weg Localanasthesie an den Gliedmassen zu erzeugen," *Arch klin Chir* 86(1908): 1007–16; C. McK. Holmes, "The History and Development of Intravenous Regional Anesthesia," *Acta anesthesiol scand* 36(Supplement 1969): 11–18.

8. Joseph L. Ransohoff, "Terminal Arterial Anesthesia," *Ann Surg* 51(1910): 453–56.

9. Holmes, "Intravenous Regional Anesthesia," *Lancet* 1(1963): 245–47.

The Fracture Table

MECHANICAL PROBLEMS INVOLVED in the reduction of fractures and dislocations in strong, healthy young adults continue to cause difficulties for today's physicians in spite of the availability of good anesthesia and muscle relaxation. It is no wonder then that surgeons have frequently turned to various types of apparatus to multiply their strength through the use of levers, screws, and pulleys. The apparatus used by Hippocrates was quite sophisticated:

It has been formerly stated by us that it will be of importance for any person who practices medicine in a populous city to get prepared a quadrangular board, about six cubits or a little more in length, and about two cubits in breadth; a fathom will be sufficient thickness for it; and then along it from the one end to the other, an excavation must be made, so that the working of the levers may not be higher than is proper; then at both sides we are to raise short, strong, and strongly-fixed posts, having axles; and in the middle of the bench five or six long grooves are to be scooped out about four inches for them, and the depth in like manner; and although the number of grooves I have mentioned will be sufficient, there is nothing to prevent their being made all over the bench. And the bench should have in its middle a pretty deep hole, of a square shape, and of about three inches in size; and into this hole, when judged necessary, is to be adjusted a corresponding piece of wood, rounded above, which, at the proper time, is to be adjusted between the perineum and the head of the thigh-bone. This upright piece of wood prevents the body from yielding to the force dragging downward by the feet; for sometimes this piece of wood serves the purpose of counter-extension upward; and sometimes, too, when extension and counter-extension are made, this piece of wood, if susceptible of some motion to this side or that, will serve the purpose of bones, or may make pressure direct on the heads along with the extension, according as it may be suitable to push inward or

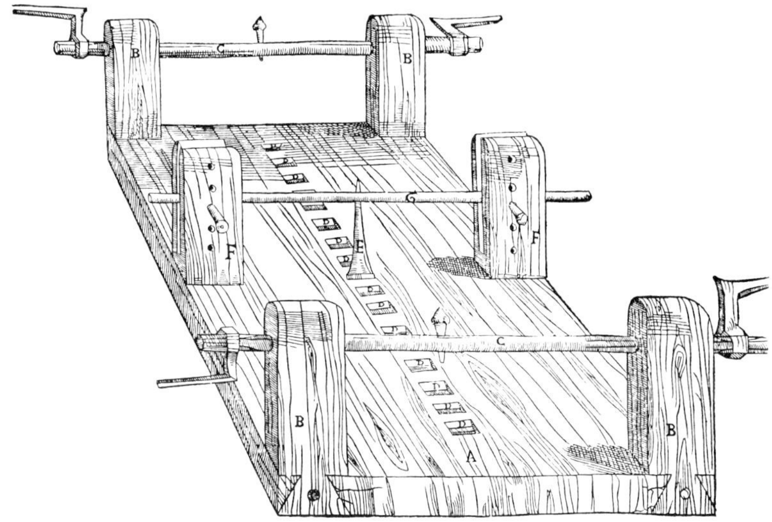

Figure B.1 The *scamnum*, or fracture table, of Hippocrates. Woodcut probably after Primaticcio. From Guido Guidi, *Chirurgia è graeco in latinum conversa* (Paris: Gaultier, 1544), 519.

outward with the lever; and the lever may be either of a round or broad form, as may be judged proper; for sometimes the one form and sometimes the other suits with the articulation. This mode of applying the lever along with extension is applicable in the reduction of all dislocations of the thigh. In the case now on hand, a round lever is proper; but in dislocations outward a flat lever will be the suitable one. By means of such machines and of such powers, it appears to me that we need never fail in reducing any dislocation at a joint.[1]

Surprisingly, we know a good deal about the fracture table used by Hippocrates (figure B.1). Passed down from antiquity in manuscript copies, the design of Hippocrates' apparatus was described and illustrated in print for the first time by Guido Guidi in 1544.[2] The table was used in many ingenious ways for the reduction of fractures and dislocations of both the upper and lower extremities as well as the back (figure B.2). In addition to the fracture table, Hippocrates described other apparatus for the reduction of dislocations of the shoulder[3] (figure B.3). The illustrations of this early fracture table excited the imagination of surgeons for centuries but did little to affect their practice. It was not until the introduction of the plaster of paris bandage and the need to support the patient during application that the modern fracture table came into being.

The modern fracture table began with a simple perineal post and sacral support that could be clamped to a sturdy table, the legs of the patient being held by assistants (figures B.4, B.5). Emphasis was on portability and convenience (figures B.6, B.7). The manual traction

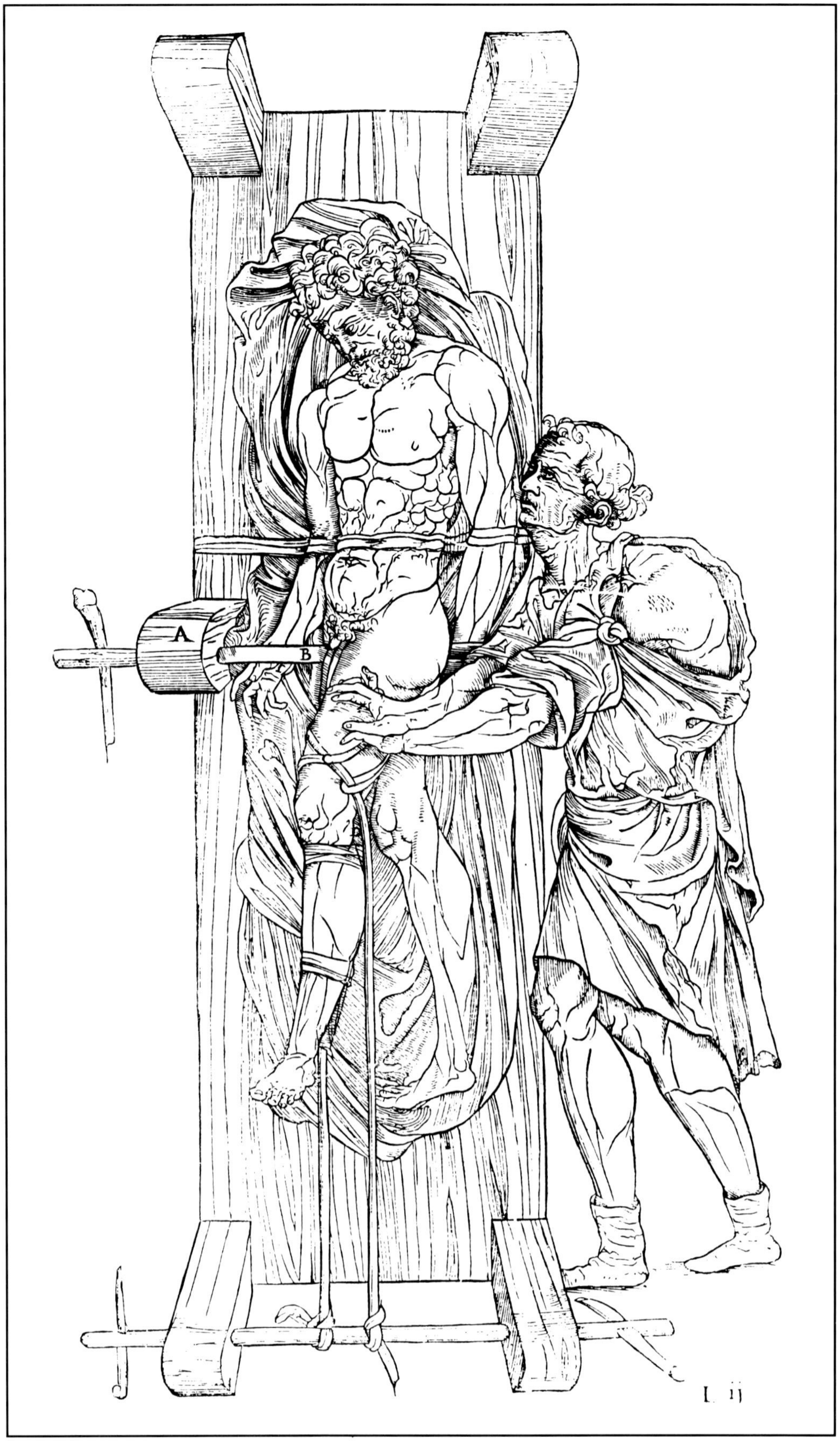

Figure B.2 The *scamnum* used to reduce a posterior dislocation of the hip. From Guidi, *Chirurgia è graeco*, 527.

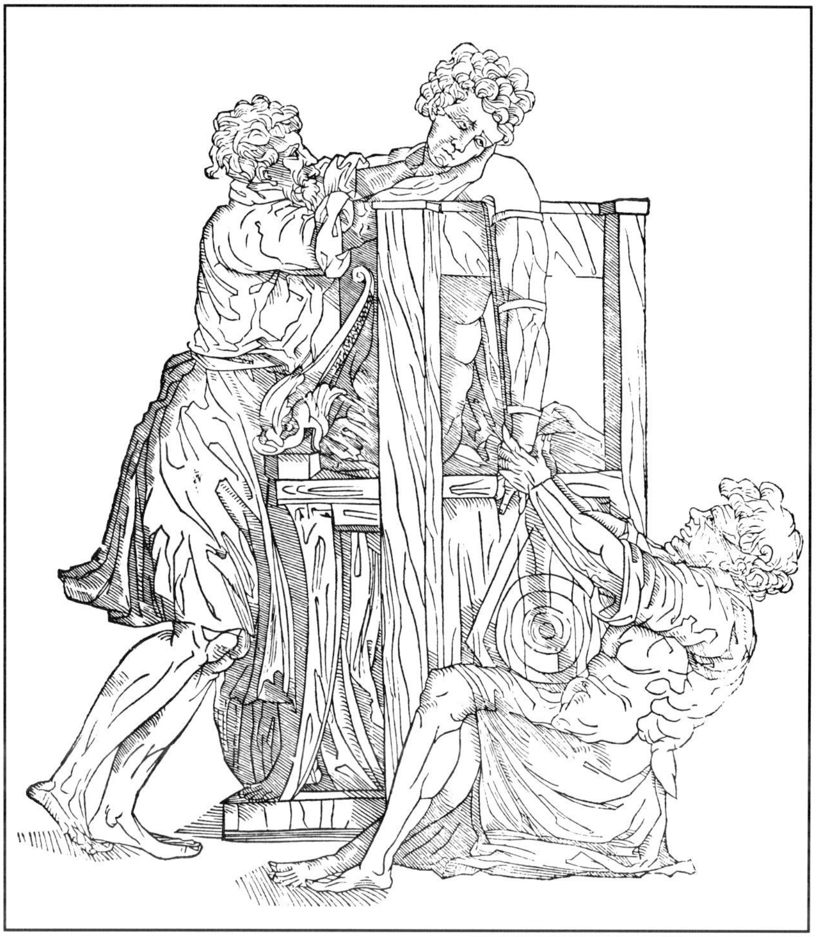

Figure B.3 The *ambe* of Hippocrates, used for reducing dislocations of the shoulder. From Guidi, *Chirurgia è graeco*, 235.

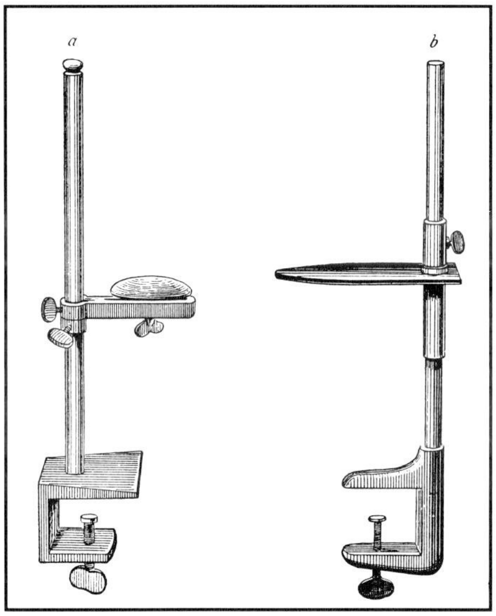

Figure B.4 Pelvic supports used in applying plaster of paris dressings for fractures of the hip and femur. From N. Senn, *Practical Surgery for the General Practictioner* (Philadelphia: W. B. Saunders, 1901), fig. 287.

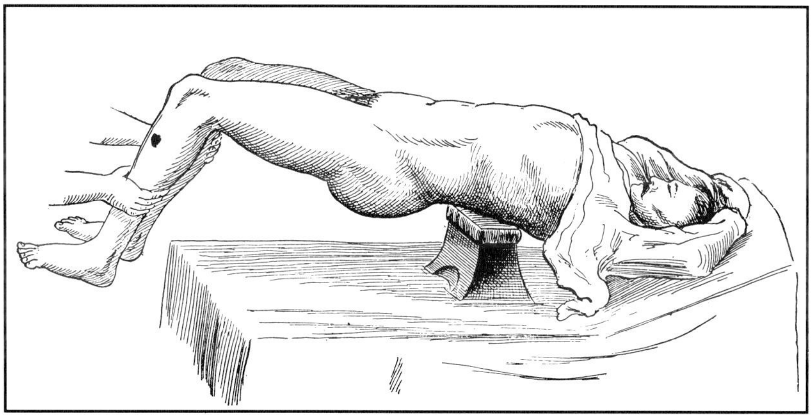

Figure B.5 Volkmann's pelvic support to be used in the application of plaster of paris dressings. From Senn, *Practical Surgery*, fig. 288.

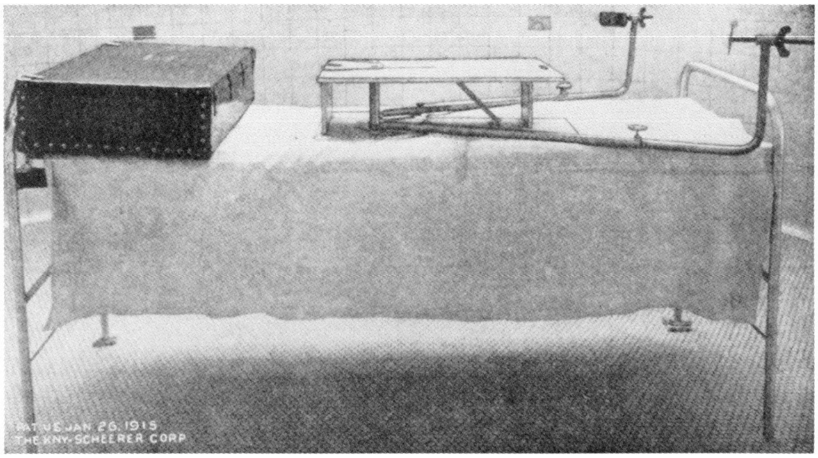

Figure B.6 A portable fracture table designed by George W. Hawley. From Charles Locke Scudder, *The Treatment of Fractures*, 10th edition (Philadelphia: W. B. Saunders, 1926), fig. 885.

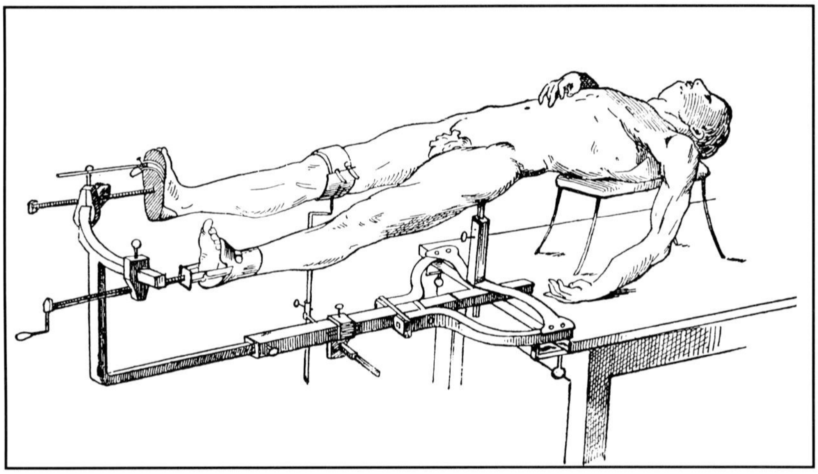

Figure B.7 Another portable fracture table. From A. Hoffa, *Lehrbuch der Orthopadischen Chirurgie*, 3d edition (Stuttgart: Ferdinand Enke, 1898), fig. 473.

and support were replaced gradually by mechanical means, and the table assumed a free-standing identity of its own (figures B.8, B.9). Special tables were sometimes used with upper extremity injuries, but they were uncommon (figure B.10). The design of fracture tables was influenced strongly by the introduction of the X ray and the need to carry out surgical procedures, particularly hip-nailing, under X-ray control (figures B.11, B.12). In this generation, we have seen modifications that continue to allow convenient use of the C-arm image intensifier.

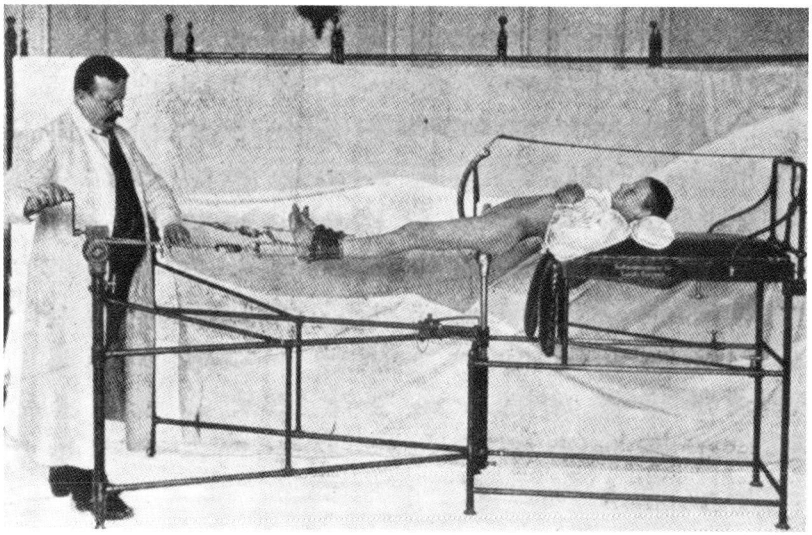

Figure B.8 Hoffa's fracture table. From Hoffa, *Lehrbuch der Orthopadischen Chirurgie*, 1898).

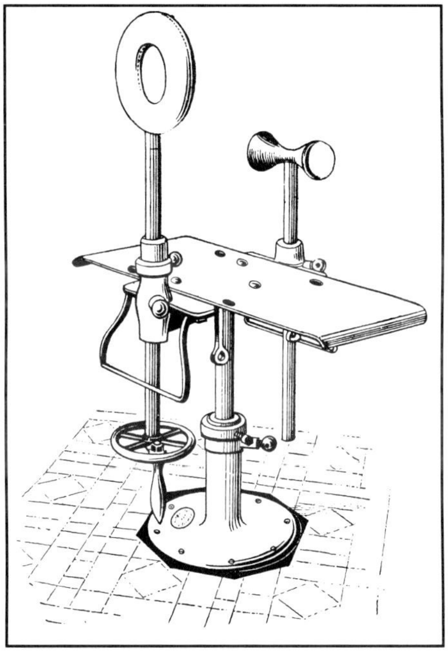

Figure B.10 The reduction chair for old dislocations of the shoulder used by Hugh Owen Thomas. From David Le Vay, *The Life of Hugh Owen Thomas* (Edinburgh: E. & S. Livingstone, 1956), fig. 2.

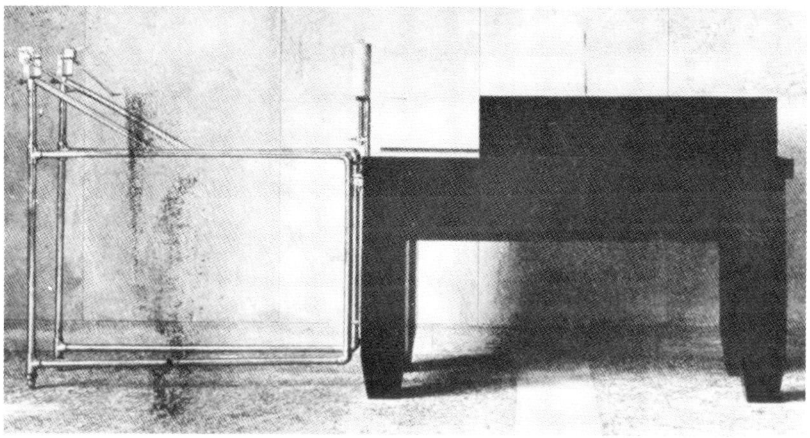

Figure B.9 A modification of Hoffa's table used at the Boston City Hospital. From F. J. Cotton, *Dislocations and Joint-Fractures*, 2d edition (Philadelphia: W. B. Saunders, 1924), fig. 929.

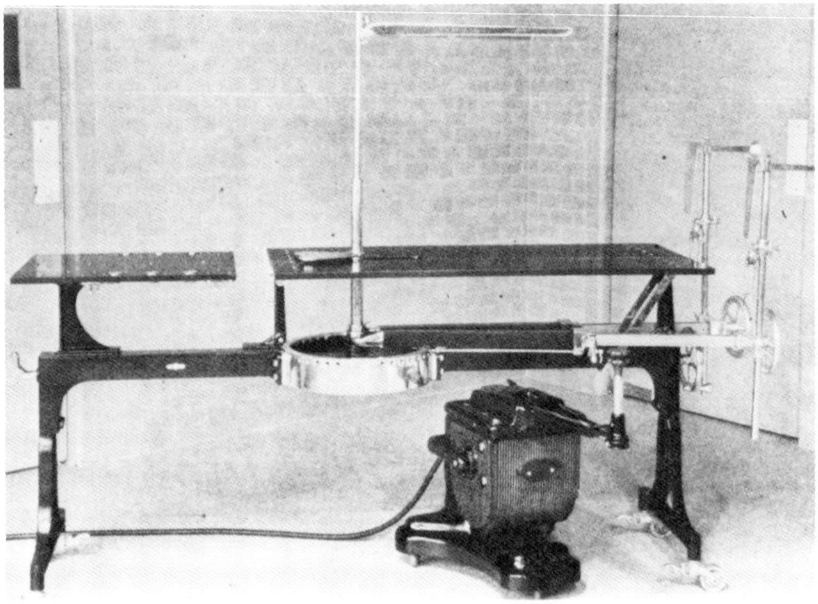

Figure B.11 The Hawley table, redesigned for the use of X rays. From George W. Hawley, "A New Fracture, X-ray and Orthopedic Table," *Am J Surg* 18(1932): 19.

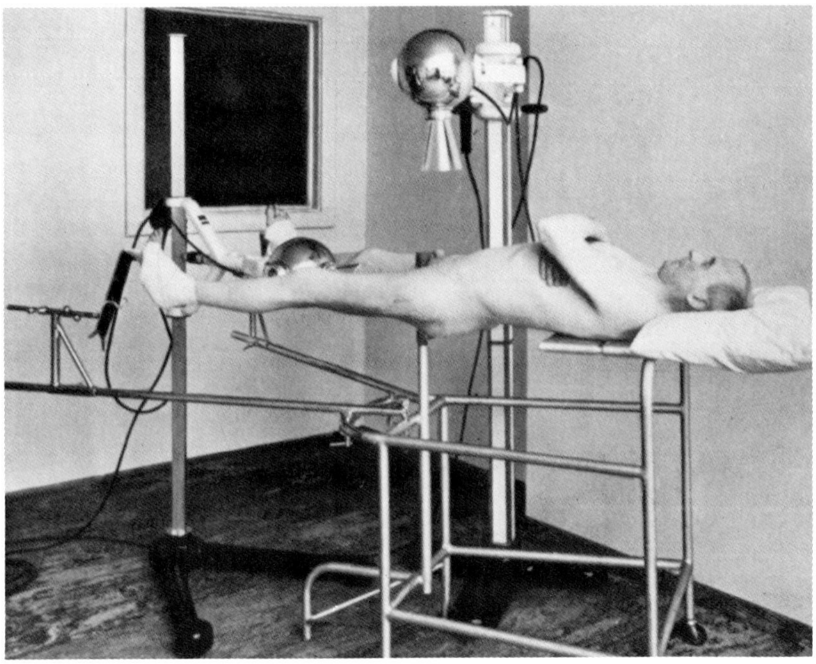

Figure B.12 The fracture table used by Watson-Jones. From R. Watson-Jones, *Fractures and Other Bone & Joint Injuries* (Baltimore: Williams & Wilkins, 1940), fig. 764.

Notes

1. Hippocrates, *The Genuine Works of Hippocrates*, trans. Francis Adams (Baltimore: Williams & Wilkins, 1939), 262–63.

2. Guido Guidi, *Chirurgie è graeco in latinum conversa* (Paris: Petrus Galterius, 1544).

3. Leonard F. Peltier, "The Continuity of Orthopedic Thought and Representation," *Clin Orthop* 89(1972): 106.

APPENDIX C

The Diagnosis of Fractures by Auscultation and Percussion

THE FIRST ATTEMPT to use the physical properties of bone as an aid to diagnosis was stimulated by the invention of the stethoscope and was based on the fact that bone is a good conductor of sound. René Théophile Hyacinthe Laennec's work on auscultation, published in 1819, made no reference to the use of the stethoscope in the diagnosis of fractures, but in 1823 his colleague Jacques Lisfranc described its use to amplify crepitus produced by moving the bone fragments.[1] Lisfranc's paper was reprinted in the *New England Journal of Medicine* the following year,[2] and the observation was noted in the works of Malgaigne and Hamilton.[3] Unfortunately, the stethoscope was not very helpful in amplifying crepitus. However, in 1840, Drs. G. P. Camman and Alonzo Clark described both the increased sound conduction across ankylosed joints and the decreased sound conduction across fractured bones.[4] They confirmed their observations by experiments carried out in the autopsy room. Both of the authors were distinguished physicians in New York City. Their observatons on sound conduction were tangential to their major interests in physical diagnosis, and they had no incentive to pursue them further. Their work therefore passed almost unnoticed by the surgical community. The use of sound conduction to diagnose fractures and dislocations has remained out of the mainstream of the literature on fractures. Instead, it has been passed down through the profession as a form of folklore, being rediscovered and described by each succeeding generation of physicians.[5]

Notes

1. René Théophile Hyacinthe Laennec, *De l'auscultation médiate* (Paris: J. A. Brosson et J. S. Chaude, 1819); Jacques Lisfranc, *Mémoire sur de nouvelles applications du stéthoscope* (Paris: Gabone, 1823).

2. Lisfranc, "Mémoire sur de nouvelles applications du stéthoscope," *N Eng J Med* (1824), 220.

3. Joseph-François Malgaigne, *Traité des fractures et des luxations* (Paris: J. B. Baillière, 1847), 1:104; Frank Hastings Hamilton, *A Practical Treatise on Fractures and Dislocations*, 3d edition (Philadelphia: Henry C. Lea, 1866), 34.

4. G. P. Camman, and A. Clark, "A New Method of Ascertaining the Dimensions, Form and Condition of Internal Organs by Percussion," *NY Quart J Med Surg*, July 1840, 62.

5. J. D. Colwell and E. H. Berg, "Auscultation as an Important Aid to the Diagnosis of Fractures," *SGO* 106(1958): 713–14; Leonard F. Peltier, "The Diagnosis of Fractures of the Hip and Femur by Auscultatory Percussion," *Clin Orthop* 123(1977): 9–11; E. Smola, "Der Perkutorische Auskultation eines Knochenbruches, Ein Hilfsmittel zum Nachweis eines Bruches ohne Roentgenbild," *Münch med Wschr* 99(1957): 701–2; F. T. Stewart, *Manual of Surgery for Students and Physicians*, 5th ed. (Philadelphia: F. T. Blakiston, 1921), 378; Lewis Atterbury Stimson, *A Practical Treatise on Fractures and Dislocations*, 8th ed. (Philadelphia: Lea & Febiger, 1917), 56.

Index

Credits

Frontispiece Jeremy Norman & Co., Inc. Plate taken from the Latin edition of Heister.
Half Title Courtesy of the Museu d'art de Catalunya, Barcelona.

CHAPTER ONE

1.1 By permission of Churchill Livingstone, Inc.
1.2 From the author's library.
1.3 From the author's library.
1.4 Courtesy Professor Tomaso Lugli, Pavia.

CHAPTER TWO

2.2 The Metropolitan Museum of Art, Rogers Fund, 1910 (10.175.132) All rights reserved. The Metropolitan Museum of Art.
2.3 Biomedical Communications, Arizona Health Services Center.
2.4 Jeremy Norman & Co., Inc.
2.5 Courtesy of the Bildarchiv Preussischer Kulturbesitz.
2.6 Courtesy of *Clinical Orthopedics and Related Research.*
2.9 - 2.10 Photographed by the author.
2.11 Jeremy Norman & Co., Inc.
2.12 Jeremy Norman & Co., Inc.
2.16 Jeremy Norman & Co., Inc.
2.20 From a print in the author's library.
2.21 Jeremy Norman & Co., Inc.
2.22 From a print in the author's library.
2.23 Courtesy of Isidor Ravdin.
2.26 Courtesy of George F. Sheldon, M.D.
2.28 From the author's library.
2.29 From the author's library.
2.31 From the author's collection.
2.32 From the author's library.
2.33 Courtesy of the National Library of Medicine.
2.35 By permission of Georg Thieme Verlag.
2.36 By permission of *Surgery, Gynecology, and Obstetrics.*
2.38 By permission of *Surgery, Gynecology, and Obstetrics.*
2.40 From the author's library.
2.42 Courtesy of Jorg Böhler.
2.44 By permission of the *Journal of Bone and Joint Surgery.*
2.46 By permission of the *Journal of Bone and Joint Surgery.*
2.48 By permission of *Transactions of the American Surgical Association.*

CHAPTER THREE

3.6 By permission of *Surgery, Gynecology, and Obstetrics.*
3.17 Reproduced by permission from Hampton, Oscar P., Jr.: *Wounds of the Extremities in Military Surgery*, St. Louis, 1951, The C. V. Mosby Co.
3.20 © MASSON Paris
3.23 Courtesy of Grune & Stratton, Inc.
3.24 Courtesy of Dr. Dehne.
3.25 By permission of the *Journal of Bone and Joint Surgery.*
3.26 Courtesy of Dr. Sarmiento.
3.27 By permission of the *Journal of Bone and Joint Surgery.*
3.29 By permission of Il Pensiero Scientifico Editore s.a.r.l.

CHAPTER FOUR

4.5 By permission of *Zentralblatt fur Chirurgie* 101; 568, 1976.
4.6 By permission of the *Journal of Bone and Joint Surgery.*
4.7 By permission of the *Journal of Bone and Joint Surgery.*
4.8 By permission of *Surgery, Gynecology and Obstetrics.*

CHAPTER FIVE

5.6 Biomedical Communications, Arizona Health Sciences Center.
5.12 Courtesy of the Historical Collections of the Library, College of Physicians of Philadelphia.
5.21 A. Moruzi, "Synthèse et prothèse osseuses. Etude clinique et radiologique des tissus osseux," Doin Editeurs, 1929.
5.23 Courtesy of Charles C Thomas, Publisher, Springfield, Illinois.
5.25 By permission of the *Journal of Bone and Joint Surgery.*
5.26 By permission of Oxford University Press.
5.28 Courtesy of the Société Belge d'Orthopédie et de Traumatologie.
5.30 Copyright 1931, American Medical Association.
5.31 By permission of Wilhelm Maudrich Verlag.
5.32 © MASSON Paris.
5.33 © MASSON Paris.
5.34 By permission of the *American Journal of Surgery.*
5.35 © MASSON Paris.
5.36 By permission of the *Journal of Bone and Joint Surgery.*
5.38 By permission of *Surgery, Gynecology and Obstetrics.*
5.39 By permission of *Surgery, Gynecology and Obstetrics.*
5.40 By permission of *Clinical Orthopaedics and Related Research.*
5.41 By permission of the *British Journal of Surgery.*
5.42 Biomedical Communications, Arizona Health Sciences Center.
5.43 Biomedical Communications, Arizona Health Sciences Center.
5.47 By permission of the *Journal of Bone and Joint Surgery.*
5.48 By permission of the *Journal of Bone and Joint Surgery.*
5.51 By permission of the *British Journal of Surgery.*
5.52 By permission of Oxford University Press.
5.53 By permission of Rush-Berivon.
5.54 By permission of Rush-Berivon.
5.55 By permission of the *Journal of Bone and Joint Surgery.*
5.57 By permission of Georg Thieme Verlag.
5.58 Courtesy of Charles C Thomas, Publisher, Springfield, Illinois.
5.61 Revue de Chirurgie Orthopédique Réparatrice de l'Appareil Moteur © MASSON.
5.63 © MASSON Paris.
5.64 © MASSON Paris.
5.65 By permission of the *Annals of Surgery.*
5.66 La Presse Médicale © MASSON Paris.
5.67 By permission of *Surgery, Gynecology, and Obstetrics.*
5.68 Courtesy of Dr. Bagby.
5.69 By permission of the *American Journal of Surgery.*
5.70 By permission of the *Mayo Clinic Bulletin.*
5.71 By permission of Springer-Verlag.
5.72 Courtesy of Dr. Allgöwer.
5.74 By permission of Ferdinand Enke Verlag.

CHAPTER SIX

6.10 By permission of the *British Journal of Surgery.*
6.13 By permission of Oxford University Press.
6.15 By permission of Hodder & Stoughton.
6.16 By permission of Hodder & Stoughton.
6.18 By permission of El Ateneo.
6.19 © MASSON Paris.
6.24 By permission of the *American Journal of Surgery.*
6.25 Biomedical Communications, Arizona Health Sciences Center.
6.26 Biomedical Communications, Arizona Health Sciences Center.

CHAPTER SEVEN

7.12 By permission of the publishers, Butterworth & Co. (Publishers) Ltd. © 1980.

7.17 By permission of Almqvist & Wiksell International.
7.18 By permission of Schwalbe & Co., A.G. Verlag.
7.19 By permission of *Annals of Surgery.*
7.20 By permission of W.B. Saunders Company.
7.21 By permission of W.B. Saunders Company.
7.23 By permission of *Surgery, Gynecology, and Obstetrics.*
7.24 By permission of the *Orthopaedic Review.*

CHAPTER EIGHT

8.4 Courtesy of Professor Yasuda.

CHAPTER NINE

9.1 Jeremy Norman & Co., Inc.
9.2a,b Jeremy Norman & Co, Inc.
9.3 By permission of C. V. Mosby Co.
9.4 From the author's collection.

CHAPTER TEN

10.8 By permission of Wilhelm Maudrich.

APPENDIX B

B.2 Jeremy Norman & Co., Inc.
B.6 By permission of the Kny-Scheerer Corp.
B.10 By permission of Churchill Livingstone, Inc.
B.11 By permission of *The American Journal of Surgery.*
B.12 By permission of *The American Journal of Surgery.*

NORMAN
PUBLISHING ™

Collaborators on the production of
Fractures: A History and Iconography of Their Treatment:

Desktop Publishing, Inc., Linotronic Output
Melanie Field, Electronic Typesetter
Steven Hiatt, Copy Editor
Elinor Lindheimer, Indexer
Jill Rotenberg, Project Manager
Seventeenth Street Studios, Designer
Martha N. Steele, Associate Editor
Thomson-Shore, Inc., Printer and Binder

The text type is Galliard,
a Postscript font from Adobe Systems.
Calligraphy by Arthur Baker.